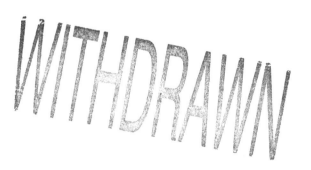

# Environmental Impacts on Reproductive Health and Fertility

# Environmental Impacts on Reproductive Health and Fertility

Edited by

**Tracey J. Woodruff**
University of California San Francisco

**Sarah J. Janssen**
University of California San Francisco

**Louis J. Guillette Jr.**
University of Florida

**Linda C. Giudice**
University of California San Francisco

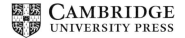
CAMBRIDGE
UNIVERSITY PRESS

CAMBRIDGE UNIVERSITY PRESS
Cambridge, New York, Melbourne, Madrid, Cape Town, Singapore,
São Paulo, Delhi, Dubai, Tokyo

Cambridge University Press
The Edinburgh Building, Cambridge CB2 8RU, UK

Published in the United States of America by Cambridge University Press, New York

www.cambridge.org
Information on this title: www.cambridge.org/9780521519526

First published 2010

Printed in the United Kingdom at the University Press, Cambridge

*A catalog record for this publication is available from the British Library*

*Library of Congress Cataloging in Publication data*
Environmental impacts on reproductive health and fertility / [edited by] Tracey J. Woodruff ... [et al.].
    p. ; cm.
  Includes bibliographical references and index.
  ISBN 978-0-521-51952-6 (hardback)
  1. Reproductive toxicology.   2. Reproductive health–Environmental aspects.
  I. Woodruff, T. J. (Tracey J.)   II. Title.
  [DNLM:  1. Reproductive Medicine.   2. Environmental Exposure–adverse effects.
  3. Infertility–chemically induced. WQ 200 E61 2010]
  RA1224.2.E683 2010
  616.6'5071–dc22        2009037855

ISBN 978-0-521-51952-6 Hardback

# Contents

Contents

# Contributors

**Lise Aksglaede**
Department of Growth and Reproduction GR, Rigshospitalet, University of Copenhagen, Copenhagen, Denmark

**Yutaka Aoki**
Department of Environmental & Occupational Health, Morgan State University School of Community Health & Policy, Baltimore, MD, USA

**Germaine M. Buck Louis**
Epidemiology Branch, Eunice Kennedy Shriver National Institute of Child Health & Human Development, Bethesda, MD, USA

**Esther L. Calderon**
Department of Physiology and Biophysics, University of Illinois at Chicago, Chicago, IL, USA

**Sylvaine Cordier**
Inserm (French Institute of Health and Medical Research) U625, Rennes, France

**Julie Damm**
Department of Growth and Reproduction GR, Rigshospitalet, University of Copenhagen, Copenhagen, Denmark

**Leo F. Doherty**
Department of Obstetrics, Gynecology & Reproductive Sciences, Yale University School of Medicine, New Haven, CT, USA

**Mary A. Fox**
Assistant Professor, Department of Health Policy and Management, Johns Hopkins Bloomberg School of Public Health, Baltimore, MD, USA

**Dori R. Germolec**
National Toxicology Program, National Institute of Environmental Health Sciences, Research Triangle Park, NC, USA

**Linda C. Giudice**
Department of Obstetrics, Gynecology & Reproductive Sciences, University of California San Francisco, San Francisco, CA, USA

**Andrea C. Gore**
Division of Pharmacology & Toxicology, Institute for Cellular and Molecular Biology and Institute for Neuroscience, The University of Texas at Austin College of Pharmacy, Austin, TX, USA

**K. Leigh Greathouse**
University of Texas M. D. Anderson Cancer Center, Smithville, TX, USA

**Louis J. Guillette Jr.**
Department of Zoology, University of Florida, Gainesville, FL, USA

**Heather J. Hamlin**
Department of Zoology, University of Florida, Gainesville, FL, USA

**Russ Hauser**
Department of Environmental and Occupational Epidemiology, Harvard School of Public Health; Vincent Memorial Obstetrics and Gynecology Service, Andrology Laboratory and In Vitro Fertilization Unit, Massachusetts General Hospital, Boston, MA, USA

**Jerrold J. Heindel**
Division of Extramural Research and Training, National Institute of Environmental Health Sciences, NIH, DHHS, Research Triangle Park, NC, USA

**Patricia Hunt**
Center for Reproductive Biology, Washington State University, Pullman, WA, USA

**Taisen Iguchi**
Okazaki Institute for Integrative Bioscience, National Institute for Basic Biology, National Institutes of Natural Sciences, and Department of Basic Biology, Graduate University for Advanced Studies (SOKENDAI), Okazaki, Japan

**Sarah J. Janssen**
Natural Resources Defense Council; University of California San Francisco, San Francisco, CA, USA

**Anders Juul**
Department of Growth and Reproduction GR, Rigshospitalet, University of Copenhagen, Copenhagen, Denmark

**Laxmi A. Kondapalli**
Department of Reproductive Endocrinology and Infertility, University of Pennsylvania, Philadelphia, PA, USA

**Robert W. Luebke**
Office of Research & Development, United States Environmental Protection Agency, Research Triangle Park, NC, USA

**Maricel V. Maffini**
Department of Anatomy and Cellular Biology, Tufts University School of Medicine, Boston, MA, USA

**John D. Meeker**
Department of Environmental Health Sciences, University of Michigan School of Public Health, Ann Arbor, MI, USA

**Pauline Mendola**
Infant, Child and Women's Health Statistics Branch, Centers for Disease Control and Prevention/National Center for Health Statistics, Hyattsville, MD, USA

**Sinichi Miyagawa**
Okazaki Institute for Integrative Bioscience, National Institute for Basic Biology, National Institutes of Natural Sciences, and Department of Basic Biology, Graduate University for Advanced Studies (SOKENDAI), Okazaki, Japan

**Annette Mouritsen**
Department of Growth and Reproduction GR, Rigshospitalet, University of Copenhagen, Copenhagen, Denmark

**Retha R. Newbold**
Developmental Endocrinology and Endocrine Disruptor Section, Laboratory of Molecular Toxicology, Division of Intramural Research, National Institute of Environmental Health Sciences, NIH, DHHS, Research Triangle Park, NC, USA

**Gail S. Prins**
Departments of Urology and Physiology & Biophysics, University of Illinois at Chicago, Chicago, IL, USA

**Richard M. Sharpe**
Professor & Research Team Leader/PI, MRC Human Reproductive Sciences Unit, Centre for Reproductive Biology, The Queen's Medical Research Institute, Edinburgh, Scotland, UK

**Niels E. Skakkebaek**
University Department of Growth & Reproduction, Rigshospitalet, Copenhagen, Denmark

**Rémy Slama**
Inserm (French Institute of Health and Medical Research) and University Joseph Fourier Grenoble U823, Grenoble, France

**Gina M. Solomon**
Natural Resources Defense Council; University of California San Francisco, San Francisco, CA, USA

**Carlos Sonnenschein**
Program in Cell, Molecular & Developmental Biology, Tufts University School of Medicine and Sackler School of Graduate Biomedical Sciences, Boston, MA, USA

**Kaspar Sørensen**
Department of Growth and Reproduction GR, Rigshospitalet, University of Copenhagen, Copenhagen, Denmark

**Ana M. Soto**
Program in Cell, Molecular & Developmental Biology, Tufts University School of Medicine and Sackler School of Graduate Biomedical Sciences, Boston, MA, USA

**Tamotsu Sudo**
Section of Translational Research and Department of Gynecologic Oncology, Hyogo Cancer Center, Akashi, Japan

**Shanna H. Swan**
Departments of Obstetrics & Gynecology and
Environmental Medicine and Community and
Preventive Medicine, University of Rochester
School of Medicine & Dentistry, Rochester,
NY, USA

**Hugh S. Taylor**
Division of Reproductive Endocrinology &
Infertility, Obstetrics, Gynecology & Reproductive
Sciences; Department of Molecular, Cellular &
Developmental Biology, Yale University School of
Medicine, New Haven, CT, USA

**Jorma Toppari**
Department of Physiology, Institute of
Biomedicine, University of Turku, Turku, Finland

**Helena E. Virtanen**
Department of Physiology, Institute of
Biomedicine, University of Turku, Turku, Finland

**Cheryl L. Walker**
The University of Texas M.D. Anderson Cancer
Center, Science Park – Research Division,
Smithville, TX, USA

**Teresa K. Woodruff**
The Oncofertility Consortium; The Institute
for Women's Health Research, Northwestern
University Feinberg School of Medicine, Chicago,
IL, USA

**Tracey J. Woodruff**
Program on Reproductive Health and the
Environment, Department of Obstetrics,
Gynecology & Reproductive Sciences, University
of California San Francisco, San Francisco,
CA, USA

**R. Thomas Zoeller**
Biology Department, University of Massachusetts
Amherst, MA, USA

# Preface

The seemingly simple question "Why"? is motivating growing awareness and concern about ubiquitous chemicals in our environment and their effect on reproductive health. Why are there fewer frogs? Why can't I get pregnant? Why do some of my patients always miscarry? Why does my child have a birth defect? Why did my young daughter get cancer? This book seeks to help us link the science of environmental health to this chorus of why. With observed increases in reproductive disorders and declines in reproductive function, a rapidly expanding body of scientific evidence indicates that a number of reproductive and developmental health problems may be caused by exposure to chemicals that are widely dispersed in our environment and with which we come into contact on a daily basis. These problems include male and female infertility, miscarriage, poor pregnancy outcomes, abnormal fetal development, early puberty, endometriosis, polycystic ovarian syndrome, uterine fibroids, and diseases and cancers of reproductive organs. The compelling nature of the collective science, with observations in humans, animal models, and wildlife, has resulted in recognition of a new field of environmental reproductive health. Environmental reproductive health focuses on exposures to environmental contaminants, particularly during critical periods in development (such as prior to conception and during pregnancy), and their potential effects on all aspects of the future reproductive life course, including conception, fertility, pregnancy, child and adolescent development, and adult health. This book reviews science in key areas of the relationship between environmental contaminants and reproductive health outcomes, integrating insights from scientific disciplines in environmental health and clinical and public health fields. It also provides recommendations on efforts toward prevention in clinical care and public policy.

If elements of the environment we create are contributing to the decline in our reproductive health and capacity, then we have, in our hands, the ability to reverse this trend. This book is intended to lay the foundation for those who want to understand the science better, whether they are scientists, clinicians, nurses and other healthcare professionals, public and environmental health practitioners, and motivates further contributions in research, clinical care, and policy toward creating healthier environments for this and future generations.

## Acknowledgements

Tracey J Woodruff
To the MIX club, and to a future of thriving children everywhere

Linda C. Giudice
To my husband, Sakis Theologis, and our sons, Alexander and Aris Theologis for their love and support, and Alison Carlson for introducing me to environmental influences and fertility

Lou Guillette
To Prof. Howard Bern and Prof. Richard E. Jones, great teachers and mentors

Sarah Janssen
To my daughter Zeo Eliabeth Avent

# Introduction

Tracey J. Woodruff and Linda C. Giudice

## Background

At the beginning of the twenty-first century, the human population is in a unique, but precarious position. Economic globalization, increasingly rapid technological change, expanding industrialization, and shifting political and religious forces have provided great opportunities and challenges for the human population. Equally, we have seen rapid changes in the health of the population. In the early part of the last century, there were great advancements in health as a result of public health interventions, particularly improved water and waste sanitation, antibiotics and vaccinations. These greatly decreased the burden of acute and infectious disease in many, but not all, parts of the world and subsequently accelerated the health of the population. As infectious and acute illnesses declined, prevalence of chronic illnesses, such as heart disease and cancer, began to rise. As we move across the boundary of the twenty-first century, chronic disease in the USA and other developed countries has brought an increasing burden to the population, and other, lesser developed countries, have not been afforded the same access to or benefits of the achievements of developed countries.

We have also seen over this time period, the emergence of the importance of the environment as a determinant of health. During the mid twentieth century, environmental pollution, primarily in air and water, emerged as a concern for acute and sudden illnesses. From the "killer smogs" in Donora, Pennsylvania, and London, UK, the mercury poisoning in Minamata, Japan, the industrial chemical releases leading to the Bhopal tragedy, to the burning water of the Cuyahoga River in Ohio – these were visceral, immediate, and tragic demonstrations of the power of chemicals in our environment with immediate impact on human health. These events also motivated demand for pioneering legislative and regulatory actions by governments, which led to reductions of pollutants in air, water, and food.

However, we now find ourselves at another critical cross road. What has become clear, focused by the steady compilation of scientific findings and books on this subject, is that reproductive health and ultimately reproductive capacity of the population are under strain, and critical indicators show that we must pay attention to the warnings ahead of us [1–4]. This is reflected by a number of concerning trends in human reproductive and developmental health. There has been a 40% increase, to about 11%, in the percent of US women who report difficulty in conceiving and maintaining pregnancy [5]. In addition, between 1982 and 2002, the percent of young women under the age of 25, a peak time of fertility, reporting difficulty in conceiving and maintaining pregnancy doubled from 4.3% to 8.3% [5, 6]. There has been a decline in the age of onset of puberty, as marked by breast development and onset of menarche, for girls in the USA between the 1940s to the mid 1990s [7].

There are also negative/adverse trends related to male reproductive health. The incidence of testicular cancer, primarily a disease of young men, has increased in Europe from 1% to 6% (depending on the country) over the past 10–40 years [8]. Testicular cancer has increased by about 60% in the USA over the last 30 years [9]. In addition, there is a relatively high prevalence of abnormally low sperm counts in several Scandinavian countries (~ 20%) [10]. Data from three cities (Boston, USA, Copenhagen, Denmark, and Turku, Finland) demonstrate a significant secular trend decrease in serum testosterone, suggesting about a 1% per year decline for the past 40–50 years [11–13]. This decline is consistent with the reduction in sperm concentration reported by Carlsen *et al.* in 1992 [14]. Also, some of the most common birth defects today

*Environmental Impacts on Reproductive Health and Fertility*, ed. T. J. Woodruff, S. J. Janssen, L. J. Guillette, and L. C. Giudice. Published by Cambridge University Press. © Cambridge University Press 2010.

**Table 1.1.** Key definitions for environmental reproductive health.

Environmental reproductive health: Interdisciplinary study of exposures to environmental contaminants, particularly during critical periods in development (such as prior to conception and during pregnancy), and their potential effects on all aspects of future reproductive health throughout the life course, including conception, fertility, pregnancy, child and adolescent development, and adult health.

Environmental contaminants: metals and synthetic chemicals in our environment, including air, water, soil, food, consumer products, and the workplace.

Reproductive health: Ability to conceive, to carry a pregnancy, pregnancy quality and outcomes, pubertal effects and adult reproductive health disorders.

are malformations of the male reproductive system, including cryptorchidism and hypospadias [15, 16]. This constellation of adverse trends suggests an overall decrease in male reproductive function.

Furthermore, there are increasing manifestations of adverse health among infants and children. Thirty percent more babies are born prematurely, and the expected gestational age of babies delivered without medical intervention is one week earlier now than 15 years ago [17]. There are increases in certain birth defects and other adverse birth outcomes, such as gastroschisis (three fold over the last 20 years in California) and hypothyroidism (138% over the past 20 years in New York) [18, 19]. And several childhood illnesses, including certain childhood cancers and neurodevelopmental disorders, such as autism, have been reported to be increasing [20], as well. While genetics comprises one important risk factor, other external influences, periconceptually, prenatally, and early in childhood are also likely contributors.

We must pay attention to these relatively rapid changes in health endpoints over the last 30–50 years, as genetic contributions could not have evolved at the same pace, indicating other external contributors such as environment and lifestyle are playing a role.

We know over roughly the same period, starting in the mid 1940s, there has been a dramatic increase in human exposure to both natural and synthetic chemicals. For example, in the USA as of 2006, there are approximately 87 000 chemical substances in commerce, with about 3000 imported or manufactured in excess of 1 million pounds each [21]. Exposures to chemicals in the environment, which are defined here as metals and synthetic chemicals in our environment, including air, water, soil, food, consumer products, and the workplace (Table 1.1), are ubiquitous. Environmental chemicals can cause a broad spectrum of effects that depend not only on route of exposure and dose, but on the susceptibility of the individual to the compound, and timing and duration of the exposure.

We know that the health of the population can be influenced by many intrinsic and extrinsic factors [22] (Fig. 1.1), in addition to chemicals in the environment. Some external factors can increase stress on the system, such as lack of access to health care, social and racial discrimination, or poverty. Other external factors can create resiliency to competing influences on health, such as good social support networks, access to services, and stable incomes. Internal factors, such as age, gender, and genotype can also influence susceptibility to diseases and disorders. The risk from environmental exposures can be enhanced or diminished by these external and internal factors [22].

Increasing concern about the role of chemicals in our environment influencing observed increases in chronic diseases and identifying chemicals that cause harm to reproductive and/or developmental health provide an opportunity to focus on preventable risk factors. To accomplish this fully, we must expand upon the scientific basis of our understanding of the links between environmental exposures and reproductive health. Furthermore, we must work across disciplines, across sectors, with those inside and outside academia, in the community, and in the policy arena to fully realize the implications of the science and translate this information into change that results in preventing exposures to harmful chemicals for individuals and populations.

It is toward this goal that we have brought together leading scientific experts from across the relevant scientific disciplines in environmental sciences, wildlife biology, clinical research, toxicology, epidemiology, and clinical and public policy translation to provide the scientific foundation for a comprehensive understanding of the intersection of environmental contaminants and reproductive and developmental health. This book provides a review of the science in key areas of the relationship between environmental contaminants and reproductive and developmental health for students and practitioners in the fields of public health,

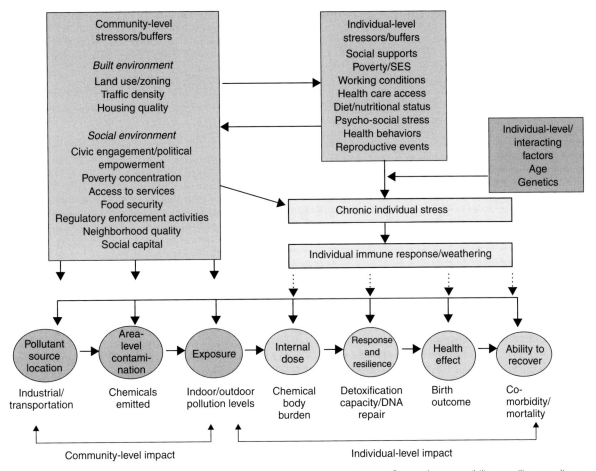

**Fig. 1.1.** External, both community level and individual level, and internal factors that can influence the susceptibility or resilience to disease. (Adapted from Morello-Frosch and Shenassa [22].)

environmental health and research, and medical and allied health professional training.

## Scope of this book

### Defining the field

Environmental reproductive health focuses on exposures to environmental contaminants (metals and synthetic chemicals), particularly during critical periods of development (such as prior to conception and during pregnancy), and their potential effects on all aspects of future reproductive health throughout the life course, including conception, fertility, pregnancy, child and adolescent development, and adult health.

### Environmental contaminants

As discussed above, environmental contaminants are metals and synthetic chemicals in our environment,

including air, water, soil, food, consumer products, and the workplace (Table 1.1). Common environmental pollutants include: pesticides and herbicides such as atrazine and chlorpyrifos; volatile organic compounds such as benzene, toluene and chloroform; heavy metals such as lead, mercury and arsenic; air contaminants such as carbon monoxide, ozone, particulate matter, and environmental tobacco smoke (ETS); and persistent organic pollutants, such as the dioxins, polychlorinated biphenols (PCBs), and the pesticide dichlorodiphenyltrichloroethane (DDT) and its breakdown product dichlorodiphenyldichloroethylene (DDE) (see Chapters 2 and 17).

There are many environmental contaminants that can affect reproductive health [4], and they can do so through diverse biological mechanisms. Historically, much of the scientific inquiry focused on genotoxic or mutagenic chemicals – i.e. those that can damage or

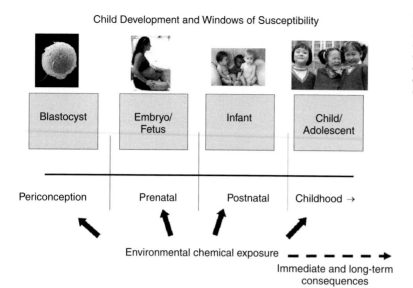

Child Development and Windows of Susceptibility

**Fig. 1.2.** Important developmental time periods during which perturbations, such as from exposure to environmental contaminants, can result in changes that can increase risk of subsequent immediate or long-term adverse health outcomes. (Modified from Louis *et al.* [32].)

interfere with the integrity of genetic material. While there are other mechanistic pathways that can contribute to disease, since the latter part of the twentieth century there has emerged emphasis on an important class of chemicals called endocrine-disrupting chemicals (EDCs), that interfere with the production, release, transport, metabolism, binding, action, or elimination of natural hormones in the body responsible for maintenance of homeostasis and regulation of developmental processes. Some of the common EDCs discussed in this book include bisphenol-A (BPA), phthalates and certain pesticides (e.g. vinclozolin, dicofol, atrazine). Many of these compounds alter estrogen, androgen, and thyroid signaling, which are essential for normal embryonic development and reproductive activity in all vertebrates studied to date [23–25]. They can also alter hormone synthesis, storage in plasma proteins, and hepatic biotransformation and clearance [26]; disrupt neural and immune signaling pathways [27–29]; and alter the regulation of gene expression (e.g. DNA methylation, RNA stability, protein degradation) (reviewed in Edwards and Myers [30]).

Much of this book focuses on the role of/implications for/potential effects of exposure to EDCs and subsequent reproductive and developmental outcomes. It is a natural area of inquiry in this field, as EDCs can interact with the hormonal system, which regulates development and maintenance of the reproductive system. Endocrine-disrupting chemicals can also target the neuroendocrine system, which plays regulatory and homeostatic roles in the control of human physiology.

As such, exposure to EDCs has broad implications for health.

## Critical and sensitive periods of development and susceptibility

Another important theme throughout the book is time periods of exposure and their influence on subsequent health risks (Fig 1.2). Key developmental stages occur throughout the life course: before and around the time of conception (gamete and blastocyst stages); prenatal development (embryo and fetal stages); and infancy, childhood, and puberty [31–33].

These time periods are marked by extensive developmental changes, such as cellular proliferation and rapidly changing metabolic and hormonal capabilities. Exposures to environmental contaminants during this period may result in adverse, permanent, and irreversible effects that can manifest immediately or later in life or even in subsequent generations. For example, it has been well established that harmful exposures during the prenatal period can result in adverse birth outcomes. Exposure to thalidomide resulted in structural limb defects, excessive alcohol intake leads to fetal alcohol syndrome, and smoking can increase risk of low birthweight babies and preterm delivery. Also, we have learned that exposures during these same critical developmental periods can result in permanent alterations to physiologic systems that may not manifest until early and late adulthood, which has been labeled the fetal origin of adult disease [34, 35].

These concepts are illustrated through the tragic episode of diethylstilbestrol (DES), a synthetic estrogen and an EDC, which is discussed in several places in the book. Diethylstilbestrol was given to pregnant women in the USA between 1938 and 1971 under the erroneous assumption that it would prevent pregnancy complications. In fact, in utero exposure to DES alters the normal programming of gene families, such as *Hox* and *Wnt*, that play important roles in reproductive tract differentiation [35–38]. As a result, female offspring exposed to DES in utero are at increased risk of clear cell adenocarcinoma of the vagina and cervix, structural reproductive tract anomalies, infertility and poor pregnancy outcomes, and male offspring have an increased incidence of genital abnormalities and a possibly increased risk of prostate and testicular cancer [39]. These observed human effects have been confirmed in numerous animal models that have also provided information on the toxic mechanisms of DES. Animal experiments have also predicted changes later found in DES-exposed humans, such as oviductal malformations [40], increased incidence of uterine fibroids [41–43], and second-generational effects [44, 45] such as increased menstrual irregularities [46] and ovarian cancer [47] in DES-exposed granddaughters and increased hypospadias in DES-exposed grandsons [48, 49].

## Sources of scientific information

Information about the potentially harmful effects of exposure to environmental contaminants comes from a variety of scientific sources, from wildlife studies, in vitro and in vivo toxicology studies, epidemiologic studies, and clinical evidence. Within each of these areas there are multiple types of testing methodologies and approaches that are used. Scientific data from animal studies, either within wildlife populations or controlled experimental settings, provide critical information to our understanding of the potential for environmental chemical exposure to result in adverse human health effects. The most extensive information comes from animal bioassays, and these are a preferable method for assessing the potential for human harm and for developing strategies for prevention of harmful exposures. Unlike pharmaceuticals, environmental contaminants were not intended for human use, and it is unethical to knowingly expose humans to these chemicals under experimental conditions to assess for harmful effects. Several studies of concordance between the perturbed developmental outcomes in experimental animal studies and the human clinical experience have been made [50–54]. In general, these studies conclude that there is concordance of developmental effects between animals and humans and that humans are *as sensitive* or *more sensitive* than the most sensitive animal species [55]. Given that there is general conservation of biological function across animal species, including humans, animal studies provide important insights into potential human harm.

However, there are limitations in how traditional toxicologic studies have been designed that decrease their utility for studying reproductive or developmental outcomes, such as insensitive strains or exposure periods, a focus on overt disease endpoints, and exposures to single chemicals at high doses rather than the mixture of low doses of chemicals more often seen by the public. While science continues to use animal studies to predict human harm, epidemiologic and clinical studies provide critical and complementary sources of information. This book covers both animal and human data to inform what we know about environmental chemicals and human reproductive and developmental health.

## Layout of this book

The book starts with a general overview of concepts: the scope of exposures to environmental contaminants and examples of typical chemicals that will be covered in this book (Chapter 2). This is followed by an overview of female and male reproductive development (Chapters 3 and 4, respectively). Presentation of scientific concepts essential to understand the relationship between exposures to environmental contaminants and biological perturbations and eventually overt disease outcomes are discussed in Chapters 5, 6 and 7. Chapters 8 through 14 review the science evaluating exposures to environmental contaminants and adverse reproductive and developmental outcomes. The book ends with two chapters discussing the implications of the science – how current knowledge informs actions that can be taken at the personal level, such as through clinical advice, and at the population level, through changes to public policy systems.

This book brings together the core environmental health sciences that form a foundation of information from which to join with other disciplines and partners in related health, social, community, legal, and policy fields to broaden our understanding of the relationship between environmental contaminants and reproductive and developmental health. It is a critical time to

5

re-energize and refocus the environmental health work that was started in the latter part of the last century to meet the new environmental health challenges of the twenty-first century, by informing our actions to prevent those exposures that may harm human health, to secure the health of this and future generations.

# References

1. Colborn T, Dumanoski D, Myers JP. *Our Stolen Future*. Penguin Books USA, Inc., 1996.

2. Crain DA, Janssen SJ, Edwards TM. *et al.* Female reproductive disorders: the roles of endocrine-disrupting compounds and developmental timing. *Fertil Steril* 2008; **90**: 911–40.

3. Schettler T, Solomon G, Valenti M, Huddle A. *Generations at Risk. Reproductive Health and the Environment*. Cambridge, MA: MIT Press, 1999.

4. Woodruff TJ, Carlson A, Schwartz JM, Giudice LC. Proceedings of the Summit on Environmental Challenges to Reproductive Health and Fertility: Executive summary. *Fertil Steril* 2008; **89**: e1–20.

5. Chandra A, Martinez G, Mosher W, Abma J, Jones J. Fertility, family planning, and reproductive health of U.S. women: Data from the 2002 National Survey of Family Growth. *Vital Health Stat* 2005; **23**: 1–160.

6. Brett K. Fecundity in 2002 NSFG women 15–24 years of age (personal communication). National Center for Health Statistics, Hyattsville, MD, 2008.

7. Euling SY, Selevan SG, Pescovitz OH, Skakkebaek NE. Role of environmental factors in the timing of puberty. *Pediatrics* 2008; **121 Suppl 3**: S167–71.

8. Bray F, Richiardi L, Ekbom A. *et al.* Trends in testicular cancer incidence and mortality in 22 European countries: continuing increases in incidence and declines in mortality. *Int J Cancer* 2006; **118**: 3099–111.

9. Shah MN, Devesa SS, Zhu K, McGlynn KA. Trends in testicular germ cell tumours by ethnic group in the United States. *Int J Androl* 2007; **30**: 206–13; discussion 213–14.

10. Jorgensen N, Asklund C, Carlsen E, Skakkebaek NE. Coordinated European investigations of semen quality: results from studies of Scandinavian young men is a matter of concern. *Int J Androl* 2006; **29**: 54–61; discussion 105–8.

11. Andersson A, Jensen TK, Petersen JH. *et al.* Trends in Leydig cell function in Danish men. *Hum Reprod* 2005; **20**: i26.

12. Perheentupa A, Laatikainen T, Vierula M. *et al.* Clear birth cohort effect in serum testosterone and SHBG levels in Finnish men. Endocrine Society Meeting 2006, Vol. Abstract OR22–3, 2006.

13. Travison TG, Araujo AB, O'Donnell AB, Kupelian V, McKinlay JB. A population-level decline in serum testosterone levels in American men. *J Clin Endocrinol Metab* 2007; **92**: 196–202.

14. Carlsen E, Giwercman A, Keiding N, Skakkebaek NE. Evidence for decreasing quality of semen during past 50 years. *Br Med J* 1992; **305**: 609–13.

15. Baskin LS, Himes K, Colborn T. Hypospadias and endocrine disruption: is there a connection? *Environ Health Perspect* 2001; **109**: 1175–83.

16. Foresta C, Zuccarello D, Garolla A, Ferlin A. Role of hormones, genes, and environment in human cryptorchidism. *Endocrine Rev* 2008; **29**: 560–80.

17. Davidoff MJ, Dias T, Damus K. *et al.* Changes in the gestational age distribution among U.S. singleton births: impact on rates of late preterm birth, 1992 to 2002. *Semin Perinatol* 2006; **30**: 8–15.

18. Harris KB, Pass KA. Increase in congenital hypothyroidism in New York State and in the United States. *Mol Genet Metab* 2007; **91**: 268–77.

19. Vu LT, Nobuhara KK, Laurent C, Shaw GM. Increasing prevalence of gastroschisis: population-based study in California. *J Pediatr* 2008; **152**: 807–11.

20. Newschaffer CJ, Falb MD, Gurney JG. National autism prevalence trends from United States special education data. *Pediatrics* 2005; **115**: e277–82.

21. US Environment Protection Agency. What is the TSCA Chemical Substance Inventory? Vol. 2007. US EPA, 2006.

22. Morello-Frosch R, Shenassa ED. The environmental "riskscape" and social inequality: implications for explaining maternal and child health disparities. *Environ Health Perspect* 2006; **114**: 1150–3.

23. Gray LE Jr, Wilson VS, Stoker T. *et al.* Adverse effects of environmental antiandrogens and androgens on reproductive development in mammals. *Int J Androl* 2006; **29**: 96–104; discussion 105–8.

24. McLachlan JA. Environmental signaling: what embryos and evolution teach us about endocrine disrupting chemicals. *Endocrine Rev* 2001; **22**: 319–41.

25. Zoeller RT, Dowling ALS, Herzig CTA. *et al.* Thyroid hormone, brain development, and the environment. *Environ Health Perspect* 2002; **110 Suppl. 3**: 355–61.

26. Guillette LJ, Jr, Gunderson MP. Alterations in the development of the reproductive and endocrine systems of wildlife exposed to endocrine disrupting contaminants. *Reproduction* 2001; **122**: 857–64.

27. Fournier M, Brousseau P, Tryphonas H, Cyr D. Biomarkers of immunotoxicity: An evolutionary perspective. In Guillette Jr LJ, Crain DA, eds. *Endocrine Disrupting Contaminants: An Evolutionary Perspective*. Philadelphia: Francis and Taylor Inc., 2000; 182–215.

28. Guillette LJ Jr. Endocrine disrupting contaminants – beyond the dogma. *Environ Health Perspect* 2006; **114** (Suppl. 1): 9–12.

29. Osteen KG, Sierra-Rivera E. Does disruption of immune and endocrine systems by environmental toxins contribute to development of endometriosis? *Sem in Reprod Endocrinol* 1997; **15**: 301–8.

30. Edwards TM, Myers JP. Environmental exposures and gene regulation in disease etiology. *Environ Health Perspect* 2007; **115**(9): 1264–70.

31. Calabrese E J. Sex differences in susceptibility to toxic industrial chemicals. *Br J Ind Med* 1986; **43**: 577–9.

32. Louis GM, Cooney MA, Lynch CD, Handal, A. Periconception window: advising the pregnancy-planning couple. *Fertil Steril* 2008; **89**: e119–21.

33. Couzin J. Quirks of fetal environment felt decades later. *Science*, 2002; **296**: 2167–9.

34. Gluckman PD, Hanson MA. Living with the past: evolution, development, and patterns of disease. *Science* 2004; **305**: 1733–6.

35. Miller C, Degenhardt K, Sassoon DA. Fetal exposure to DES results in de-regulation of Wnt7a during uterine morphogenesis. *Nat Genet* 1998; **20**: 228–30.

36. Pavlova A, Boutin E, Cunha G, Sassoon D. Msx1 (Hox-7.1) in the adult mouse uterus: cellular interactions underlying regulation of expression. *Development* 1994; **120**: 335–45.

37. Taylor HS, Vanden Heuvel GB, Igarashi P. A conserved Hox axis in the mouse and human female reproductive system: late establishment and persistent adult expression of the Hoxa cluster genes. *Biol Reprod* 1997; **57**: 1338–45.

38. Woodruff TK, Walker CL. Fetal and early postnatal environmental exposures and reproductive health effects in the female. *Fertil Steril* 2008; **89**: e47–51.

39. Schrager S, Potter BE. Diethylstilbestrol exposure. *Am Fam Physician* 2004; **69**: 2395–400.

40. Newbold RR, Tyrey S, Haney AF, McLachlan JA. Developmentally arrested oviduct: a structural and functional defect in mice following prenatal exposure to diethylstilbestrol. *Teratology* 1983; **27**: 417–26.

41. Baird DD, Newbold R. Prenatal diethylstilbestrol (DES) exposure is associated with uterine leiomyoma development. *Reprod Toxicol* 2005; **20**: 81–4.

42. Cook, JD, Davis BJ, Cai SI. *et al.* Interaction between genetic susceptibility and early-life environmental exposure determines tumor-suppressor-gene penetrance. *Proc Nat Acad Sci USA* 2005; **102**: 8644–9.

43. McLachlan JA, Newbold RR, Bullock BC. Long-term effects on the female mouse genital tract associated with prenatal exposure to diethylstilbestrol. *Cancer Res* 1980; **40**: 3988–99.

44. Newbold RR, Hanson RB, Jefferson WN. *et al.* Increased tumors but uncompromised fertility in the female descendants of mice exposed developmentally to diethylstilbestrol. *Carcinogenesis* 1998; **19**: 1655–63.

45. Newbold RR, Hanson RB, Jefferson WN. *et al.* Proliferative lesions and reproductive tract tumors in male descendants of mice exposed developmentally to diethylstilbestrol. *Carcinogenesis* 2000; **21**: 1355–63.

46. Titus-Ernstoff L, Troisi R, Hatch EE. *et al.* Menstrual and reproductive characteristics of women whose mothers were exposed in utero to diethylstilbestrol (DES). *Int J Epidemiol* 2006; **35**: 862–8.

47. Blatt, J, Van Le L, Weiner T, Sailer S. Ovarian carcinoma in an adolescent with transgenerational exposure to diethylstilbestrol. *J Pediatr Hematol Oncol* 2003; **25**: 635–6.

48. Brouwers MM, Feitz WF., Roelofs LA. *et al.* Hypospadias: a transgenerational effect of diethylstilbestrol? *Hum Reprod* 2006; **21**: 666–9.

49. Klip H, Verloop J, van Gool JD. *et al.* Hypospadias in sons of women exposed to diethylstilbestrol in utero: a cohort study. *Lancet* 2002; **359**: 1102–7.

50. Francis EZ, Kimmel CA, Rees DC. Workshop on the qualitative and quantitative comparability of human and animal developmental neurotoxicity: summary and implications. *Neurotoxicol Teratol* 1990; **12**: 285–92.

51. Hemminki K, Vineis P. Extrapolation of the evidence on teratogenicity of chemicals between humans and experimental animals: chemicals other than drugs. *Teratog Carcinog Mutagen* 1985; **5**: 251–318.

52. Kimmel CA, Holson JF, Hogue CJ, Carlo G. *Reliability of Experimental Studies for Predicting Hazards to Human Development*. NCTR Technical Report for Experiment No. 6015, Jefferson, AR, 1984.

53. Newman LM, Johnson EM, Staples RE. Assessment of the effectiveness of animal developmental toxicity testing for human safety. *Reprod Toxicol* 1993; **7**: 359–90.

54. Nisbet ICT, Karch NJ. *Chemical Hazards to Human Reproduction*. Park Ridge, NJ: Noyes Data Corp., 1983.

55. National Research Council. *Scientific Frontiers in Developmental Toxicology and Risk Assessment*. Washington, DC: National Academy Press, 2000.

# Chapter 2

# Environmental contaminants and exposure

Mary A. Fox and Yutaka Aoki

## Introduction

People come into contact with potentially hazardous chemical contaminants as part of daily life. Chemical contaminants arise from natural and anthropogenic sources. Chemical contaminants occur in the ambient environment such as outdoor air, surface water and soil, and in the air, dust on surfaces, food, water, and products found and used in indoor environments, e.g. workplaces, schools, and homes.

Contact or exposure to a hazardous chemical contaminant is necessary but not sufficient in itself to result in an adverse health effect. A sufficient amount of the chemical contaminant must be absorbed into the body and must reach the relevant site within the body where it may change or disrupt normal function. Absorption (or uptake) is influenced by properties of the body and properties of the chemical contaminant. Once inside the body the contaminant may be altered by metabolism, stored, or eliminated as waste.

This chapter reviews concepts of exposure and dose; identifies sources of contaminants; and describes the circumstances of human exposures. The range of contaminants of concern for reproductive health is discussed in Chapter 1. Selected examples highlighting exposure and dose topics are provided below.

## Understanding exposure and dose

### Basic definitions of exposure and dose

The following definitions are adapted from Zartarian et al. [1]. Exposure is defined as contact between a contaminant and the target (for our purposes the target of interest is the human body). Dose is defined as the amount of contaminant that enters the target over a specified time period by crossing a contact boundary. The contact boundary is a point or area of the body where exposure occurs. Dose as defined here is difficult to measure because a dose of contaminant at the contact boundary is then processed in the body, as discussed later. Body burden – the amount of a contaminant that enters the body and *remains inside* – can be more easily measurable and is used as a dose measure. Understanding exposure to environmental contaminants entails understanding the contaminants – their physical and chemical properties and where they are found – as well as the human activities that result in contact with contaminants. Various determinants of exposure to environmental contaminants are summarized in Table 2.1 and reviewed below. A discussion of dose follows.

## Sources of contaminants and circumstances of exposure

### Contaminant sources and disposition in the environment

Contaminants are introduced into outdoor and indoor environments from multiple sources such as manufacturing and energy production (contaminants used during production and retained in products or released as wastes or emissions), vehicular emissions, and consumer product use (e.g. insecticide applications to pets). The ultimate disposition of a contaminant in the environment will depend on its physical form (solid, liquid, or gas), chemical properties (e.g. solubility in water and reactivity) and its interactions with other natural processes. Some contaminants may be broken down quickly in ambient environments, while others persist.

Contaminants may be introduced into one or more media and may move between media. The chemical form of a contaminant may be changed as it moves through the environment. For example, mercury is found in the environment as metallic mercury and in

*Environmental Impacts on Reproductive Health and Fertility*, ed. T. J. Woodruff, S. J. Janssen, L. J. Guillette, and L. C. Giudice. Published by Cambridge University Press. © Cambridge University Press 2010.

**Table 2.1.** Important determinants of exposure.

| | |
|---|---|
| Contaminants | Physical and chemical properties of contaminants |
| | Single or multiple contaminant(s) |
| | Amount or concentration of contaminants |
| Sources of contaminants | Naturally occurring or man-made |
| | Emissions including industrial and automotive |
| | Consumer products including foods and food containers, toys, electronics, lotions, cosmetics |
| Environmental media | Air |
| | Water |
| | Soil |
| | Dust |
| | Food |
| | Consumer products |
| | Multiple media |
| Exposure pathways/routes | Eating or drinking/ingestion |
| | Breathing/inhalation |
| | Touching/dermal absorption |
| | Combinations of pathways/routes |
| Exposure settings | At home |
| | At work |
| | At school |
| | In transit |
| | Indoors and outdoors |
| Exposure frequency and duration | Frequency: one-time, intermittent, continuous |
| | Duration: seconds or minutes up to lifetime |
| Population(s) of concern | Adult |
| | Adolescent |
| | Child |
| | Fetus |
| | Other special populations or individuals, such as those with underlying chronic conditions |

organic and inorganic forms. Mercury changes forms as it moves through different environmental media. Conversion of inorganic mercury to methylmercury (organic form) occurs primarily in microorganisms in aquatic environments [2].

An important concept regarding movement of contaminants in the environment is bioaccumulation – where an organism retains contaminants at a concentration higher than that in its environment. Most often contaminants that bioaccumulate are lipophilic (fat-loving) and not easily broken down; they accumulate in fatty tissues. Biomagnification occurs when many species in the food chain bioaccumulate. Biomagnification may result in concentration increases by orders of magnitude, from environmental media to the top of the food chain. Contaminants released into the environment in only minute amounts may be biomagnified to be health hazards. Methylmercury is

biomagnified up the food chain and contaminates food fish [2].

Multiple contaminants may be found in a given medium and may also occur in multiple media. For example, Fox *et al.* (2002) evaluated health risks for estimated concentrations of 148 hazardous air pollutants for a study area in Philadelphia [3]. The US EPA analyzes exposure to groups of related pesticides that are found in food and water (resulting from agricultural practices) and also used in and around the home [4]. Total exposure to a given contaminant must consider multiple sources, pathways, and routes of exposure. Total exposure to an individual or population must consider multiple contaminants in multiple media.

## Humans and their environments

People interact with multiple environmental media every day, contacting indoor and outdoor air, surface

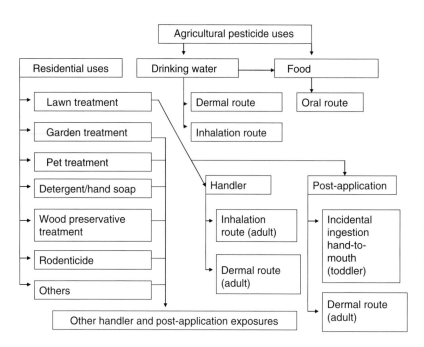

**Fig. 2.1.** Examples of sources, pathways, and routes of exposure to pesticides (adapted from EPA [80]).

and drinking water, soil and dust, food, and consumer products. The contaminated media people contact through breathing, eating and drinking, and touching are called exposure pathways. Exposure pathways correspond to exposure routes of inhalation, ingestion, and dermal absorption. Figure 2.1 contains some examples of exposure pathways and exposure routes resulting from agricultural and residential pesticide uses. For example, after applying a pesticide to a lawn a child playing in the grass may ingest some pesticide residue due to hand-to-mouth behavior. Exposure settings are the places where people spend time and include homes, gardens, workplaces, schools, and cars. Occurrence of contaminants will vary by setting and humans are exposed to multiple contaminants simultaneously or sequentially.

### Timing of exposure: frequency and duration

Frequency and duration of exposure to environmental contaminants depends on human activities and on the occurrence of contaminants. People move through multiple exposure settings on a daily basis and will likely contact many environmental media in different geographic locations over a lifetime. Contaminants, as mentioned above, may move through multiple media and may persist in some media and not in others. Characterizing the timing of exposure requires understanding how often and how long a person is in contact

with a contaminated medium and the occurrence of contaminants in that medium.

### Populations of concern

Human activities and exposure settings and subsequent contaminant exposure change by age and life stage. For example, a child has greater incidental soil ingestion than an adult. A child also consumes more food and drink per unit of body weight than an adult to meet its growth and developmental needs. The workplace is an exposure setting relevant for reproductive-age adults. Table 2.2 includes information on a number of contaminants of concern for reproductive health, many of which are used in commercial production and other workplace settings. Exposures to the developing fetus through blood and amniotic fluid will depend on the mother's exposures and how the contaminants are distributed and processed in her body (more detail is given in the dose and body burden sections). In the first few months of life a breast-fed infant's exposure through food will be largely determined by its mother's body burden and a formula-fed infant will be exposed to any contaminants in the formula, in the water used to prepare its formula, or contaminants that may leach from the bottle, e.g. bisphenol-A[5]. Mouthing and crawling bring an infant into contact with contaminants in toys and house dust. Lifestyle differences such as consumption of traditional diets by indigenous populations also

**Table 2.2.** Selected examples of contaminants linked to reproductive, fertility or developmental problems.

| Types of contaminants and examples | Sources and exposure circumstances |
| --- | --- |
| Metals | |
| *Mercury* | Occurs from energy production emissions and naturally. Enters the aquatic food chain through a complex system. Primary exposure by consumption of contaminated seafood |
| *Lead* | Found in older homes where lead-based paints were used and in or on some toys and children's jewelry. Exposure by incidental ingestion |
| Organic compounds | |
| Ethylene oxide | Occupational exposure to workers sterilizing medical supplies or engaged in manufacturing |
| Pentachlorophenol | Wood preservative for utility poles, railroad ties, wharf pilings; formerly a multi-use pesticide. Found in soil, water, food, breast milk |
| Bisphenol A | Chemical intermediate for polycarbonate plastic, resins. Found in consumer products and packaging. Exposure through inhalation, ingestion, dermal absorption |
| *PCBs* | Used as industrial insulators and lubricants. Banned in the 1970s but persistent. Present in the aquatic and terrestrial food chains resulting in exposure by ingestion |
| *Dioxins* | Byproducts of manufacture and combustion of chlorine-containing products. Persistent in the environment; present in the aquatic and terrestrial food chains resulting in exposure by ingestion |
| *PFOS* | Perfluorinated compound used in consumer products as stain- and water-repellant. Persists in the environment. Occupational exposure to workers and general population exposure by inhalation, ingestion, dermal contact |
| DEHP | Phthalates are plasticizers in consumer products and used as solvents for personal care products. Exposures occur by inhalation, ingestion and dermal absorption |
| Pesticides | |
| Chlorpyrifos | Organophosphate pesticide used in agricultural production and for home pest control (home uses are now restricted [75]). Exposure routes include inhalation, dietary and non-dietary ingestion, and dermal contact. |
| *DDT* | Organochlorine insecticide banned in USA in the 1970s but still used abroad. Persistent in soil. Enters the food chain resulting in ingestion exposures. |
| Air contaminants | |
| ETS Common air pollutants (e.g. PM, ozone, Pb) | Burning of tobacco products. Exposure by inhalation from active or passive smoking. Sources include combustion of wood and fossil fuels, and industrial production. Exposure by inhalation |
| Glycol ethers | Used in enamels, paints, varnishes, stains, electronics, cosmetics. Occupational and general population exposure by inhalation, ingestion, dermal contact |

Notes: Contaminants in *italics* are persistent and/or bioaccumulative.
Source and exposure data: [76, 77].
Health effects information: [51, 77–79].
Abbreviations: DDT, dichlorodiphenyltrichloroethane; DEHP, di-(2 ethyl hexyl) phthalate; ETS, environmental tobacco smoke; Pb, lead; PCB, polychlorinated biphenyl; PFOS, perfluorooctane sulfonate; PM, particulate matter.

may result in increased exposures. For example, a number of persistent organic contaminants are present in the traditional diets consumed in northern Alaska[6].

The location, nature, and extent of contamination present in the environmental media people contact is the other determinant of human exposure. Studies investigating environmental injustices have shown exposure disparities to poor communities and communities of color due to circumstances such as: proximity to a greater number of contaminant sources (see, for example, Perlin *et al.* [7]); exposure to contaminants at higher concentrations (see, for example, environmental tobacco smoke or lead in Rauh *et al.* [8]); or exposure to mixtures of chemicals with greater overall toxicity (see, for example, Fox *et al.* [3]).

# Distinguishing exposure and dose

The terms exposure and dose are often used interchangeably. It is advisable, however, to distinguish these conceptually. Dose information is more relevant than

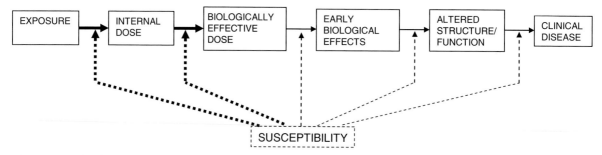

**Fig. 2.2.** Simplified flow chart of classes of biomarkers (indicated by boxes). (Adapted from *Environ Health Perspect* 1987; **74**: 3–9, with permission [9].)

exposure information in studying the health effects of contaminants since as a component of disease etiology it is more proximal to the health outcome. On the other hand, measuring dose tends to be more difficult than determining exposure. Dose estimates are often calculated using exposure information.

## Understanding dose in relation to the disease process

The widely accepted "biomarker" (biological marker) paradigm (Fig. 2.2)[9] is useful in conveying a better understanding of exposure and dose. "Exposure" to a human host (a target) could result in an "internal dose," which in turn would result in exposing a "target organ" to the contaminant. Once transferred into the target organ, the contaminant becomes a "biologically effective dose" to a "target site" (e.g. organ, group of cells, or molecule). Quantified as a concentration, both internal dose and biologically effective dose are body-burden measures. The successive process of exposure becoming dose to the next enclosed entity is reminiscent of a set of Matryoshka nesting dolls. Once a contaminant reaches an ultimate target molecule, distinction between exposure and dose blurs with no further boundary to cross.

As an example, consider ingestion of dioxin-contaminated soil. A relatively easy way to estimate dioxin dose through this exposure route would be to measure dioxin concentration in the soil (or estimate it through modeling) and multiply the concentration with typical consumption rates of soil. The estimated dose is not equivalent to a biologically relevant dose because the bioavailability of the dioxin (i.e. how much of it is absorbed by the gastrointestinal [GI] tract) is much lower than 100% and not easily measured or estimated. With some extra effort we can measure concentrations of dioxins in human serum – "internal dose" – and

epidemiologically study the health effects of dioxin exposure. To study dioxin hepatotoxicity, we can measure dioxin concentration in homogenized liver – biologically effective dose at the target organ. Note that the dioxin concentration in serum and liver would be different. This is primarily because serum and liver differ in concentration of lipids, where most dioxins are present due to their high lipophilicity. Even after adjusting for lipid content the two – serum vs. liver – concentrations still may differ potentially because dioxins may be moving between the blood and liver as well as be metabolized in the liver. Conceptually, biologically effective dose at the target molecule, e.g. the arylhydrocarbon (Ah)-receptor (receptor for dioxin), would be a better predictor of hepatic adverse effects. But because the Ah-receptor is in the cytosol (which is hard to isolate), the biologically effective dose for the Ah-receptor is difficult to measure.

Various processes act on contaminants to affect their ultimate fate and distribution within the body and the biologically effective dose relevant to the health outcome of concern. These toxicokinetic processes are known as ADME: Absorption, Distribution, Metabolism, and Excretion [10–12]. Each of these processes may be influenced by inherited or acquired factors. In a population with the same level of exposure, some individuals may be more susceptible to the toxic effects of contaminants due to differences in ADME. In Fig. 2.2, the first two upward dashed arrows on the left coming from the box labeled "Susceptibility" represent the kinds of ADME-related susceptibility factors discussed in this chapter. The other three upward dashed arrows represent susceptibility regarding toxicodynamics, i.e. the study of what chemicals do to the body, and are beyond the scope of this chapter. In general, we need to be concerned about potentially high-risk subgroups of individuals with ADME-related susceptibilities. They include pre-existing illness (e.g. chronic liver disease leading to low detoxifying capacity), sub-optimal nutrition (e.g. low antioxidant intake), and other specific conditions to be mentioned below.

# Determinants of dose: absorption, distribution, metabolism, and excretion

## From exposure to dose: intake and absorption

Intake means that contaminants have passed through a nominal body boundary such as the mouth or nose. Absorption occurs at the contact boundaries between the body and the environment, e.g. gastrointestinal tract, respiratory tract, and skin. Absorption occurs either through passive diffusion (contaminants move according to a concentration gradient without requiring energy input) or active transport (energy-dependent movement sometimes against a concentration gradient) or both. Rates of absorption may be affected by many factors. For instance, absorption of a contaminant on skin may increase dramatically in the presence of open wounds, an acquired condition. Some toxic metals (e.g. lead) are similar in their chemical properties to necessary metals (e.g. calcium). If the body is deficient in calcium or iron, lead absorption is increased [13]. Polymorphism in the genes coding proteins involved in the active transport system may also affect absorption [14].

## Distribution and storage in the body

Distribution refers to the movement of agents from the absorption site(s) to potential targets and other components of the host. In the developed human body, distribution occurs primarily through the bloodstream. Once transported to a target organ boundary, compounds enter the organ either through passive diffusion or active transport. Organisms have some barriers designed to keep unwanted compounds from reaching sensitive target organs. Agents in a pregnant mother's body may transfer across the placenta to the fetus. In the past, the placenta was considered (or, desired, rather) to be a perfect protective barrier. This optimistic view has been proven wrong through such unfortunate examples as fetal alcohol syndrome [15], fetal Minamata disease (from mercury exposures) [16], thalidomide-induced limb defects [17], and the trans-generational reproductive effects of diethylstilbestrol (DES) (see Chapter 1). The blood–brain barrier has some, albeit limited, ability. Some toxic agents, such as methylmercury, cross the blood–brain barrier easily [11]. The blood–brain barrier is underdeveloped in

fetuses, making them especially susceptible to central nervous system toxicity [18]. Many exogenous compounds bind to carrier molecules in plasma, such as albumin and lipoprotein, through interaction with amino acid residues, lipophilicity, ionic interaction, etc. Individuals with higher concentrations of any of these carrier molecules, e.g. those with hyperlipidemia, as an inherited or acquired condition, thus may retain higher concentration of agents in plasma.

Some contaminants are "stored" in the body. For instance, lipophilic compounds such as organochlorine pesticides and dioxin-like compounds may be taken up by adipose tissues and stored for a long period of time[19]. Certain toxic metals (e.g. lead [11] and cadmium [20]) are stored in bone. Contaminants are not permanently stored; they can be mobilized (e.g. increased blood lead level during pregnancy due to greater bone turnover) [13]. Other contaminants pass through the body quickly (e.g. perchlorate). Stopping exposure to such contaminants results in immediate reduction in body burden.

## Metabolism

Metabolism or biotransformation (as reviewed extensively by Parkinson [12]) of contaminants may occur in any part of the body including the site of absorption, blood, and target or non-target tissues. In general, living organisms including humans deal with absorbed contaminants by changing them into a more water-soluble form through enzymatic reaction, thereby facilitating their eventual removal in urine. Often metabolites are less toxic than the parent compound, but metabolism may also enhance toxicity. Biotransformation reactions are generally divided into two phases. In phase I reactions (catalyzed by enzymes such as carboxylesterases and the cytochrome P450 family), agents undergo hydrolysis, reduction, or oxidation, revealing or creating a residue(s) that renders them water-soluble or allows them to undergo phase II reaction. In phase II (e.g. glucuronidation and methylation), additional component(s) are conjugated to the agents or their metabolites, also increasing water solubility, which easily allows excretion from the body.

For many of the genes that code the phase I and II enzymes, genetic polymorphisms have been documented. These polymorphisms may influence enzyme phenotypes in terms of catalytic capacity or quantity present (either through changes in enzyme production or removal). Sometimes between-individual distribution of biotransformation enzyme activity in tissue

13

shows bimodal (or even trimodal) distribution, allowing us to group individuals clearly into slow or fast metabolizers. Depending on the toxicity of intermediate and ultimate metabolites, either slow or fast metabolizers are more susceptible. A classical example of this is the higher risk of bladder cancer among slow acetylators (Phase II) in White populations [21]. Polymorphism in genes coding biotransformation enzymes as a susceptible factor has been studied for childhood leukemia [22], for which an in utero origin and environmental etiology have been reported [23].

As an example of a phase I reaction, some organophosphate compounds are oxidized by cytochrome P450 isozymes to become a more toxic form called oxons [24]. Some organophosphates are detoxified by serum paraoxonase (a Phase I enzyme), which is found in lower concentrations in the fetus and neonates than in adults [25]. There is emerging evidence that low activity paraoxonase phenotype is a susceptibility factor for organophosphate toxicity [26]. Parkinson (2001) describes many phase II examples [12].

Biotransformation enzymes are distributed throughout the body, but they are most abundant in the liver, the main initial site of biotransformation for chemicals absorbed through the GI-tract. Liver clearance of contaminants by neonates is considerably reduced compared with adults [27], making neonates potentially more susceptible. Acquired deficiency in liver function of pregnant women, e.g. from cirrhosis, may also result in a higher dose of such agents to the fetus. Activity of some biotransformation enzymes are increased or decreased as a result of exposure to an inducer or suppressor, which sometimes is the compound(s) metabolized by the enzyme. Inducers and suppressors are often found in the diet. Some contaminants known as "hormone mimics" may be biotransformed by hormone-metabolizing enzymes due to their molecular similarity to an endogenous hormone.

## Excretion

Excretion is the process that eliminates contaminants from the body. Perhaps the most important route of excretion is through the kidneys, where water-soluble forms of contaminants or their metabolites are filtered and pumped out in the urine. Some contaminants are excreted in bile through the liver after undergoing a phase II conjugation reaction. Highly volatile contaminants are often eliminated via exhalation. Depending upon their chemical properties contaminants may be excreted through other glands including sweat, saliva, tears, as well as breast milk, which is important in reproductive health. Since breast milk has a high fat content, many lipophilic contaminants and their metabolites are excreted in breast milk in relatively high concentrations. Excretion also occurs through continuously or periodically departing parts of the body including hair, nail, dead skin, and other epithelial cells, e.g. gastrointestinal lining.

Because of easy access, samples of urine and hair (sometimes nails) are collected from individuals and analyzed for contaminants. Often measurements of contaminants in these samples are interpreted as markers of exposure or dose. In a strict sense, though, they are markers of excretion. To interpret them as markers of exposure (or body burden) at the population level, it is necessary to assume that all subjects involved are similar in terms of ADME processes (or excretion rate is universally proportionate to body burden). However, when a high concentration of a contaminant is detected in the urine of an individual, it could represent very different scenarios, characterized by high or low risk for adverse effects. The individual may have: high exposure (increased risk); enhanced ability to excrete the contaminant through urine (perhaps signaling decreased risk); or lower capacity to store the contaminant in adipose tissue or bone (either increased or decreased risk depending on other factors including the fate of stored contaminants). Contaminant concentrations in excreta must be interpreted with care.

The capacity to excrete a contaminant varies individually, again according to heritable or acquired conditions. For instance, rates of excretion through the kidney are affected by the relative size of kidney, perfusion rate, anatomic and molecular characteristics of the kidney related to its filtering and reabsorption capacity, etc. Pregnancy itself transfers contaminants from the mother's body to the fetus.

## How reproductive and developmental functions affect exposure and dose

In reproductive environmental health, a fetus is arguably the most important target, with the placenta acting as an absorption barrier. Fetal dose thus may be estimated using data on maternal internal dose (serum concentration of a contaminant), the characteristics of placenta as an absorption barrier and amnion as a reabsorption site. A more direct measurement would come from the contaminant concentration in umbilical cord blood, which is readily accessible primarily at the time of delivery. Many active transport systems operate at high capacity during fetal and neonatal developmental periods potentially increasing absorption of contaminants.

Exposure to eggs and sperm may affect reproductive health as damage to the egg or sperm can increase the risk of adverse health effects in subsequent offspring. Eggs experience the lifetime exposure history of a female. Sperm mature over a 72-day period and are potentially exposed to agents between the time of ejaculation and the time of conception. Damage to cells involved in sperm production/maturation, e.g. Sertoli cells, may result in infertile or otherwise compromised sperm. A fertilized egg does not benefit from the placental barrier until it fully develops.

## Time-varying nature of exposure and dose

So far, our discussion has focused on fixed exposures and how various factors, heritable and acquired, may change the consequence of the exposure. Now we consider how the level of exposure and dose for a given individual could change over time and the implications of such changes. The time-varying nature of exposure and dose is especially important for reproductive health since a high dose that occurs at a critical time in development may have devastating effects, as documented for example for thalidomide embryopathy [17] and DES (see Chapter 1).

Consider an infant ingesting breast milk containing lead. On a given day, the baby might consume more or less breast milk. Lead concentration in the breast milk would increase or decrease per changes in the maternal blood lead. One day the baby may ingest a small piece of chipped paint containing lead from a recalled toy or house dust. If the baby goes to a country where leaded gasoline is still used, she will be exposed to lead in the air. As this example shows, the level of exposure of an individual to a given contaminant changes continuously. Internal dose and biologically effective dose arising from the exposure change accordingly.

Depending upon the physicochemical properties of a contaminant, current body burden may be determined predominantly by current (or recent) exposure. This would be the case for carbon monoxide in air at relatively low concentrations. On the other hand, for contaminants such as polychlorinated biphenyls (PCBs), which are lipophilic and stable, with a long retention time in our body (plausible estimates of the biological half-life for PCBs in humans range from a few to several years [28]), the predominant determinant of the current body burden is past exposure from contaminated food. Eating a PCB-free diet would not result in an immediate decrease in the internal dose of PCBs. Even over a period when PCB exposure changes little, the internal dose of PCBs may increase as a result of changes in the host characteristics, e.g. mobilization of contaminant stored in adipose tissue following dieting or increased physical activity.

## Quantifying dose by estimation or measurement

### Overview of methods

Exposure assessments for epidemiological research or human health risk assessment purposes produce estimates of dose. Data collection for exposure assessments includes monitoring of environmental media and surveys of human activity patterns. These data are combined mathematically by multiplying the concentration of a contaminant in media by the rate of contact with media to develop dose estimates. For example, if a baby drinks 0.7 liter per day of breast milk containing 2 µg per liter of lead, her dose of lead is 1.4 µg per day. Assuming 100% bioavailability, this figure is typically interpreted as the dose. Usually estimates like this are divided by body weight as a way of standardization allowing comparisons. (Think of a pill ingested by an infant or adult. If the same amount of drug is taken and is instantaneously distributed throughout the body, the infant with lower body weight would have a higher dose than the larger adult.) If the baby's weight is 5 kg, her estimated dose is 0.56 µg per kg body weight per day ($2 \times 1.4/5 = 0.56$). Simple dose estimates of this form can be further refined with data on the contaminant bioavailability. When estimating dose for a population, a standard practice is to assume a typical contact rate and weight corresponding to the population of interest, rather than collecting data on each specific case. Population-level information on various determinants of exposure has been compiled by the US EPA. Further information on exposure assessment methods can be found in the EPA's *Guidelines for Exposure Assessment* [29], *Child-specific Exposure Factors Handbook* [30] and Paustenbach [31]. Qualitative assessments of exposure, e.g. whether or not pesticides are used in the home, are also used in epidemiological research.

Many contaminants of concern (and their metabolites) can be measured in body tissues such as blood or serum, urine, hair, saliva, etc. Sources of such biomonitoring data in the USA (the National Health and

Nutrition Examination Survey, discussed later) and Europe have emerged in recent years as important tools for environmental health research and policy [32]. As one relevant example, analyses of banked Swedish breast-milk samples revealed an alarming increase in body burden of flame retardants since the 1960s [33]. Biomarker measurements establish that contaminant exposure and absorption have occurred. However, the relationship between contaminants measured in body tissues and disease may not be well understood. Interpretation of biomarkers as measures of internal dose or biologically effective dose requires an understanding of ADME and disease processes.

### Strengths and limitations of available methods

#### What we can measure vs. what we want to measure

The distinction between what we can measure (or estimate) and the disease-relevant entity that we intend to measure is important for interpreting scientific findings. Due to practical difficulties the available dose estimate or measurement may not approximate the latter well, but it is all that is available. In studying effects of difficult-to-measure exposures and doses (e.g. low-level, highly time-varying), continued improvement in measurement is crucial.

#### When high exposures are of concern

Toxic agents typically have monotonically increasing dose–response relationships. Highly exposed individuals are at higher risk for adverse health effects. Variation in intake or contact rates with certain media may be large: high-end contact rates observed in surveys or specially designed studies are used when estimating high-end exposure level. Often exposure data are provided in the form of a population average. Average exposure level tells little about the high-end exposure (unless exposure is highly homogeneous) and may be of limited use for assessing exposure-related risks. Wherever possible, attempts to assess variation in exposure, e.g. providing percentiles or standard deviation of the distribution, should be made.

Sometimes a single massive, short-term exposure results in a dose that has profound adverse effects. For instance, a brief exposure to a high concentration of carbon monoxide in air could be fatal. Again, a time-averaged exposure will not be useful in studying this kind of exposure-effect relationship if the averaging time is too long (e.g. 8 or 24 hours). An exposure or dose index that reflects short-term peak exposures, e.g. maximum of average for each 10-minute period

recorded over one day (or during a critical period of development), is often relevant.

## Obtaining data on exposure and dose

Large nationally representative surveys are great sources of data on exposure and dose.

The National Health and Nutrition Examination Survey (NHANES) contains multiple items relevant to contaminant exposure and dose. Most notably, the laboratory component of the survey includes an "environmental health profile." In the 1999–2006 survey, blood and urine from subsamples of participants were assayed for numerous contaminants of reproductive health concern. Interpretation of these biomonitoring data as measures of exposure or dose are subject to the caveats mentioned above. The survey also includes: a 2-day dietary recall; questions on use of pesticides in the home; and questions on industry and occupation.

Investigation of contaminant sources may be difficult using NHANES data, with the possible exception of dietary exposure. If exposures are primarily through diet, the two-day dietary recall and food frequency questionnaire may adequately capture the necessary information. On the other hand, the data available on occupation and industry are based on rather broad categories and the only contaminant included with the occupation questions is environmental tobacco smoke [34].

## Case examples

Table 2.2 summarizes source and exposure information for a selection of important contaminants linked to reproductive and fertility problems or adverse birth or developmental outcomes. Three of these selected contaminants are discussed in more detail to highlight exposure sources, circumstances, and health outcomes of concern.

## Mercury

### Uses and exposure sources, pathways, and routes

Mercury and its compounds have been used in many ways – industrial, pesticidal, medicinal, and cosmetic – many of which have been discontinued. Remaining uses account for a small portion of the mercury released into the environment. Historically, mercury in the industrial processes (e.g. mercury amalgam in the chloralkali process and as a catalyst for acetaldehyde production) accounted for a significant source of mercury discharge to a local body of water. Currently the main anthropogenic sources of mercury in the environment include combustion of fossil fuel, which has naturally occurring mercury, and incineration of medical waste [2]. Mercury takes one of three valence states: $Hg^0$, Hg+, Hg++. Biomagnification and methylation of mercury have been mentioned earlier. Acidification of the environment occurring on a global scale may cause release of mercury in the sediment into a body of water. Elemental mercury ($Hg^0$) is used in dental amalgam, which gives low-level, long-term inhalation exposure. High-level exposure to elemental mercury through inhalation has happened in occupational settings, e.g. hat-making and gold mining.

### Absorption and markers of internal dose

Inhaled elementary mercury in vapor form is easily absorbed. Absorption of organic mercury in seafood is facilitated through amino acid carriers with cysteine residues. The thiol group of cysteine has high affinity for mercury. The main source of exposure in humans is through contaminated seafood [2]. Elemental mercury and organic mercury easily cross the placental and blood–brain barriers. Hair is the most common specimen analyzed for an internal dose marker of mercury, followed by blood and, much less frequently, urine. A desiccated piece of umbilical cord, a common keepsake in the Asia–Pacific region, has been used to determine fetal internal dose. Methylmercury concentrations in umbilical cord blood tend to be higher than that in maternal blood [35].

### Reproductive and developmental outcomes of concern

Neurologic effects in the fetus and neonate have been documented for high-level organic mercury exposure from poisoning incidents in Japan, Iraq, and other places [2]. Recent studies from the Farrow Islands documented neurocognitive effects from seafood consumption, which have been recognized as developmental effects by the National Academy of Sciences and the US EPA [2]. A recent concern was the possibility that the mercury-containing preservative thimerosal in vaccines caused autism. In 2004 an Institute of Medicine Committee studied the issue and concluded that "the evidence favors rejection of a causal relationship" [36]. Inorganic mercury has estrogenic effects [37] and might adversely affect viability of male fetuses. A US government-funded review found no convincing evidence for any adverse health effects from dental amalgam other than rare hypersensitivity [38]. Danish researchers concluded that dental amalgam is unsuitable for medical reasons [39].

### Minamata disease

In the 1950s a massive outbreak of methylmercury poisoning occurred among residents living near Minamata Bay in southern Kyushu Island in Japan. The source of exposure was contaminated seafood. Congenital or pediatric cases would have received the mercury dose in utero and/or via ingestion of breast milk or seafood. In the 1930s the Chisso factory started to discharge into the bay wastewater containing methylmercury, a catalytic by-product. The discharge continued until 1968, when the national government officially recognized the cause of the outbreak as the wastewater from the factory. Despite this recognition, no official restrictions on catching or selling seafood from Minamata Bay have ever been implemented. The 1968 recognition incorrectly stated that the ban had been in place and that no new cases had occurred since 1960.

Minamata disease is commonly described as a "neurological disorder," in which various senses (hearing, vision, smell, taste, and touch) and motor coordination including speech are impaired [2]. Yet the evidence for non-neurological effects, such as decreased live male births [40] and elevated leukemia mortality [41], is emerging. Unfortunately, except for one cross-sectional study [42], no population-based epidemiological study of the disease has been conducted in Minamata to date. Formation of a cohort for prospective follow-up at an earlier time would have been immensely useful for investigating a broad range of potential health effects from methylmercury. A second incident of mercury poisoning occurred in Agano in Honsyu Island in the mid 1960s. In Agano pregnant women were screened based on hair mercury concentration. Those with hair mercury at 50 parts per million or greater were given advice on "birth control."

# Organophosphate pesticides

### Uses and exposure sources, pathways, and routes

Organophosphates are a class of insecticides that act on the nervous system by inhibiting enzyme function. Organophosphates are used in food production and for control of residential insects and pathogen-carrying mosquitoes. Organophosphates are not persistent in the environment and came into wide use as the organochlorine pesticides (which do persist in the environment) were phased out [43]. Nonetheless, organophosphates are found in indoor and outdoor environments. Lu *et al.* (2004) evaluated multiple pathways of exposure in agricultural and non-agricultural communities and found detectable levels of organo-phosphate pesticides in indoor air, house dust, soil, food and on children's hands and toys [44]. Pesticide applicators and agricultural workers may be exposed by inhalation, dermal absorption, dietary and non-dietary ingestion at work and can introduce organophosphates into their home environments [45]. Organophosphate residues on foods are the most important contributor to exposure for the general population [46].

### Absorption and markers of internal dose

Organophosphates are absorbed into the body through inhalation, ingestion, and dermal routes of exposure [47,48]. Metabolites of organophosphates have been measured in blood, urine, saliva, breast milk, amniotic fluid, umbilical cord blood, and meconium [49,50]. Environmental sampling such as air monitoring does not always correlate well with metabolite levels in biological tissues [49].

### Reproductive and developmental outcomes of concern

Pesticide exposures (including organophosphates) to male agricultural workers are associated with various measures of poor semen and sperm quality including reduced seminal volume and percentage motility, and decreased sperm count per ejaculate and reduced percentage of viable sperm [51, 52]. Pesticide exposures (including organophosphates) to female agricultural workers are associated with reproductive effects such as menstrual cycle disturbances, longer time to pregnancy as well as spontaneous abortion, stillbirths, and developmental effects in offspring [52,53]. In utero exposures have been associated with neurodevelopmental abnormalities in animals (see, for example, Lazarini *et al.* [54]); and neurodevelopment and growth abnormalities in humans. Outcomes observed in epidemiological studies include pervasive developmental disorder; decreased gestational duration; intrauterine growth restriction; and reduced head circumference, birthweight, and length [55–59].

## Phthalates

### Uses and exposure sources, pathways, and routes

Phthalates are a class of chemicals used in the commercial production of plastic items such as bags, food packaging, medical tubing and blood-storage bags, and toys, and in soaps, lotions, and personal care products as well as many other common products [60]. In addition to exposure due to use of consumer products containing phthalates, people are exposed to phthalates in multiple environmental media including ambient air, water and soil, indoor air and house dust. People come into contact with phthalates through all routes of exposure: ingestion, inhalation, and dermal absorption.

### Absorption and markers of internal dose

Phthalates are absorbed into the body and metabolites of multiple phthalates are found in urine, maternal and fetal serum, amniotic fluid, and breast milk [60–62]. The relative contribution of any particular source or route of exposure to total human exposure and to internal dose remains unclear. Inhalation and ingestion are thought to be important routes of exposure for the general population [60]. Sathyanarayana *et al.* report on research showing that the use of lotions, shampoos, and powders on infants (dermal exposure) is associated with increased concentrations of phthalate metabolites in infant urine [63].

### Reproductive and developmental outcomes of concern

There is a substantial body of literature on the reproductive and developmental effects of certain phthalates in animals. In utero exposures to di-(2-ethylhexyl) phthalate (DEHP), di-*n*-butyl phthalate (DBP), benzyl butyl phthalate (BBP), and or diisononyl phthalate (DINP) affect male reproductive development with outcomes such as reduced ano-genital distance, nipple retention, hypospadias, and undescended testes [64]. In utero exposure to individual phthalates and mixtures of phthalates reduces testosterone production in fetal rats[65–67]. Testicular lesions were found in pubertal and adult rats exposed to DINP [68]. Reduced ovarian hormone production, anovulation, and failure to maintain pregnancy were observed in female rats exposed to DEHP [69,70].

Epidemiological evidence of the reproductive effects of phthalates is limited. Examples of outcomes observed in human studies include: reduced male fertility through altered semen quality in men with higher urinary concentrations of mono-*n*-butyl phthalate and monobenzyl phthalate [71], and altered male reproductive development represented by shorter ano-genital distance in infants with prenatal exposure to phthalates [72].

## Discussion of case examples

Considering the Minamata Bay contamination in comparison to exposures to phthalates exemplifies a shift in the focus of environmental health from major ambient pollution events to everyday contact with consumer products. Environmental health policies enacted by the US government over the past 30–40 years have succeeded in reducing contamination in the ambient environment in many cases, although there are certain notable exceptions, for example a documented increase in polybrominated diphenyl ethers (PBDEs) [73].

Protecting reproductive and developmental health is a daunting task. Reproductive system function is complex, as is the developing organism. There are multiple types of contaminants of concern found in multiple environmental media. The populations of concern include men and women of reproductive age, and the fetus, infant, and child.

# Environmental contaminants and exposure: science and policy issues

It is important to have information on sources of contaminants and the circumstances of exposure. Exposure may be demonstrated through biomonitoring of human tissues but reducing exposure through individual or public policy change will be impossible without knowledge of contaminant sources and exposure circumstances.

People are exposed to multiple contaminant mixtures. However, research on mixture exposures and potential health effects is scant. Research on the developmental effects of in utero exposure to phthalates is a notable exception.

The time-varying nature of an individual's exposure implies that a single measurement does not accurately reflect the average exposure level of that individual. A high level of within-individual, across-time variation in exposure may artificially inflate between-individual variation. In order to accurately estimate intrinsic between-individual variation, contribution of within-individual variation needs to be removed. Failure to properly remove it results in overestimation of the intrinsic between-individual variation and the proportion of individuals with exposures at or above critical levels. (Nonetheless, we generally are more concerned about underestimation arising from failure to capture data on highly exposed individuals or high-exposure situations.)

Within-individual variation in contaminant exposure and dose over time makes it difficult to study its health effects. In an ideal epidemiological study, we would follow subjects prospectively over time, repeatedly measuring their exposure (dose), and determine their health status periodically. A *prospective* study

like this is very costly and would take a long time to conduct. A *retrospective* study, which investigates associations between past exposure and existing health effects, may avoid the extended time requirement, but past exposure is difficult or impossible to measure. Studies of health effects of persistent organic pollutants (POPs) are an exception, since POPs tend to remain in the body for a long time. Internal doses of these contaminants measured at a single time point often are considered to be a good measure of the internal dose experienced in the past.

In experimental animal studies controlled doses of potentially harmful substances are used. These studies are basically free of the problems stemming from the difficulties in estimating dose and exposure in humans. There are other advantages to animal experiments (e.g. primary prevention before large-scale human exposure and potential to inform mechanism of toxicity). The main disadvantage is difficulty in inter-species extrapolation. Thus, human observational and animal experimental studies complement each other in the assessment of potential reproductive effects from environmental exposure.

Many chemicals currently used are non-persistent, and chemicals to be introduced will be increasingly non-persistent because of regulations. The need to study these non-persistent chemicals poses a challenge for epidemiologists because of their transient nature in the environment and in the body.

Certain exposures could be reduced instantaneously through personal efforts. For instance, since seafood is a major source of exposure to PCBs, a mother can reduce PCB exposure considerably by eliminating seafood from her diet. This does not, however, achieve rapid reduction in her PCB internal dose. If she is breastfeeding, the diet modification does not immediately reduce exposure of her baby to PCBs through breast milk, either.

While reducing seafood consumption could lower PCB levels, it can also reduce intake of beneficial components of seafood such as omega-3 fatty acid. It is necessary to go beyond personal efforts and regulate contaminants in the environment. PCBs have been banned in major industrial countries since the 1970s [74]. PCB concentrations in the environment have been declining, but older individuals have substantial body burdens while younger individuals still are exposed, albeit at lower levels. It can take a long time for regulatory actions to achieve meaningful reductions in ambient contaminant concentrations.

## Summary

Contaminants with links to problems with reproduction, fertility and birth outcomes, as well as developmental disorders and fetal origins of adult disease are found in all types of environmental media from ambient air and water to foods, to personal care products such as soaps and lotions. Multiple contaminants are present in our environment and humans are exposed to mixtures of contaminants. Exposures can take place in any setting, indoors and out. Human exposure and absorption of contaminants depend on properties of the contaminant and the medium in which it is present, as well as human activities, which change over the lifespan. The nature of reproductive system function and human development presents challenges to quantitative measurement of contaminant exposure and dose and subsequent study of health effects. Effective public policies to reduce exposure and health risks will require information on sources and circumstances of exposure to contaminants.

## References

1. Zartarian V, Bahadori T, McKone T. Adoption of an official ISEA glossary. *J Expo Anal Environ Epidemiol* 2005; **15**: 1–5.

2. National Research Council. *Toxicological Effects of Methylmercury*. Washington, DC: The National Academies Press; 2000.

3. Fox MA, Burke T, Groopman I. Evaluating cumulative risk assessment for environmental justice: a community case study. *Environ Health Perspect* 2002; **110**: 203–9.

4. Environmental Protection Agency (EPA). *Assessing Pesticide Cumulative Risk* [Internet]. Environmental Protection Agency 2008 June 16 Available from: URL: http://www.epa.gov/oppsrrd1/cumulative/ (Accessed Aug 31, 2008.)

5. Le HH, Carlson EM, Chua JP. *et al*. Bisphenol A is released from polycarbonate drinking bottles and mimics the neurotoxic actions of estrogen in developing cerebellar neurons. *Toxicol Lett* 2008; **176**: 149–56.

6. Hoekstra PF, O'Hara TM, Backus SM. *et al*. Concentrations of persistent organochlorine contaminants in bowhead whale tissues and other biota from northern Alaska: implications for human exposure from a subsistence diet. *Environ Res* 2005; **98**: 329–40.

7. Perlin SA, Wong D, Sexton K. Residential proximity to industrial sources of air pollution: interrelationships among race, poverty, and age. *J Air Waste Manag Assoc* 2001; **51**: 406–21.

8. Rauh VA, Landrigan PJ, Claudio L. Housing and health: intersection of poverty and environmental exposures. *Ann N Y Acad Sci* 2008; **1136**: 276–88.

9. Anonymous. Biological markers in environmental health research. Committee on Biological Markers of the National Research Council. *Environ Health Perspect* 1987; **74**: 3–9.

10. Rodricks JV. *Calculated Risks: The Toxicity and Human Health Risks of Chemicals in our Environment*. 2nd Edition. Cambridge: Cambridge University Press, 2007.

11. Rozman KK, Klaassen CD. Absorption distribution and excretion of toxicants. In Klaasen C, ed. *Casarett and Doull's Toxicology: The Basic Science of Poisons*. 6th Edition. New York: McGraw-Hill, 2001: 107–32.

12. Parkinson A. Biotransformation of xenobiotics. In Klaasen C, ed. *Casarett and Doull's Toxicology: The Basic Science of Poisons*. 6th Edition. New York: McGraw-Hill, 2001: 133–224.

13. Goyer RA. Lead toxicity: current concerns. *Environ Health Perspect* 1993; **100**: 177–87.

14. Kang HJ, Song IS, Shin HJ. *et al*. Identification and functional characterization of genetic variants of human organic cation transporters in a Korean population. *Drug Metab Dispos* 2007; **35**: 667–75.

15. Calhoun F, Warren K. Fetal alcohol syndrome: historical perspectives. *Neurosci Biobehav Rev* 2007; **31**: 168–71.

16. Ekino S, Susa M, Ninomiya T. *et al*. Minamata disease revisited: an update on the acute and chronic manifestations of methyl mercury poisoning. *J Neurol Sci* 2007; **262**: 131–44.

17. Miller MT, Stromland K. Teratogen update: thalidomide: a review, with a focus on ocular findings and new potential uses. *Teratology* 1999; **60**: 306–21.

18. Rodier PM. Developing brain as a target of toxicity. *Environ Health Perspect* 1995; **103**: 73–6.

19. Kutz FW, Wood PH, Bottimore DP. Organochlorine pesticides and polychlorinated biphenyls in human adipose tissue. *Rev Environ Contam Toxicol* 1991; **120**: 1–82.

20. Jarup L. Cadmium overload and toxicity. *Nephrol Dial Transplant* 2002; **17**: 35–9.

21. Rothman N, Garcia-Closas M, Hein DW. Commentary: Reflections on G. M. Lower and colleagues' 1979 study associating slow acetylator phenotype with urinary bladder cancer: meta-analysis, historical refinements of the hypothesis, and lessons learned. *Int J Epidemiol* 2007; **36**: 23–8.

22. Sinnett D, Labuda D, Krajinovic M. Challenges identifying genetic determinants of pediatric cancers – the childhood leukemia experience. *Fam Cancer* 2006; **5**: 35–47.

23. Smith MT, McHale CM, Wiemels JL. *et al*. Molecular biomarkers for the study of childhood leukemia. *Toxicol Appl Pharmacol* 2005; **206**: 237–45.

24. Sams C, Mason HJ, Rawbone R. Evidence for the activation of organophosphate pesticides by

cytochromes P450 3A4 and 2D6 in human liver microsomes. *Toxicol Lett* 2000; **116**: 217–21.

25. Furlong CE, Holland N, Richter RJ. *et al.* PON1 status of farmworker mothers and children as a predictor of organophosphate sensitivity. *Pharmacogenet Genomics* 2006; **16**: 183–90.

26. Costa LG, Cole TB, Furlong CE. Polymorphisms of paraoxonase (PON1) and their significance in clinical toxicology of organophosphates. *J Toxicol Clin Toxicol* 2003; **41**: 37–45.

27. Gow PJ, Ghabrial H, Smallwood RA. *et al.* Neonatal hepatic drug elimination. *Pharmacol Toxicol* 2001; **88**: 3–15.

28. Shirai JH, Kissel JC. Uncertainty in estimated half-lives of PCBs in humans: impact on exposure assessment. *Sci Total Environ* 1996; **187**: 199–210.

29. Environmental Protection Agency (EPA). *Guidelines for Exposure Assessment*. Environmental Protection Agency, Risk Assessment Forum, Washington, DC, 600Z-92/001, 1992. Available from: URL: http://oaspub.epa.gov/eims/eimscomm.getfile?p_download_id=429103 (Accessed Aug 31, 2008.)

30. Environmental Protection Agency (EPA). *Child-specific Exposure Factors Handbook* (Interim Report). Environmental Protection Agency 2002. Available from: URL: http://cfpub.epa.gov/ncea/cfm/recordisplay.cfm?deid=55145 (Accessed Aug 31, 2008.)

31. Paustenbach DJ. The practice of exposure assessment: a state-of-the-art review. *J Toxicol Environ Health B Crit Rev* 2000; **3**: 179–291.

32. Angerer J, Bird MG, Burke TA. *et al.* Strategic biomonitoring initiatives: moving the science forward. *Toxicol Sci* 2006; **93**: 3–10.

33. Noren K, Meironyte D. Certain organochlorine and organobromine contaminants in Swedish human milk in perspective of past 20–30 years. *Chemosphere* 2000; **40**: 1111–23.

34. Centers for Disease Control and Prevention (CDC). *Documentation, Codebook, and Frequencies, Occupation, Questionnaire, Survey Years: 2003 to 2004*. Centers for Disease Control and Prevention 2008 January. Available from: URL: http://www.cdc.gov/nchs/data/nhanes/nhanes_03_04/ocq_c.pdf (Accessed Aug 31, 2008.)

35. Stern AH, Smith AE. An assessment of the cord blood: maternal blood methylmercury ratio: implications for risk assessment. *Environ Health Perspect* 2003; **111**: 1465–70.

36. Institute of Medicine. *Immunization Safety Review: Vaccines and Autism*. Washington, DC: The National Academies Press, 2004.

37. Zhang X, Wang Y, Zhao Y. *et al.* Experimental study on the estrogen-like effect of mercuric chloride. *Biometals* 2008; **21**: 143–50.

38. Brownawell AM, Berent S, Brent RL. *et al.* The potential adverse health effects of dental amalgam. *Toxicol Rev* 2005; **24**: 1–10.

39. Mutter J, Naumann J, Walach H. *et al.* [Amalgam risk assessment with coverage of references up to 2005]. *Gesundheitswesen* 2005; **67**: 204–16.

40. Sakamoto M, Nakano A, Akagi H. Declining Minamata male birth ratio associated with increased male fetal death due to heavy methylmercury pollution. *Environ Res* 2001; **87**: 92–8.

41. Yorifuji T, Tsuda T, Kawakami N. Age standardized cancer mortality ratios in areas heavily exposed to methyl mercury. *Int Arch Occup Environ Health* 2007; **80**: 679–88.

42. Yorifuji T, Tsuda T, Takao S. *et al.* Long-term exposure to methylmercury and neurologic signs in Minamata and neighboring communities. *Epidemiology* 2008; **19**: 3–9.

43. National Research Council (NRC). *Pesticides in the Diets of Infants and Children*. Washington, DC: National Academy Press; 1993.

44. Lu C, Kedan G, Fisker-Andersen J. *et al.* Multipathway organophosphorus pesticide exposures of preschool children living in agricultural and nonagricultural communities. *Environ Res* 2004; **96**: 283–9.

45. Curl CL, Fenske RA, Kissel JC. *et al.* Evaluation of take-home organophosphorus pesticide exposure among agricultural workers and their children. *Environ Health Perspect* 2002; **110**: A78792.

46. Environmental Protection Agency (EPA). *Organophosphate Pesticides (OP) Cumulative Assessment – 2006 Update* [Internet]. Environmental Protection Agency 2008 June 16. Available from: URL: http://www.epa.gov/oppsrrd1/cumulative/2006-op/index.htm (Accessed Aug 31, 2008.)

47. Garfitt SJ, Jones K, Mason HJ. *et al.* Oral and dermal exposure to propetamphos: a human volunteer study. *Toxicol Lett* 2002; **134**: 115–18.

48. Aprea C, Terenzoni B, De A, V. *et al.* Evaluation of skin and respiratory doses and urinary excretion of alkylphosphates in workers exposed to dimethoate during treatment of olive trees. *Arch Environ Contam Toxicol* 2005; **48**: 127–34.

49. Fenske RA, Bradman A, Whyatt RM. *et al.* Lessons learned for the assessment of children's pesticide exposure: critical sampling and analytical issues for future studies. *Environ Health Perspect* 2005; **113**: 1455–62.

50. Samarawickrema N, Pathmeswaran A, Wickremasinghe R. *et al.* Fetal effects of environmental exposure of pregnant women to organophosphorus compounds in a rural farming community in Sri Lanka. *Clin Toxicol (Phila)* 2008; **46**: 489–95.

51. Hanke W, Jurewicz J. The risk of adverse reproductive and developmental disorders due to occupational pesticide exposure: an overview of current epidemiological evidence. *Int J Occup Med Environ Health* 2004; **17**: 223–43.

52. Peiris-John RJ, Wickremasinghe R. Impact of low-level exposure to organophosphates on human reproduction and survival. *Trans R Soc Trop Med Hyg* 2008; **102**: 239–45.

53. Bretveld R, Brouwers M, Ebisch I. *et al.* Influence of pesticides on male fertility. *Scand J Work Environ Health* 2007; **33**: 13–28.

54. Lazarini CA, Lima RY, Guedes AP. *et al.* Prenatal exposure to dichlorvos: physical and behavioral effects on rat offspring. *Neurotoxicol Teratol* 2004; **26**: 607–14.

55. Eskenazi B, Harley K, Bradman A. *et al.* Association of in utero organophosphate pesticide exposure and fetal growth and length of gestation in an agricultural population. *Environ Health Perspect* 2004; **112**: 1116–24.

56. Eskenazi B, Marks AR, Bradman A. *et al.* Organophosphate pesticide exposure and neurodevelopment in young Mexican-American children. *Environ Health Perspect* 2007; **115**: 792–8.

57. Eskenazi B, Rosas LG, Marks AR. *et al.* Pesticide toxicity and the developing brain. *Basic Clin Pharmacol Toxicol* 2008; **102**: 228–36.

58. Perera FP, Rauh V, Tsai WY. *et al.* Effects of transplacental exposure to environmental pollutants on birth outcomes in a multiethnic population. *Environ Health Perspect* 2003; **111**: 201–5.

59. Whyatt RM, Rauh V, Barr DB. *et al.* Prenatal insecticide exposures and birth weight and length among an urban minority cohort. *Environ Health Perspect* 2004; **112**: 1125–32.

60. Centers for Disease Control and Prevention (CDC). *Third National Report on Human Exposure to Environmental Chemicals*. Atlanta, GA, 2005.

61. Fennell TR, Krol WL, Sumner SC. *et al.* Pharmacokinetics of dibutylphthalate in pregnant rats. *Toxicol Sci* 2004; **82**: 407–18.

62. Dostal LA, Weaver RP, Schwetz BA. Transfer of di(2-ethylhexyl) phthalate through rat milk and effects on milk composition and the mammary gland. *Toxicol Appl Pharmacol* 1987; **91**: 315–25.

63. Sathyanarayana S, Karr CJ, Lozano P. *et al.* Baby care products: possible sources of infant phthalate exposure. *Pediatrics* 2008; **121**: e260–8.

64. Gray LE, Jr., Ostby J, Furr J. *et al.* Perinatal exposure to the phthalates DEHP, BBP, and DINP, but not DEP, DMP, or DOTP, alters sexual differentiation of the male rat. *Toxicol Sci* 2000; **58**: 350–65.

65. Parks LG, Ostby JS, Lambright CR. *et al.* The plasticizer diethylhexyl phthalate induces malformations by decreasing fetal testosterone synthesis during sexual differentiation in the male rat. *Toxicol Sci* 2000; **58**: 339–49.

66. Mylchreest E, Sar M, Wallace DG. *et al.* Fetal testosterone insufficiency and abnormal proliferation of Leydig cells and gonocytes in rats exposed to di(n-butyl) phthalate. *Reprod Toxicol* 2002; **16**: 19–28.

67. Howdeshell KL, Wilson VS, Furr J. *et al.* A mixture of five phthalate esters inhibits fetal testicular testosterone production in the Sprague-Dawley rat in a cumulative, dose-additive manner. *Toxicol Sci* 2008; **105**: 153–65.

68. Foster PM, Foster JR, Cook MW. *et al.* Changes in ultrastructure and cytochemical localization of zinc in rat testis following the administration of di-n-pentyl phthalate. *Toxicol Appl Pharmacol* 1982; **63**: 120–32.

69. Davis BJ, Maronpot RR, Heindel JJ. Di-(2-ethylhexyl) phthalate suppresses estradiol and ovulation in cycling rats. *Toxicol Appl Pharmacol* 1994; **128**: 216–23.

70. Gray LE, Jr., Laskey J, Ostby J. Chronic di-n-butyl phthalate exposure in rats reduces fertility and alters ovarian function during pregnancy in female Long Evans hooded rats. *Toxicol Sci* 2006; **93**: 189–95.

71. Duty SM, Silva MJ, Barr DB. *et al.* Phthalate exposure and human semen parameters. *Epidemiology* 2003; **14**: 269–77.

72. Swan SH, Main KM, Liu F. *et al.* Decrease in anogenital distance among male infants with prenatal phthalate exposure. *Environ Health Perspect* 2005; **113**: 1056–61.

73. Hale RC, Alaee M, Manchester-Neesvig JB.*et al.* Polybrominated diphenyl ether flame retardants in the North American environment. *Environ Int* 2003; **29**: 771–9.

74. Ceccarini A, Giannarelli S. Polychlorobiphenyls. In Nollet LML, ed. *Handbook of Water Analysis*. 2nd Edition. Boca Raton: CRC Press, 2007; 537–8.

75. Environmental Protection Agency (EPA). *Reregistration Eligibility Decision for Chlorpyrifos.* Environmental Protection Agency 2006 July 31 Available from: URL: http://www.epa.gov/pesticides/reregistration/REDs/chlorpyrifos_red.pdf

76. Library of Medicine. *Hazardous Substances Data Bank* [Internet]. United States Library of Medicine 2008 Available from: URL: http://toxnet.nlm.nih.gov/cgi-bin/sis/htmlgen?HSDB

77. Woodruff TJ, Carlson A, Schwartz JM. *et al.* Proceedings of the Summit on Environmental Challenges to Reproductive Health and Fertility: executive summary. *Fertil Steril* 2008; **89**: e1–20.

78. Hauser R, Sokol R. Science linking environmental contaminant exposures with fertility and reproductive health impacts in the adult male. *Fertil Steril* 2008; **89**: e59–65.

79. Perera FP, Rauh V, Whyatt RM,.*et al.* A summary of recent findings on birth outcomes and developmental effects of prenatal ETS, PAH, and pesticide exposures. *Neurotoxicology* 2005; **26**: 573–87.

80. Environmental Protection Agency (EPA). General Principles For Performing Aggregate Exposure And Risk Assessments. Environmental Protection Agency, Office of Pesticide Programs, Washington, DC, November 14, 2001. Available from: http://www.epa.gov/pesticides/trac/science/aggregate.pdf (Accessed Oct 27, 2008.)

# Chapter 3

# Development and maturation of the normal female reproductive system

## 3.1 Ovary

Laxmi A. Kondapalli and Teresa K. Woodruff

The ovaries are paired, ovoid structures measuring approximately $30 \times 20 \times 10$ mm in adulthood and weighing 3–5 g [1]. They contain the female gametes or germ cells. The ovaries are situated posterior and lateral to the uterus. Medially, they are attached to the uterus by a thick muscular uterovarian ligament. The infundibulopelvic ligament, containing the primary ovarian vasculature, suspends the lateral aspect of the ovary to the pelvic sidewall. The body of the ovary is attached to the posterior broad ligament by the mesovarium, a thin peritoneal fold.

A single layer of cells, originating from the coelomic epithelium, creates a serosal sheath over the ovary. Once known as the "germinal epithelium," the serosa now is more appropriately termed the surface epithelium and gives rise to 90% of human ovarian neoplasms [2, 3]. The cortex exists beneath the serosa and is divided into an outer, fibrous, acellular layer known as the tunica albuginea and an inner cellular, yet avascular, region of active cortex. The active cortex contains follicles of varying stages of maturation, including those comprising the ovarian reserve, the pool of primordial and primary follicles awaiting the signal for development. In addition, the cortical stroma weaves a network of spindle-shaped cells and reticular fibers around the follicles. The central region of the ovary, the medulla, is highly vascularized and consists of growing and atretic follicles as well as involuting corpora lutea. Interspersed among the follicles is a network of dense connective tissue, blood vessels, and lymphatic tissue [4].

The ovary has two main functions: to provide mature female gametes at the time of ovulation and to secrete steroid hormones and a variety of peptide and growth factors. The ovarian hormones stimulate the development of the reproductive system, induce the development of secondary sexual characteristics, and promote a receptive endometrium for the growth and development of the proconceptus. Follicle-stimulating hormone (FSH) and luteinizing hormone (LH) released by the anterior pituitary in a cyclic fashion control ovarian function. These hormones are regulated by the pulsatile release of gonadotropin-releasing hormone (GnRH) from the hypothalamus and the gonadal peptide hormone, inhibin. Thus, a highly coordinated series of positive and negative feedback systems comprise this hypothalamic–pituitary–ovarian axis.

### Embryonic development of the follicle

In the human, gametes are derived from primordial germ cells that develop in the wall of the yolk sac at 4 weeks gestation [5]. The primordial germ cells originate within the primitive ectoderm, but the specific cells of origin are yet to be determined [6]. These primordial germ cells migrate from the yolk sac to the budding gonads by ameboid movement between 4–6 weeks gestation. The genital ridge is a thickened region along the ventral cranial mesonephros which gives rise to the embryonic ovary. The factors that signal and direct the migration of the primordial germ cells to the genital ridge remain unknown [7]. The mesodermal epithelium of the urogenital sinus proliferates to produce the epithelium and stroma of the gonad and envelope the dividing germ cells to form the ovary [1].

In the absence of a testis-determining factor from the Y chromosome, which coordinates the release of anti-müllerian hormone by 4–6 weeks gestation in males, the germ cells differentiate into primitive oogonia [8]. Once the primordial germ cells arrive at the gonads, they differentiate into oogonia at 6–8 weeks gestation and begin mitosis, or process of rapid cell

*Environmental Impacts on Reproductive Health and Fertility*, ed. T. J. Woodruff, S. J. Janssen, L. J. Guillette, and L. C. Giudice. Published by Cambridge University Press. © Cambridge University Press 2010.

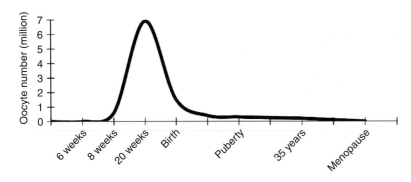

**Fig. 3.1.** Female reproductive potential across the lifespan. Primordial germ cells migrate, proliferate, and populate the evolving ovaries. Germ cell numbers dramatically increase in utero, development reaching maximal potential of 6–7 million at 20 weeks gestation. Equally impressive is the rapid decline due to follicle atresia shortly after 20 weeks, resulting in 400 000 at puberty. Of note, only 300–400 [less than 1%] from the original follicle pool are destined for ovulation, making this process highly inefficient.

division. As mitosis continues, the oogonia arrange into clusters surrounded by flat epithelial cells, granulosa cells, by 9 weeks gestation. The oogonia pass through a series of mitotic cycles before entering meiosis, the discrete mechanisms directing this transition remain unknown. The number of germ cells rapidly increases from 600 000 oogonia at 8 weeks and reaches a maximum of 6–7 million by 20 weeks gestation [6, 9]. Mitotic activity, the number and rate of cell divisions, is a major determinant of the oocyte pool [9]. The first meiotic division commences at approximately 15 weeks, thus marking the transformation of oogonia to oocytes. Oocytes arrest in prophase I until the signal for recruitment into the follicular phase of the menstrual cycle is received. Although the specific mechanisms for this arrest are still under investigation, anti-müllerian hormone could be one factor responsible for maintaining primordial follicles in the resting pool [10, 11]. This period of quiescence can last for 40 years or more and ends with ovulation or more commonly, atresia.

## Folliculogenesis

The female reproductive system is exceptionally inefficient. As the number of germ cells rapidly duplicates early in fetal development, the corresponding atresia results in an exponential fall in oocytes prior to birth. The maximum reproductive potential, or maximum number of germ cells, is achieved in the developing female in utero and from that point onward, the process of oocyte death ensues reducing the number of oocytes in the fetal ovary from 6–7 million at 20 weeks gestation, to approximately 1–2 million oocytes at birth (Fig. 3.1). Several mechanisms contribute to this depletion including oocyte and follicular atresia, errors in the normal development of some oogonia, oocyte regression, and improper packaging of oocytes with supportive cells [7]. The process of rapid decline occurs into puberty leaving an ovarian pool

of 300 000–400 000 follicles. Of these, only 300–400 oocytes will ovulate during a woman's reproductive lifetime until she is left with roughly 1000 at menopause. As a result of this inefficient sequence, less than 1% of the maximal reproductive potential is destined for ovulation and possible fertilization [7, 9, 12].

The oocytes that remain in the ovary at the time of birth are in prophase of meiosis I. The first meiotic prophase consists of five stages: leptotene, zygotene, pachytene, diplotene, and diakinesis [7]. At birth, all primary oocytes have entered and remain in prophase I, specifically the diplotene phase, a resting stage in prophase. Most ovarian follicles become atretic during the prepubertal period resulting in 400 000 oocytes total in both ovaries at puberty [6, 7, 9]. Primary oocytes remain arrested in prophase I and do not complete the first meiotic division until stimulated to develop sometime after puberty.

The ovarian follicle, the functional unit of the ovary, is composed of the oocyte surrounded by one or more layers of somatic cells, known as granulosa cells (Fig. 3.2). Follicles at rest within the ovarian cortex are known as primordial follicles and these follicles become activated by unknown factors. The first observable phenotype associated with activation is that the surrounding squamous follicular cells develop into cuboidal granulosa cells and proliferate [13, 14]. The granulosa cells rest on a basement membrane that separates the evolving follicle from surrounding stromal cells, which differentiate into the thecal cells. The oocyte and granulosa cells secrete glycoproteins onto the surface of oocyte inducing the formation of the zona pellucida [15]. Small, finger-like processes, called transzonal projections, originate from the granulosa cells and traverse through the zona pellucida [16, 17]. The transzonal projections interdigitate with the microvilli of the oocyte plasma membrane and allow for transfer of nutrients

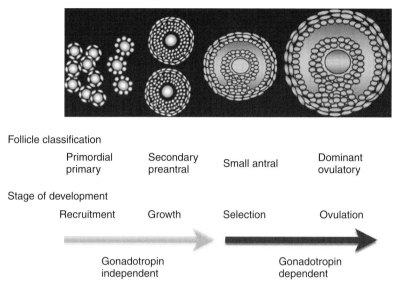

Follicle classification

| Primordial primary | Secondary preantral | Small antral | Dominant ovulatory |

Stage of development

| Recruitment | Growth | Selection | Ovulation |

Gonadotropin independent          Gonadotropin dependent

**Fig. 3.2.** Folliculogenesis. Follicles are the functional unit of the ovary, consisting of an oocyte surrounded by one or more layers of somatic cells known as granulosa cells. The process of folliculogenesis encompasses the formation of primordial follicles to the development of a mature, fertilizable oocyte. *Primordial follicles* remain at the earliest stage of development in a quiescent state. They consist of a primary oocyte surrounded by a single layer of flattened pregranulosa cells, ranging from 30–50 μm. *Primary follicles* (50–100 μm) are characterized by a single layer of cuboidal granulosa cells and may receive a signal for recruitment into the growth follicle pool. With the expansion of a second layer of granulosa cells, the follicle progresses as a *secondary follicle* (100–200 μm). Mitotic activity is high at this point, resulting in rapid proliferation of granulosa cells. The *preantral follicle* is marked by a fully grown oocyte surrounded by a zona pellucida, multiple layer of granulosa cells, basal lamina and theca cells (200 μm – 2 μm). Follicles are capable of growth up to the preantral stage in the absence of gonadotropin (*gonadotropin-independent*). The formation of a fluid-filled cavity adjacent to the oocyte [antrum] denotes an *antral follicle* (2–10 mm). The impressive growth in follicle size occurs as the granulosa and theca cells continue mitotic proliferation along with expansion of the antrum. In addition, antral follicles become responsive to gonadotropins, specifically FSH (*gonadotropin-dependent*). In the natural cycle, usually one antral follicle is selected for further development and ultimately reaches ovulation.

and communication between the two compartments. Fluid-filled spaces appear between granulosa cells as they develop into an antral follicle.

Although a group of follicles are recruited in each cycle, only one oocyte normally reaches full maturity while the others degenerate and become atretic. As the follicle matures, the oocyte resumes meiosis I shortly before ovulation. With ovulation, the maturing oocyte divides – first meiotic division – forming two daughter cells of unequal size, the secondary oocyte and a polar body. The secondary oocyte receives most of the cytoplasm and 23 diploid chromosomes whereas the first polar body receives 23 diploid chromosomes and minimal cytoplasm. After meiosis I, the oocyte enters meiosis II where chromosomes are aligned along the metaphase plate, the meiotic spindle forms within the secondary oocyte and the oocyte is released from the ovary during ovulation. Meiosis II is completed at fertilization and in the absence of fertilization it undergoes degeneration 24–36 hours after ovulation.

# Reproductive modulators

In humans, the size of the ovarian reserve decreases dramatically with age (Fig. 3.1). The ovarian reserve is variable among individual women as is the rate of follicular depletion. Variability in the initial size of the follicular pool and the rate of depletion contributes to the onset of menopause [9, 18]. A number of factors are thought to influence the age of menopause including race, parity, environmental factors, nutrition, socioeconomic status, and lifestyle exposures such as tobacco use [19, 20].

Although understanding the endogenous endocrine modulators and their impact on reproductive function is a rapidly evolving area of inquiry, there is a growing need for a better understanding of ovarian regulation given the expanding literature on the potential and real influence of environmental contaminants and occupational risks to ovarian function and fertility. Further, an awareness of these risks is growing as they are discussed regularly in women's magazines and are becoming a major concern for patients. In addition, physicians commonly use medical therapies, such as chemotherapeutic agents, in the management of their patients' conditions without clear knowledge of the reproductive consequences of such treatment. Environmental toxins have been linked to a variety of adverse reproductive outcomes such as bleeding irregularities, precocious or delayed puberty, premature ovarian failure, infertility or subfertility, pregnancy loss and congenital malformations, among others [21–26]. Human studies that explore the causal relationship between environmental exposures and resulting reproductive outcomes face a variety of challenges. For instance, it is difficult to estimate the dose of exposure or even to know when the period of critical exposure occurs for many adverse reproductive outcomes. A growing literature suggests that exposure to contaminants early in development – prenatal and neonatal periods – can be associated with a range of adverse reproductive outcomes that do not appear until after puberty or even later in life [26]. Further, in humans, it is difficult to determine the baseline prevalence of various adverse reproductive phenomena, for example, estimates of baseline infertility vary greatly depending on a number of variables, including STD prevalence, age structure and nutrition in a population. In addition, further confounding variables such as genetic predisposition, racial or ethnic differences, and socioeconomic influences likely impact reproductive outcomes.

Reproductive modulators affect reproductive function at many different levels. Oocytes enter the first meiotic division while in utero and remain arrested in prophase I until ovulation begins. Maternal exposure to toxins can impact the in utero development of the ovaries and oocytes in the growing female fetus. These fetuses can experience impaired fertility or even premature ovarian insufficiency as adults. Additionally, exposure to environmental toxins during a woman's lifetime can irreparably damage the resting cohort of follicles by inducing genetic mutations or cytotoxic effects [27]. Reproductive toxins can disrupt endocrine hormone production thus manifesting as menstrual or ovulatory dysfunction. The hypothalamic–pituitary–ovarian axis is exquisitely regulated to synchronize the menstrual cycle and interference at any point along this axis can result in loss of cyclicity or ovulation.

One example of such an effect of exogenous agents on reproductive potential is seen in chemotherapy patients. It has been well documented that children and women of reproductive age with cancer exhibit reduced or total loss of ovarian function and oocyte number following treatment with chemotherapy, radiation therapy, or both [28, 29]. In particular, germ cells are very sensitive to the dose and duration of cytotoxic chemotherapeutic drugs [28, 30]. The elimination of ovarian function is associated with absent or infrequent menstrual bleeding, decreased ovarian size, lower antral follicle counts, and increased circulating gonadotropin levels [31, 32]. As a result, these individuals suffer from an inability to achieve or maintain pregnancy and experience premature ovarian insufficiency.

The primary type of chemotherapeutic agents that damage the ovary are the alkylating agents: cyclophosphamide, melphalan, chlorambucil, and drugs like cis-platinum and vinca alkaloids [33]. Histological sections of ovaries, which have been exposed to cytotoxic drugs, have shown a wide spectrum of changes ranging from decreased numbers of follicles, total follicle absence, and fibrosis. In vivo studies demonstrate that exposure of oocytes to cyclophosphamide metabolites adversely affects oocyte function [34]. In addition, cyclophosphamide destroys the primordial follicle pool and has deleterious effects on the somatic cells. The destruction of both oocyte and surrounding cells might be due to the interdependence of the granulosa cells and the oocyte, which communicate through gap junctions. Providing options to young women and girls with a cancer diagnosis prior to treatment is an important way to avoid drug exposures that can be fertility threatening [35–37].

## Summary

In summary, the development of the ovary is dependent on local and endocrine factors that can be the target of endocrine disruptors. Endocrine disruptors may be harder to manage because of our inability to control the environment in which we develop, live, and nurture offspring. On the other hand, iatrogenic effects of agents such as chemotherapeutics can be mitigated, but only if physicians (both oncologists and reproductive specialists) are willing to offer knowledge and technologies that can spare the reproductive potential of young women facing a life-preserving but fertility-threatening cancer agent.

## References

1. Fauser BCJM. Follicle pool depletion: Factors involved and implications. *Fertil Steril* 2000; **74**: 629–30.

2. Williams TI, Toups KL, Saggese DA. *et al.* Epithelial ovarian cancer: Disease etiology, treatment,

detection, and investigational gene, metabolite, and protein biomarkers. *J Proteome Res* 2007; **6**: 2932–62.

3. Permuth-Wey J, Sellers TA. Epidemiology of ovarian cancer. *Methods Mol Biol* 2009; **472**: 413–37.

4. Sinclair AH, Berta P, Palmer MS. *et al.* A gene from the human sex-determining region encodes a protein with homology to a conserved DNA-binding motif. *Nature* 1990; **346**: 240–4.

5. Byskov AG, Hoyer PE. Embryology of mammalian gonads and ducts. In Knobil E, Neill J, eds. *The Physiology of Reproduction*. New York: Raven Press, 1988: 265–302.

6. Baker TG. A quantitative and cytological study of germ cells in human ovaries. *Proc Roy Soc Lond* 1963; **158**: 417–33.

7. Speroff L, Fritz MA. *Clinical Gynecologic Endocrinology and Infertility*. 7th Edition. Philadelphia: Lippincott Williams & Wilkins, 2005; 97–111.

8. Jost A, Vigier B, Prepin J, Perchellet JP. Studies on sex differentiation in mammals. *Recent Prog Horm Res*. 1973; **29**: 1–41.

9. Oktem O, Oktay K. The ovary: Anatomy and function throughout human life. *Ann NY Acad Sci* 2008; **1127**: 1–9.

10. Durlinger AL, Kramer P, Karels B. *et al.* Control of primordial follicle recruitment by anti-Müllerian hormone in the mouse ovary. *Endocrinology* 1999; **140**: 5789–96.

11. Durlinger AL, Gruijter MJ, Kramer P. *et al.* Anti-Müllerian hormone inhibits initiation of primordial follicle growth in the mouse ovary. *Endocrinology* 2002; **143**: 1076–84.

12. Broekmans FJ, Knauff EAH, te Velde ER, Macklon NS, Fauser BC. Female reproductive ageing: current knowledge and future trends. *Trends Endocrinol Metab* 2007; **18**: 58–65.

13. Hirshfield AN. Development of follicles in the mammalian ovary. *Int Rev Cytol* 1991; **124**: 43–101.

14. Braw-Tal R. The initiation of follicle growth: The oocyte or the somatic cells? *Mol Cell Endocrin* 2002; **187**: 11–18.

15. Wassarman PM. Zona pellucida glycoproteins. *J Biol Chem* 2008; **283**: 24 285–9.

16. Albertini DF, Barret SL. Oocyte-somatic cell communication. *Reprod Suppl* 2003; **61**: 49–54.

17. Albertini DF, Rider V. Patterns of intercellular connectivity in the mammalian cumulus-oocyte complex. *Microsc Res Tech* 1994; **27**: 125–33.

18. Santoro N. The menopause transition. *Am J Med* 2005; **118**: 8–13.

19. Westhoff C, Murphy P, Heller D. Predictors of ovarian follicle number. *Fertil Steril* 2000; **74**: 624–8.

20. Gougeon A. Dynamics of human follicular growth: Morphologic, dynamic, and functional aspects. In Leung PCK, Adashi EY, eds. *The Ovary*. San Diego: Elsevier Academic Press, 2004; 25–43.

21. Drbohlav P, Bencko V, Masata J, Jirsova S. Effect of toxic substances in the environment on reproduction. *Ceska Gynekol* 2004; **69**: 20–6.

22. Environmental Working Group. Body burden-the population in newborns: A benchmark investigation of industrial chemicals, pollutants and pesticides in umbilical cord blood. 2005. http://ewg.org/reports/bodyburden2/execsumm.php.

23. Mlynarcikova A, Fickova M, Scsukova S. Ovarian intrafollicular processes as a target for cigarette smoke components and selected environmental reproductive disruptors. *Endocr Regul* 2005; **39**: 21–32.

24. Sugiura-Ogasawara M, Ozaki Y, Sonta S. *et al.* Exposure to bisphenol A is associated with recurrent miscarriage. *Hum Reprod* 2005; **20**: 2325–9.

25. Tsutsumi O. Assessment of human contamination of estrogenic endocrine-disrupting chemicals and their risk for human reproduction. *J Steroid Biochem Mol Biol* 2005; **93**: 325–30.

26. Crain DA, Jansenn SJ, Edwards TM. *et al.* Female reproductive disorders: the role of endocrine-disrupting compounds and developmental timing. *Fertil Steril* 2008; **90**: 911–40.

27. Goldman RH. Occupational and environmental risks to reproduction in females. *Up to Date Online* 2008. http://uptodateonline.com.

28. Meirow D, Nugent D. The effects of radiotherapy and chemotherapy on female reproduction. *Hum Reprod Update* 2001; **7**: 535–43.

29. Wallace WH, Thomson AB, Saran F, Kelsey TW. Predicting age of ovarian failure after radiation to a field that includes the ovaries. *Int J Radiat Oncol Biol Phys* 2005; **62**: 738–44.

30. Goodwin PJ, Ennis M, Pritchard KI. *et al.* Risk of menopause during the first year after breast cancer diagnosis. *J Clin Oncol* 1999; **17**: 2365–70.

31. Mackie EJ, Radford M, Shalet SM. Gonadal function following chemotherapy for childhood Hodgkin's disease. *Med Pediatr Oncol* 1996; **27**: 74–8.

32. Papadakis V, Vlachopapadopoulou E, Van Syckle K. *et al.* Gonadal function in young patients successfully treated for Hodgkin disease. *Med Pediatr Oncol* 1999; **32**: 366–72.

33. Abir R, Fisch B, Raz A. *et al.* Preservation of fertility in women undergoing chemotherapy: current approach and future prospects. *J Assist Reprod Genet* 1998; **15**: 469–77.

34. Pydyn EF, Ataya KM. Effect of cyclophosphamide on mouse oocyte in vitro fertilization and cleavage: recovery. *Reprod Toxicol* 1991; **5**: 73–8.

35. Woodruff TK. The emergence of a new interdiscipline: oncofertility. *Cancer Treat Res* 2007;**128**: 3–11.

36. Backhus LE, Kondapalli LA, Chang RJ. *et al.* Oncofertility consortium consensus statement: guidelines for ovarian tissue cryopreservation. *Cancer Treat Res.* 2007; **138**: 235–9.

37. Nieman CL, Kinahan KE, Yount SE. *et al.* Fertility preservation and adolescent cancer patients: lessons from adult survivors of childhood cancer and their parents. *Cancer Treat Res* 2007; **138**: 201–17.

# 3.2 Oviduct and uterus

Leo F. Doherty and Hugh S. Taylor

## Introduction

The development of the internal female reproductive tract, namely the fallopian tubes (oviducts), uterus, cervix, and upper vagina, is a coordinated process influenced directly by specific gene expression and indirectly by hormone activity. The early human embryo is phenotypically identical in both sexes. Differences in sexual development between males and females occur as a result of specialization of organ systems in response to a chromosomal complement that is determined at the time of conception. The genotype of an embryo, specifically the presence or absence of a Y chromosome, is responsible for gonadal development. Differentiation of the gonad into either an ovary or a testis directs the development of the internal genital structures. Knowledge of the normal development of the female genital tract is an essential foundation to be able to understand abnormalities of the reproductive tract.

During the 6th week of embryonic development the müllerian (paramesonephric) ducts develop lateral to the wolffian (mesonephric) ducts in both males and females (see Fig. 3.3). The mesonephric ducts are remnants of renal development that persist to affect the development of the internal genitalia. The müllerian ducts arise from an invagination of the dorsal coelomic epithelium on the surface of the mesonephric duct in the urogenital ridge. The development of the müllerian ducts is thought to be influenced by the wolffian ducts [1]. The müllerian ducts extend from the level of the 3rd thoracic segment to the posterior wall of the urogenital sinus. The caudal portion of each müllerian duct apposes the contralateral duct before the pair of ducts contact the urogenital sinus. The cranial ends of the müllerian ducts open into the coelomic cavity. At the end of the 6th week of development, the genital systems of male and female embryos appear similar [2]. By the 7th week of development, however, the presence or absence of a testis (and testis-derived hormones) determines the subsequent developmental fate of both the müllerian and wolffian ducts.

The presence of a Y chromosome, in genetic males, and expression of the SRY gene lead to a series of events that result in further development of the wolffian ducts

and regression of the müllerian ducts. SRY expression leads to the development of Sertoli cells. Sertoli cells influence ductal development in two ways. First, Sertoli cells produce anti-müllerian hormone (AMH), also known as müllerian inhibiting substance (MIS), which induces degeneration of the müllerian ducts. Anti-müllerian hormone is a 560-amino-acid glycoprotein belonging to the transforming growth factor β (TGF-β) family of proteins [3, 4]. Anti-müllerian hormone exerts its effect upon the müllerian duct by binding to the MIS-specific type II (Misr2) receptor. Misr2 is upregulated by Wnt-7a. Mutations in AMH, Misr2, or Wnt-7a result in persistence of the müllerian ducts in males [5]. Second, the Sertoli cells recruit mesenchymal cells into the gonadal ridge that differentiate into testosterone-secreting Leydig cells. Under the influence of testosterone, the wolffian ducts develop into the seminal vesicles, vas deferens, and epididymis. See Chapter 4 for a more detailed explanation of the development of the male reproductive system.

Female embryos lack the SRY gene and therefore do not develop Sertoli cells. Therefore, no AMH is secreted in female embryos and the müllerian ducts persist and continue development. Because there is no Sertoli cell-induced development of Leydig cells, there is insufficient testosterone production to further stimulate the development of the wolffian ducts. The wolffian ducts therefore regress in females, with the exception of some vestiges. The epoöphoron and paraoöphoron (found in the mesentery of the ovary) and the Gartner's ducts (found between the broad ligament and the vagina) are the remnants of the wolffian duct that persist in females. There is controversy regarding a potential role of wolffian duct-derived tissue in vaginal development that will be discussed below.

The müllerian ducts, in the absence of AMH, develop into fallopian tubes, uterus, cervix, and upper vagina. Estrogen, produced by granulosa cells in the ovary, is necessary to attain a fully developed uterus. Estrogen receptor α (ER-α) is expressed in mesenchyme of the developing human uterus beginning in the early second trimester [6]. The differentiation into unique (albeit smaller) morphologic structures does not require estrogen or the estrogen receptor. This is in sharp contrast to the wolffian ducts, which regress in the absence of testosterone or a functional testosterone receptor. Mice with a targeted disruption of ER-α have

*Environmental Impacts on Reproductive Health and Fertility*, ed. T. J. Woodruff, S. J. Janssen, L. J. Guillette, and L. C. Giudice. Published by Cambridge University Press. © Cambridge University Press 2010.

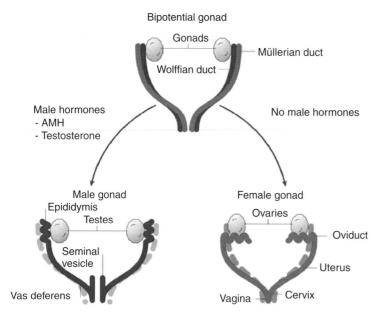

Bipotential gonad

Gonads

Wolffian duct

Müllerian duct

Male hormones
- AMH
- Testosterone

No male hormones

Male gonad
Epididymis
Testes

Seminal
vesicle

Vas deferens

Female gonad
Ovaries

Oviduct

Uterus

Vagina

Cervix

**Fig. 3.3.** Prior to sexual differentiation of the gonad, the müllerian and wolffian ducts are present in both sexes. The müllerian ducts develop lateral to the wolffian ducts. As the paired müllerian ducts extend toward the urogenital sinus, they cross medial to the wolffian ducts where they meet and appose one another. After gonadal differentiation is complete, the secreted hormone products influence the further development and/or regression of the ducts. Testes secrete anti-müllerian hormone (AMH) and testosterone, causing the müllerian ducts to degenerate and the wolffian ducts to develop into the seminal vesicles, vas deferens, and epididymis. Ovaries do not secrete AMH or testosterone, and therefore the müllerian duct persists and develops into the fallopian tubes, uterus, cervix, and upper vagina. In the absence of testosterone, the wolffian ducts regress. (Adapted from Kobayashi and Behringer, *Nat Rev Genet* 2003; **4**: 969–80 [42].)

rudimentary genitalia with a distinct oviduct, uterus, cervix, and vagina [7].

## Genetic basis of müllerian duct development

The female reproductive system arises from a uniform müllerian duct and differentiates into distinct segments with unique structure and function. The genetic basis of this differential pattern of segmentation has been described [8, 9]. Developmental patterning genes have been highly conserved throughout evolution. Multi-cellular animals share the same genes that determine the body plan along undifferentiated developmental axes. The conservation of the genetic pathways that regulate reproductive tract development among animals underscores the importance of animal models in evaluating the effects of chemicals such as endocrine disruptors on the human reproductive tract.

Many genes have been found necessary for normal development of the müllerian ducts. Some genes are involved in early development of the reproductive tract and have effects on the development of both sexes. The importance of these various genes is often best understood by examination of the phenotype of mice with targeted disruption of each individual gene. *Lim1* is a transcription factor involved in the development of the urogenital system that is found in the developing müllerian duct as early as embryonic day 11.5. The importance of *Lim1* in the developing reproductive tract is shown by the fact that mice with mutations in *Lim1* have absent fallopian tubes, uterus, and upper vagina in females and absent wolffian duct derivatives in males [10]. *Pax2* is a homeodomain containing transcription factor critical to the development of the urogenital tract in both sexes. *Pax2*-null mice show degeneration of the reproductive tracts (wolffian and müllerian) and absence of the ureters and kidneys. While mice with mutations in *Lim1* have complete absence of the ducts, *Pax 2*-null mice initially form wolffian and müllerian ducts, which later degenerate [11]. Another homeobox containing transcription factor, called *Emx2*, is expressed in the epithelial components of the developing urogenital system [12]. *Emx2*-null mice lack all components of the urogenital system, specifically the kidneys, ureters, gonads, and genital tracts. Although the wolffian duct initially forms in *Emx2* mutant mice on embryonic day 10.5, it degenerates on embryonic day 11.5. The müllerian duct never forms in *Emx2*-null mice [13].

Genetic factors influencing sex-specific reproductive tract development have also been described. The mammalian homologues of the *Drosophila* gene wingless, known as *Wnt* genes, encode glycoproteins that are important in many aspects of embryonic development. *Wnt-4* is required for normal development of the müllerian duct in both sexes [14]. *Wnt-4*-null males are phenotypically normal, while females are masculinized with absent müllerian ducts. *Wnt-4* also functions in the ovary

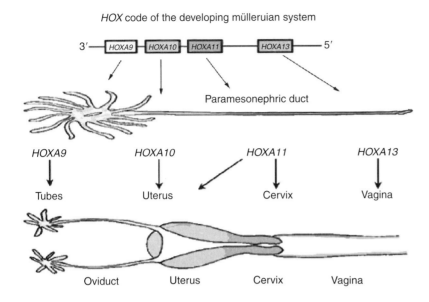

HOX code of the developing mülleruian system

**Fig. 3.4.** *HOX* genes give segmental identity to the developing müllerian duct. Expression of a particular *HOX* gene in a segment of this duct leads to appropriate development of adult structures.

to prevent development of testosterone-producing Leydig cells, thus *Wnt-4*-null females secrete more testosterone due to development of Leydig cells within the ovary [15].

The *HOX* genes establish cellular identities along undifferentiated axes in all higher multi cellular animals [16]. The müllerian and wolffian duct systems are two such seemingly uniform undifferentiated tissue axes. *HOX* genes give differential identity to the various segments of these developmental axes (see Fig. 3.4). In women, the expression of *HOX* genes leads to the development of distinct female reproductive structures (fallopian tubes, uterus, cervix, and upper vagina) from the previously uniform müllerian duct.

Homeobox (*HOX*) genes are the homologues of the homeotic genes in *Drosophila*. In humans, 39 *HOX* genes are clustered into four unlinked genomic loci designated *HOXA-D*. They are located on chromosomes 7, 17, 12, and 2. Position within the cluster reflects both the timing and spatial position of developmental expression [17–19]. Genes that are more 3' are expressed earlier and more cranially than their 5' neighbors (which are expressed later and more caudally). These genes give rise to tissue identity along several body axes, including the central nervous system, vertebrae, limbs, and the reproductive tract.

*HOX* genes are transcription factors that regulate gene expression to determine appropriate body segment identity. The order and differential expression of *HOX* genes along previously undifferentiated axes lead to proper development of appropriate region-specific body structures. *HOX* genes of groups 9–13

are expressed in restricted domains along the axes of the developing wolffian and müllerian ducts [20, 21]. *HOXA9* is expressed in areas destined to become the fallopian tube. *HOXA10* is expressed in the developing uterus. *HOXA11* is expressed in the primordia of the lower uterine segment and cervix. *HOXA13* is expressed in the ectocervix and upper vagina. There is no *HOXA12* gene. The expression of these *HOX* genes in the designated location along müllerian ducts leads to the development of appropriate adult structures (Fig. 3.4). Similar *HOX* expression in males leads to segmental identity of the wolffian duct [22].

Alterations in *HOX* genes help illustrate their developmental importance. Hand-foot-genital syndrome is a rare dominantly inherited condition associated with mutations in the *HOXA13* gene [23,24]. Both men and women with mutations in the *HOXA13* gene have reproductive tract anomalies. Genital abnormalities in this syndrome include hypospadias in males and müllerian fusion defects (described later in this chapter) in females.

Reproductive tract development is altered by the non-steroidal estrogen diethylstilbestrol (DES). Diethylstilbestrol alters the expression of *HOXA* genes in the müllerian duct [25]. In utero DES exposure shifts *HOXA9* expression from the oviducts to the uterus and decreases both *HOXA10* and *HOXA11* expression in the uterus. The typical uterine structure (driven by *HOXA10* and *HOXA11*) is lost and the uterus displays a developmental identity more similar to those structures

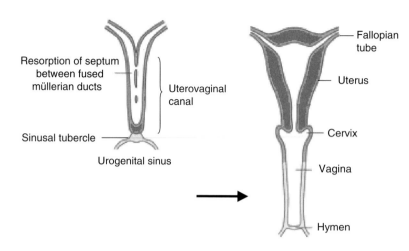

**Fig. 3.5.** After the two müllerian ducts fuse together, the vertical septum between the two ducts is resorbed to form the single uterovaginal canal. The uterovaginal canal will then differentiate further into the uterus, cervix, and upper vagina.

in which *HOXA9* is usually expressed (the fallopian tube). The T-shaped uterus seen in women exposed to DES could represent a narrow and more branched structure, similar to the structure of the fallopian tube. As mentioned above in the discussion on AMH, *Wnt-7a* is necessary for müllerian duct regression in males (by increasing expression of *Misr2*). *Wnt-7a* also functions in normal female development. It is expressed in the fallopian tube and uterine epithelium, and mice with mutations in the gene show abnormal fallopian tube coiling and uterine gland development [26]. Diethylstilbestrol decreases uterine expression of *Wnt-7a* [27]. It is therefore likely that the anomalies associated with in-utero DES exposure are due to alteration of *HOX* and other developmental gene expression.

Diethylstilbestrol is not the only estrogen-like compound (xenoestrogen) to affect *HOX* gene expression. Methoxychlor (MXC) is a pesticide and xenoestrogen that has been shown to decrease *HOX* gene expression in a similar fashion to DES [28]. Methoxychlor exposure in utero leads to adverse reproductive outcomes in mice. *HOXA10* is permanently repressed in the uteri of mice exposed to MXC in utero [29]. Bisphenol A (BPA) is a xenoestrogen that causes adverse reproductive outcomes in both humans and animals. *HOXA10* levels are increased in adult mice that were exposed to BPA in utero [30]. Alterations in the normally precise temporal regulation of *HOXA10*, either increased or decreased, appear to have implications for reproductive success.

## Maturation of the müllerian ducts

As mentioned above, the müllerian ducts begin lateral to the wolffian ducts. As they extend caudally and

medially, they cross medial to the wolffian ducts where they meet and appose one another. As the ducts come into contact with one another, they form a Y-shaped structure which serves as the primordium of the fallopian tubes, uterus, cervix, and upper vagina [31]. The upper, non-apposing portions of the duct will develop into the fallopian tubes. As the müllerian ducts grow caudally, they make contact with a thickening of the posterior wall of the urogenital sinus known as the sinusal tubercle (also known as the müllerian tubercle) [32]. When two müllerian ducts contact the sinusal tubercle, the apposing ducts begin to fuse into a single tubular structure. Fusion begins at the caudal aspect of the müllerian ducts and continues cranially. The apposing walls of the müllerian ducts initially form a vertical septum between the two ducts. This septum degenerates in the caudal-cranial direction (see Fig. 3.5). Once the septum between the two fused müllerian ducts has been completely resorbed, a tubular structure with a single lumen is formed. This tubular structure is known as the uterovaginal canal, which will become the uterus and cervix, as well as part of the upper vagina (there is controversy regarding the development of the vagina, which will be mentioned below) [33]. The two caudal openings of the unfused portions of the müllerian ducts will develop into the uterine openings of the fallopian tubes. The two cranial openings of the müllerian ducts, which open into the coelomic cavity, will develop into fimbria of the fallopian tubes.

The epithelium of the uterovaginal canal is derived from the coelomic epithelium (mesothelium). As the caudal portion of the uterovaginal canal contacts the sinusal tubercle of the urogenital sinus, a mesenchymal thickening surrounds its walls. The epithelium of the cervix, uterus (including the endometrial glands), and

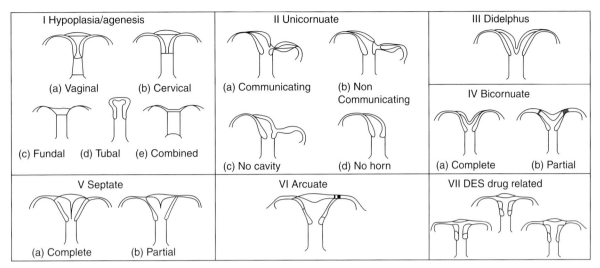

**Fig. 3.6.** The spectrum of clinically observed abnormalities of the female reproductive tract as classified by the American Society for Reproductive Medicine. (Reproduced from Allen and Feste, *Fertil Steril* 1989; **51**: 199–201 [43].)

fallopian tubes originate from the epithelium of the utero-vaginal canal. The cervical stroma, endometrial stroma, and smooth muscle of the myometrium are derived from the mesenchymal thickening that surrounds the utero-vaginal canal as it contacts the urogenital sinus [34].

## Development of the vagina

Despite many years of research, the embryology and development of the vagina remains controversial. The commonly accepted theory of vaginal development, made popular by Koff in 1933, will be described first. Koff proposed that as the uterovaginal canal develops, the sinusal tubercle of the urogenital sinus thickens and forms a pair of tissue swellings known as the sinovaginal bulbs [34]. These bulbs fuse together to form a solid tissue known as the vaginal plate. The vaginal plate is thought to develop into the lower portion of the vagina, with the upper vagina developing from the uterovaginal canal. The vaginal plate is canalized by desquamation of cells to form the vaginal lumen. A membrane of endodermal tissue separates the lumen of the vagina from the base of the urogenital sinus. The membrane partially degenerates during vaginal development. The remaining tissue persists as the hymen of the vagina [2].

Prior to the largely popular theory of vaginal development described by Koff, work done by Hart and Mijsberg in the early twentieth century suggested that the sinovaginal bulbs originate from the wolffian ducts (not the urogenital sinus) [35]. This theory was largely abandoned after the work of Koff. In 1970, Witschi's work again suggested a wolffian origin of the sinovaginal bulbs [36]. Using monoclonal antibodies to wolffian duct-specific antigens, Acien found staining within the sinovaginal bulbs [37]. This finding is strongly suggestive of a wolffian origin of the sinovaginal bulbs. In XY mice that are insensitive to testosterone (a model for androgen insensitivity syndrome), the sinovaginal bulbs were found to be under negative control by testosterone [38]. The shortened vaginas seen in patients with androgen insensitivity syndrome are thought to originate from the sinovaginal bulbs.

Further research is needed to completely understand the development of the vagina. Despite controversy in the literature regarding the origin of the sinovaginal bulbs, the remaining development of the vagina (fusion of the sinovaginal bulbs, development of the vaginal plate, and canalization of the vaginal plate) is well understood.

## Abnormal müllerian development

Although the scope of this chapter is to describe normal female reproductive development, a brief survey of common müllerian abnormalities is helpful to reinforce an understanding of normal development. Müllerian duct anomalies can be separated into three broad categories: (1) agenesis or hypoplasia of the müllerian tract, (2) failure of müllerian duct fusion, and (3) failure to resorb the intervening tissue between the fused müllerian ducts. The American Society for Reproductive Medicine (ASRM) has established the most widely used classification system for müllerian anomalies (see Fig. 3.6) [39]. Class I defects involve hypoplasia or agenesis of segments of the müllerian tract. These segmental defects may arise from aberrant control of developmental identity of individual müllerian duct components; this identity is regulated by *HOX* genes. Class II defects (unicornuate) involve the unilateral hypoplasia or agenesis of structures derived from a single müllerian duct. Class III defects (didelphus) arise from the failed fusion of the müllerian ducts. The didelphic uterus consists of two completely separate hemi-uteri and two cervixes. Class IV defects (bicornuate) result from incomplete fusion of the müllerian ducts. Bicornuate uteri demonstrate the fact that fusion of the müllerian ducts occurs in a caudal to cranial fashion since the unfused portion of a bicornuate uterus is always at the fundal (cranial) portion of the uterus. Class V defects (septate) occur due to failure of resorption of the median tissue between the two müllerian ducts. Again, this tissue degenerates in a caudal to cranial direction. These septa vary in length. Short septa originate at the fundus and extend into the uterine cavity, terminating at various distances from the fundus. Complete septa can extend the entire length of the uterus, divide the cervix, and extend into the vagina. Any longitudinal septum in the vagina should prompt evaluation of the uterus, since persistence of a longitudinal vaginal septum will always indicate a septate uterus (since the resorption occurs from caudal to cranial). Class VI defects describe the arcuate uterus, in which most (but not all) of the dividing septum between the two müllerian ducts is resorbed. Class VII consists of DES-induced anomalies.

Understanding vaginal anomalies can also reinforce an understanding of normal vaginal development, regardless of the theory of vaginal development to which one subscribes. As mentioned in the previous paragraph, longitudinal vaginal septa are indicative of a complete failure of resorption of the septum between the fused müllerian ducts. Transverse vaginal septa occur when either the vertical fusion of the caudal portion of the fused müllerian ducts (the uterovaginal canal) and the vaginal plate fails or the canalization of the vaginal plate fails. Transverse vaginal septa typically occur in the upper portion of the vagina, but can develop in any portion of the vagina [40]. Transverse vaginal septa vary widely in size and range from thin obstructing membranes to thick septa that extend through more than half the length of the vagina causing vaginal atresia [41].

In summary, müllerian development is dependent on coordinated gene expression and hormone exposure [30]. The genes that control normal patterning of the reproductive tract are beginning to be identified. The development induced by appropriate hormone exposure persists throughout adult life and inappropriate exposure can lead to uterine anomalies. An understanding of the normal developmental program that regulates reproductive tract patterning will undoubtedly allow us to better understand how exposure to environmental factors may perturb this process.

# References

1. Gruenwald P. The relation of the growing Mullerian duct to the Wolffian duct and its importance for the genesis of malformations. *Anat Rec* 1941; **81**: 1–19.
2. Schoenwolf G, Bleyl S, Brauer P, Francis-West P. *Larsen's Human Embryology*. 4th edition. Philadelphia: Elsevier Churchill Livingstone, 2009.
3. Cate R, Mattaliano R, Hession C, *et al*. Isolation of the bovine and human genes for Müllerian inhibiting substance and expression of the human gene in animal cells. *Cell* 1986; **45**: 685–98.
4. Tran D, Muesy-Dessole N, Josso N. Anti-Müllerian hormone is a functional marker of foetal Sertoli cells. *Nature* 1977; **269**: 411–12.
5. Yin Y, Ma L. Development of the mammalian female reproductive tract. *J Biochem* 2005; **137**: 677–83.
6. Glatstein IZ, Yeh J. Ontogeny of the estrogen receptor in the human fetal uterus. *J Clin Endocrinol Metab* 1995; **80**: 958–64.
7. Mueller S, Korach K. Immortalized testis cell lines from estrogen receptor (ER) alpha knock-out and wild-type mice expressing functional ERalpha or ERbeta. *J Androl* 2001; **22**: 652–64.
8. Yin Y, Ma L. Development of the mammalian female reproductive tract. *J Biochem* 2005; **137**: 677–83.
9. Kobayashi A, Behringer RR. Developmental genetics of the female reproductive tract in mammals. *Nat Rev Genet* 2003; **4**: 969–80.
10. Kobayashi A, Shawlot W, Kania A, Behringer RR. Requirement of Lim1 for female reproductive tract development. *Development* 2004; **131**: 539–49.
11. Torres M, Gomez-Pardo E, Dressler GR, Gruss P. Pax-2 controls multiple steps of urogenital development. *Development* 1995; **121**: 4057–65.
12. Pellegrini M, Pantano S, Lucchini F, Fumi M, Forabosco A. Emx2 developmental expression in the primordia of the reproductive and excretory systems. *Anat Embryol* 1997; **196**: 427–33.
13. Miyamoto N, Yoshida M, Kuratani S, Matsuo I, Aizawa S. Defects of urogenital development in mice lacking Emx2. *Development* 1997; **124**: 1653–64.
14. Yin Y, Ma L. Development of the mammalian female reproductive tract. *J Biochem* 2005; **137**: 677–83.

15. Vainio S, Heikkila M, Kispert A, Chin N, McMahon AP. Female development in mammals is regulated by Wnt-4 signalling. *Nature* 1999; **397**: 405–9.

16. McGinnis W, Krumlauf R. Homeobox genes and axial patterning. *Cell* 1992; **68**: 283–302.

17. Hunt P, Krumlauf R. Hox codes and positional specification in vertebrate embryonic axes. *Annu Rev Cell Biol* 1992; **8**: 227–56.

18. Krumlauf R. Hox genes in vertebrate development. *Cell* 1994; **78**: 191–201.

19. Taylor HS, Vanden Heuvel GB, Igarashi P. A conserved Hox axis in the mouse and human female reproductive system: late establishment and persistent adult expression of the Hoxa cluster genes. *Biol Reprod* 1997; **57**: 1338–45.

20. Taylor HS. The role of HOX genes in the development and function of the female reproductive tract. *Semin Reprod Med* 2000; **18**: 81–9.

21. Warot X, Fromental-Ramain C, Fraulob V, Chambon P, Dolle P. Gene dosage-dependent effects of the Hoxa-13 and Hoxd-13 mutations on morphogenesis of the terminal parts of the digestive and urogenital tracts. *Development* 1997; **124**: 4781–91.

22. Mortlock DP, Innis JW. Mutation of HOXA13 in hand-foot-genital syndrome. *Nat Genet* 1997; **15**: 179–80.

23. Goodman FR, Bacchelli C, Brady AF *et al.* Novel HOXA13 mutations and the phenotypic spectrum of hand-foot-genital syndrome. *Am J Hum Genet* 2000; **67**: 197–202.

24. Block K, Kardana A, Igarashi P, Taylor HS. In utero diethylstilbestrol (DES) exposure alters *Hox* gene expression in the developing mullerian system. *FASEB J* 2000; **14**: 1101–8.

25. Miller C, Pavlova A, Sassoon DA. Differential expression patterns of Wnt genes in the murine female reproductive tract during development and the estrous cycle. *Mech Dev* 1998; **76**: 91–9.

26. Miller C, Degenhardt K, Sassoon DA. Fetal exposure to DES results in de-regulation of Wnt7a during uterine morphogenesis. *Nat Genet* 1998; **20**: 228–30.

27. Taylor HS. Endocrine disruptors affect developmental programming of HOX gene expression. *Fertil Steril* 2008; **89**: e57–8.

28. Fei X, Chung H, Taylor HS. Methoxychlor disrupts uterine Hoxa10 gene expression. *Endocrinology* 2005; **146**: 3445–51.

29. Smith C, Taylor H. Xenoestrogen exposure imprints expression of genes (Hoxa10) required for normal uterine development. *FASEB J* 2007; **21**: 239–46.

30. Acien P. Embryological observations on the female genital tract. *Hum Reprod* 1992; **7**: 437–45.

31. Drews U, Sulak O, Schenck PA. Androgens and the development of the vagina. *Biol Reprod* 2002; **67**: 1353–9.

32. Kurita T, Cooke PS, Cunha GR. Epithelial-stromal tissue interaction in paramesonephric (Mullerian) epithelial differentiation. *Dev Biol* 2001; **240**: 194–211.

33. Koff AK. Development of the vagina in the human fetus. *Contrib Embryol* 1933; **24**: 59–91.

34. Hart DB. Preliminary note on the development of the clitoris, vagina, and hymen. *J Anat Physiol* 1896; **31**: 18–28.

35. Witschi E. Development and differentiation of the uterus. In Mack H, ed. *Prenatal Life; Biological and Clinical Perspectives, Proceedings*. Detroit: Wayne State University, 1970; 11–34.

36. Acien P. Embryological observations on the female genital tract. *Hum Reprod* 1992; **7**: 437–45.

37. Drews U, Sulak O, Schenck PA. Androgens and the development of the vagina. *Biol Reprod* 2002; **67**: 1353–9.

38. Golan A, Langer R, Bukovsky I, Caspi E. Congenital anomalies of the mullerian system. *Fertil Steril* 1989; **51**: 747–55.

39. Spence JE. Vaginal and uterine anomalies in the pediatric and adolescent patient. *J Pediatr Adolesc Gynecol* 1998; **11**: 3–11.

40. Rock J, Jones H. *Te Linde's Operative Gynecology*. 9th Edition. Philadelphia: Lippincott Williams & Wilkins, 2003.

41. Kobayashi A, Behringer RR. Developmental genetics of the female reproductive tract in mammals. *Nat Rev Genet* 2003; **4**: 969–80.

42. Allen S, Feste Jr. Pelvic disease classifications. *Fertil Steril* 1989; **51**: 199–201.

# 3.3 Breast

Maricel V. Maffini, Carlos Sonnenschein, and Ana M. Soto

## Normal development of the human breast

The breast is comprised of two main compartments: (1) the parenchyma, i.e. the epithelial cells, representing the functional part of the organ, and (2) the connective tissue or stroma which is the scaffolding of the organ. The stroma is composed of many different cell types (including fibroblasts, fat cells, immune cells, blood vessels, etc.) and an extracellular fibrotic matrix of which the main component is collagen fibers.

The breast parenchyma is arranged into ducts whose main function is to conduct milk to openings in the nipple. At the distal end of the small ducts there are lobules composed of very small sacs or alveoli where milk is produced in response to hormonal signals. These lobules are populated by the ductal epithelial, lobular epithelial, and myoepithelial cells (Fig. 3.7).

The mammary gland is a versatile, plastic organ that undergoes growth, differentiation, secretory activity and regression, primarily postnatally. These complex and at times rapid changes are the result of the harmonious interactions between cells, between cells and extracellular matrix, and between cells and hormones. The tremendous capacity of the mammary gland to remodel the connective tissue and re-shape itself, especially during puberty, pregnancy, and post-lactation involution is remarkable and appears to be comparable in all mammals.

## Fetal and infantile breast development

The first sign of breast development appears as a thickening of the epidermis (milk lines) on the ventral surface of the 5-week-old human fetus. By the 15th week of gestation, the breast buds extend, producing cords of epithelium which invade the underlying mesenchyme. The collagenous mesenchyme differentiates into fatty stroma between weeks 20 and 32. The epithelial cords become hollow, forming a lumen, during the last 2 months of gestation; at this time ductal and lobuloalveolar branching also occurs. Near birth, the nipple is formed by evagination of the mammary surface [1]. Both male and female mammary glands develop in a similar manner and no morphological differences are observed during fetal development and during the first 2 years of age [2]. After birth, the mammary gland remains in a resting state until puberty.

## Pubertal and adult breast

With the onset of puberty and its cyclical secretion of estrogen and progesterone, the ducts grow by invading the adjacent connective tissue; lobuloalveolar differentiation and growth also occur at this time. Other hormones contributing to the growth and differentiation of the gland are growth hormone, insulin, and glucocorticoids [1]. These organizational changes occur through interactions between the stroma and the epithelium [3].

The adult breast is composed of 15–25 defined lobes of functional tissue associated with each of the major lactiferous ducts that open in the nipple [1]. The smallest functional unit of the resting non-pregnant breast is the terminal ductal lobular unit (TDLU) (fig 3.7); this unit consists of a group of alveoli connected by ductules that drain into a larger duct. Changes in cell proliferation, cell size, and tissue appearance are observed throughout the menstrual cycle.

## Pregnancy, lactation, and involution

Other massive architectural changes occur during pregnancy and post-lactation. Similar to the changes observed during puberty, these are also tightly regulated by stromal–epithelial interactions and hormones. During the first trimester of pregnancy, terminal ducts and lobules grow rapidly at the same time that the stroma is reduced. Lobular growth continues during the second and third trimesters with secretion accumulating in the lumen; the amount of stroma relative to the amount of parenchyma continues to decrease [1].

After the cessation of lactation, the breast undergoes involution. The number and size of lobules decrease, and fat and collagen reappear in the stroma. After several months, the morphology of the breast resembles that of the resting gland.

## Development of the rodent mammary gland

The rodent mammary gland develops similar to the human breast, which makes these animals suitable surrogate models to study mammary gland biology.

*Environmental Impacts on Reproductive Health and Fertility*, ed. T. J. Woodruff, S. J. Janssen, L. J. Guillette, and L. C. Giudice. Published by Cambridge University Press. © Cambridge University Press 2010.

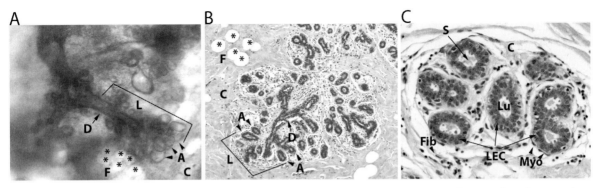

**Fig. 3.7.** Representative images of the adult human breast. (A) Whole-mount preparation of human breast showing a three-dimensional terminal ductal lobular unit. (B) Cross-section of the structure showed in (A). (C) High-power image showing alveoli in detail. Staining: A, carmine-alum; B–C, hematoxylin and eosin; D, duct; F(*), fat; L, lobule; A, alveoli; C, collagen fibers; LEC, luminal epithelial cells; Myo, myoepithelial cells; Fib, fibroblasts; S, secretion; Lu, lumen. The area labeled L in (A) corresponds to the area labeled L in (B).

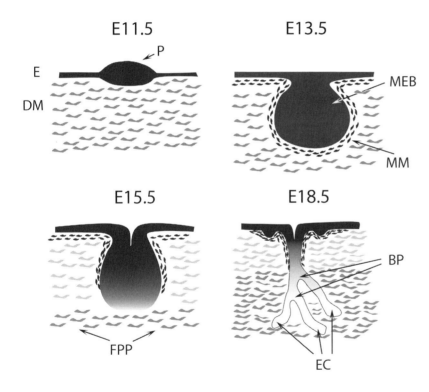

**Fig. 3.8.** Schematic representation of mouse fetal mammary gland development. E, epithelium; DM, dermal mesenchyme; P, mammary placode; MEB, mammary epithelial bud; MM, mammary mesenchyme; FPP, presumptive fat pad; BP, branching points; EC, epithelial cords.

The mouse mammary gland development begins at embryonic day 10.5 (E10.5) with the appearance of presumptive mammary lines. Mammary placodes invaginate into the dermis at E13.5 as the mammary mesenchyme surrounding the epithelium becomes increasingly dense [4]. At E15.5 the precursor to the underlying fat pad is invaded by the mammary bud as it elongates into a cord called the mammary sprout. By E18, the mammary sprout has begun to branch

and develop a lumen [5] (Fig. 3.8). At this point, the growth of the mammary gland parallels the growth of the organism as a whole until puberty, at which time the gland undergoes substantial remodeling.

At puberty, rising levels of estrogens cause a rapid increase in ductal growth (Fig. 3.9) characterized by high levels of both cellular proliferation and apoptosis (cell death) at the terminal end buds (TEB); the bulbous TEB lead the migration of the ducts into the

37

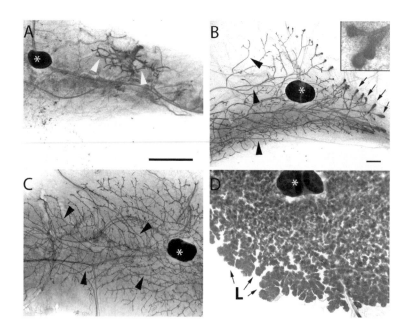

**Fig. 3.9.** Mouse mammary gland at different stages of development. (A) PND10: small ductal tree. (B) PND30 (puberty): ductal tree extension and presence of terminal end buds (TEB); the inset is a close-up of TEB.(C) Adult resting mammary gland: complex network of ducts and absence of TEB. (D) Full-term pregnant gland: abundance of milk-producing lobules. Arrowheads, ducts; arrows, TEB; L, lobules; asterisk, lymph node. Scale bars: 1 mm.

stroma. The combination of proliferation and apoptosis is essential for the development of a lumen [6]. The ductal tree develops into a network of ducts, terminal ducts, and alveolar buds as it completely fills the stroma. Pregnancy stimulates a period of dramatic proliferation of the epithelium and development of lobules where milk will be produced (Fig. 3.9). After birth the mammary gland undergoes widespread apoptosis as it returns to a morphology resembling the pre-pregnancy state [7].

## Hormone receptors during mammary gland development

The most important hormones regulating mammary gland development are estrogen and progesterone. During pregnancy and lactation, prolactin also contributes to lobular differentiation and milk production. We will concentrate on estrogen and progesterone because of their fundamental role during puberty to develop a normal adult breast.

Estrogen and progesterone are steroid hormones that act on target cells through their receptors. The classical estrogen receptors (ER) and progesterone receptors (PR) are located in the cell's nucleus, where the hormone-receptor complex binds to the DNA and modulates gene expression. In addition, membrane-bound ER and PR have been described [8,9]; in these cases, the hormones produce rapid effects through non-genomic actions.

## Estrogen receptor expression in the fetal and infant breast

The earliest stages of fetal breast formation appear to be independent of steroid hormones. ER-α protein has been detected using immunohistochemical techniques in epithelial cell nuclei in the fetal breast starting at gestation week 30 [10]. From birth to puberty, this receptor was heterogeneously expressed in the breast epithelial cells [10, 11].

## Estrogen receptor expression in the adult breast

The most abundant ER in the non-pregnant adult breast is ER-β which is expressed in approximately 70% of the epithelial cells [12]. ER-α is expressed in only 4–15% of the ductal and lobular epithelial cells in the adult breast. The number of ER-α positive cells, however, increases with age reaching the highest percentage in post-menopausal women [11]. The presence of ER-β remains constant in most cases. Unlike ER-β, ER-α is not expressed in the breast stroma [13]. Once the menstrual cycle is established, ER expression in the adult breast is also cyclical. During pregnancy and lactation, ER-α levels decrease [11].

## Progesterone receptor expression in the human breast

The earliest that PR has been detected in the human breast is between 3 and 7 years of age in the epithelial cells. Progesterone receptor was also detected in the pubescent breast [11]. The pattern of progesterone receptor expression is heterogeneous in the epithelial cells and absent in the stromal cells [14]. Contrary to the cyclicity observed in ER expression, PR did not vary with menstrual phases. Progesterone receptor is present during early pregnancy; it is rare in late pregnancy and re-appears post-partum. The breast of postmenopausal women shows high level of PR expression in the luminal epithelial cells [11].

## Estrogen receptors in the rodent mammary gland

Saji and collaborators examined ER expression in rat mammary gland from post-anatal week 1 through pregnancy, lactation, and involution. Similar to what has been observed in the human breast, ER-α expression was low from birth to adulthood, increased during lactation, and decreased again during involution. In contrast with the fluctuating expression of ER-α, ER-β was observed in all stages and remained relatively constant with approximately 50% of epithelial cells expressing it. Estrogen receptors-beta is also expressed in the nuclei of stromal cells [12]. In mice, ER-α and ER-β are first expressed at E12.5 in the mesenchyme surrounding the bud [15]. By E16 these receptors were shown to be functional [16]. However, at post-natal time points, ER-α expression is mainly localized to the epithelium [17]. We have observed a punctate expression of ER in the epithelium at E18 which could be interpreted as a transition from mesenchyme-only to epithelial-only expression [5].

## Impact of environmental insults in mammary gland development: Windows of vulnerability

There are critical times in the lifespan of an individual that appear to be crucial for eliciting developmental mishaps. This vulnerability window differs depending upon the time at which specific developmental events occur in particular tissues or organs. The perinatal period and puberty are the most susceptible stages during mammary gland development because of the complex tissue organization that takes place at both ages. Epidemiologic and laboratory animal data have shown that exposure to environmental toxins such as endocrine disruptors, radiation, or other carcinogens during the critical periods of organogenesis (gestation) and organ growth and differentiation (puberty) have long-lasting consequences that usually correlate with the development of diseases during adulthood [18–21]. Breast development during pregnancy could also be considered a third period of susceptibility. Interruption or alterations of the processes leading to a functional lactation could result in mortality or malnourishment of the offspring [22].

## Susceptibility of the mammary gland during the perinatal period

### Perinatal exposure to endocrine disruptors

The developing organism is critically sensitive to both endogenous and exogenous hormones, a phenomenon that led Dr. Howard Bern to coin the phrase the "fragile fetus" [23]. For instance, it is well accepted that some of the developmental alterations mediated by estrogens occur at significantly lower doses than those necessary for causing estrogenic effects in adults. Thus, the developing organism seems to be far more sensitive to minute variations of hormone levels than the adult organism.

### Perinatal exposure to diethylstilbestrol

Beginning in the 1940s, the potent synthetic estrogen diethylstilbestrol (DES) was administered to pregnant women as a treatment to decrease the risk of miscarriage, although it was later proven to be ineffective. Women exposed in utero to DES have experienced functional deficits in fertility as well as malformations of the genital tract. Diethylstilbestrol treatment produced similar effects in mice, establishing the mouse as a useful model for developmental toxicity of xenoestrogens (xeno meaning foreign) and its underlying mechanisms [24].

Diethylstilbestrol studies in rodents demonstrated that the chemical exerted effects on mammary gland development at doses much lower than those to which so-called DES daughters had been exposed [25] and than those necessary to produce estrogenic effects in adults [26]. Numerous studies examined a link between DES and cancer. Regarding prenatal exposure to DES and risk of mammary cancer, between 1979 and 1987 it was first reported that rodents exposed to DES had an increased propensity to develop tumors compared with unexposed animals [27, 28, 29]. The offspring of CD1 mice exposed in utero to DES had a higher incidence of ovarian and mammary tumors than offspring of non-exposed females, suggesting transgenerational effects of exposure to the synthetic estrogen [30].

More importantly, many of the so-called DES daughters are now reaching the age of high detection of breast cancer. This unfortunate episode in medical history offers the unique opportunity to test the hypothesis that, in humans, in utero exposure to estrogens increases the risk of breast cancer in adulthood. Using a cohort of almost 5000 exposed and 2000 unexposed daughters, Palmer and collaborators showed that "women with prenatal exposure to DES have an increased risk of breast cancer after age 40" [18]. In summary, laboratory animal experiments predicted several decades ago what the current epidemiologic data are now demonstrating.

## Bisphenol-A, a ubiquitous xenoestrogen

Bisphenol-A (BPA) is a ubiquitous chemical used as the building block of polycarbonate plastics and epoxy resins. Bisphenol-A is found in countless products we use or come in contact with on a daily basis including food containers, baby bottles, water pipes, dental sealants, optical lenses, water storage tanks, the lining of aluminum cans, and milk containers. In addition, approximately 100 tons of BPA are released into the atmosphere each year as a consequence of its production [31].

Bisphenol-A has been known to be estrogenic since 1936 [32]. It was not until the 1990s however, that it was accidentally discovered that BPA leaches from polycarbonate plastics in concentrations sufficient to induce cell proliferation in estrogen-target MCF7 cells via binding to ER. Subsequent studies have demonstrated that incomplete polymerization of BPA during the manufacturing process as well as depolymerization due to high temperature (such as exposure to microwaves, hot water, or sunlight) causes BPA to migrate into foods [33], beverages [34], infant formula [34], saliva (from dental sealants) [35], etc. BPA has also been found in dust particles [36], leachates from waste water treatment plants, river water [37], and surface and drinking water [38].

The developing fetus is at risk of exposure to BPA via its mother, while the neonate is at particular risk via ingestion of BPA from infant formula (sold in epoxy-resin lined cans) or breast milk [39]. In fact, recent data conclude that the ubiquitous nature of BPA means that fetal and neonatal exposure to BPA is all but ensured. A recently published study by the Centers for Disease Control and prevention found BPA in the urine of 92.6% of Americans, with higher concentrations found in children and adolescents than in adults [40]. Bisphenol-A has been measured in maternal and fetal plasma as well as placental tissue in humans, in milk from lactating mothers and in amniotic fluid [41, 42]. Similarly, BPA has been shown to cross the placenta in rodents [43].

## Effects of perinatal exposure to BPA in the mammary gland

Bisphenol-A, like many endocrine disruptors, has substantial effects on fetal development even at extremely low doses due to its interaction with the endocrine system. Exposure of pregnant mice to 250 and 25 ng BPA/kg body weight (bw)/day for 14 days beginning on gestational day 8 affected numerous aspects of the development of their female offspring. These doses are *200 and 2000 times lower*, respectively, than the safe daily intake of BPA of 50 μg BPA/kg bw/day established by the US EPA. When examined on E18, mammary glands of the fetuses of mothers exposed to 250 ng BPA showed altered growth parameters, including an altered stroma, with more advanced fat pad maturation and altered localization of fibrous collagen [5]. Maturation of the fat pad drives ductal growth and branching, and the mammary glands of the BPA-exposed females had increased ductal area compared with unexposed mice. The mammary epithelium of the 250 ng BPA-exposed fetuses also displayed decreased cell size and delayed lumen formation [5].

Developmental differences in the mammary gland from control groups were detected also after birth. At PND10 (postnatal day 10), the percentage of proliferating epithelial cells was significantly decreased compared with controls in BPA-exposed mice. At PND30, BPA-exposed offspring had an increased number and area of TEB relative to the total gland ductal area, with a decreased incidence of cell death in these structures when compared with controls. This reduced cell death is a likely cause of the observed delay in ductal growth as cell death is essential for the hollowing and outward extension of subtending ducts. These effects can collectively be attributed to an increased sensitivity to estradiol at the age of puberty in BPA-exposed animals [44].

The BPA-exposed offspring also showed a significant increase in the number of PR positive cells in the

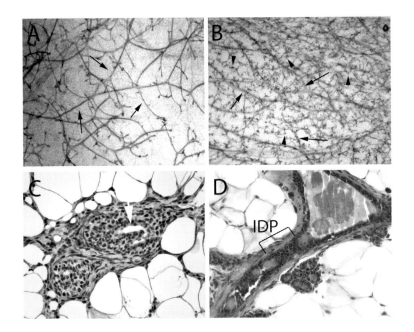

**Fig. 3.10.** Perinatal exposure to BPA causes alteration in the mammary gland. (A) Three-month-old unexposed mouse (arrows: ducts). (B) Three-month-old BPA-exposed mouse. Note the abundance of epithelial structures (arrows: ducts; arrowheads: alveolar buds). (C) Carcinoma *in situ* developed in rats perinatally exposed to BPA. The arrow points at the lumen that is almost filled with epithelial cells. (D) Intraductal proliferation was observed in perinatally exposed mice. The lines mark intraductal proliferation (IDP).

ductal epithelium at puberty. The clustered localization of these PR positive cells suggested them as possible sites of future branching points, a notion supported by the increase in lateral branching found in the offspring at 4 months of age [44]. By 6 months of age, the virgin mammary glands of these perinatally exposed mice demonstrate such a large increase in ducts, terminal ends, and alveolar buds that they resemble the mammary glands of untreated pregnant mice [45]. By 12–15 months of age, these mice developed precancerous lesions called intraductal proliferation (i.e. epithelial cells proliferate into the ductal lumen) [46] (Fig. 3.10).

To explore the links between prenatal BPA exposure and mammary gland neoplasia, we used a rat model, because it closely resembles the human disease regarding estrogen dependency and histopathology. BPA was administered to pregnant dams at doses of 2.5, 25, 250, and 1000 µg/kg bw/day. Fetal exposure to BPA, from E9 to postnatal day 1, resulted in the development of carcinomas *in situ* in the mammary glands of 33% of the rats exposed to 250 µg/kg bw/day while none of the unexposed animals developed neoplasias [20] (Fig. 3.10). These cancers were only observed once the animals had reached young adult age. Fetal exposure to BPA also significantly increased the number of precancerous lesions, specifically intraductal proliferation, by three to four times, an effect also observed in puberty and during

adult life. The lesions observed in the BPA-exposed animals were highly proliferative and contained abundant ER-positive cells, suggesting that the proliferative activity in these lesions may be estrogen mediated [20].

In conclusion, these results indicate that perinatal exposure to environmentally relevant doses of BPA results in persistent alterations in mammary gland morphogenesis, development of precancerous lesions, and carcinoma *in situ*. Moreover, the altered growth parameters noted in the developing mammary gland on E18 suggest that the fetal gland is a direct target of BPA, and that these alterations cause the mammary gland phenotypes observed in perinatally exposed mice at puberty and adulthood.

### Perinatal exposure to other environmental toxins and its effect on the mammary gland

Fluoropolymers have been used since the 1940s in the manufacture of consumer and industrial products such as weather- and stain-resistant materials (fabrics, carpets), non-stick cookware, electrical materials, etc. Perfluorooctanoic acid (PFOA) has, in itself, broad applications but is also a degradation product of other perfluorinated compounds [47]. It is very persistent and its presence is widespread in the population [48]. A recent study by White *et al.* [49] showed that pregnant mice exposed to PFOA during gestation experienced reduction in the dam's mammary gland differentiation, delay in involution after weaning, and alteration in milk protein gene expression. They have also observed that the female offspring had stunted mammary ductal growth [49]. The mechanisms by which PFOA is affecting the mammary gland are unknown; however, these results suggest that PFOA may be acting in a different manner in an adult than in a developing individual.

Atrazine is a commonly used herbicide used to control the growth of weeds and grass in crops. It has been detected in ground and surface waters throughout the USA, and recent studies showed that atrazine and its derivatives are present in the urine of the general population, not just farmers [50, 51]. Using the Long–Evans rat model, Enoch et al. showed that gestational exposure to an atrazine metabolite mixture induced a significant delay in the development of the offspring mammary glands that persisted for 2 months after birth [52]. Interestingly, there was a persistence of terminal end buds (TEB) in the 2-month-old rats while no TEB were observed in the control animals. The untimely persistence of epithelial structures suggests that the communication between the stroma and the epithelium and the reciprocal signals necessary to maintain the homeostasis of the tissue may have been compromised during the gestational exposure.

Dioxin or 2,3,7,8-tetrachlorodibenzo-*p*-dioxin (TCDD) is a member of the polyhalogenated hydrocarbons (PHAHs) family. It is a very potent toxin that affects many systems during development and adulthood, including the endocrine system. The most complete epidemiological data regarding non-occupational exposure to TCDD of a human population originated in Seveso, Italy. In 1976 a chemical factory explosion released several kilograms of dioxin into the environment; serum and tissue samples of the exposed population were collected at the time and have been used to analyze the long-term effects of dioxin exposure. Recently a significant correlation was found between high levels of serum dioxin and increased incidence of breast cancer in the exposed population compared with those unexposed [53]. A continued follow-up of the exposed population will help in identifying whether time of exposure, i.e. gestational, pubertal, adulthood, also correlates with breast cancer incidence.

Animal studies have shown similarities with the epidemiological data. Rats exposed prenatally to TCDD developed many more mammary tumors than non-exposed animals when challenged with a chemical carcinogen at puberty [54]. Moreover, it was reported that TCDD had a persistent effect on the morphology and functionality of the mammary gland of the second generation of exposed animals [55]. In a more detailed study using rats, female offspring exposed in utero to TCDD had a reduced number of primary ducts and their ability to invade the mammary stroma was stunted. These offspring also had decreased lateral branching and the number of TEB was reduced but they persisted longer compared with non-exposed animals [22]. The extended presence of the highly proliferative TEB could be interpreted as a prolongation of the window of susceptibility to potential carcinogens [56]. The mechanisms by which TCDD acts on the mammary gland are still unknown; however, based on the laboratory animal experiments it is likely that dioxin acts both directly on the mammary gland and systemically by affecting several targets in the endocrine system [56].

## Susceptibility of the mammary gland during puberty

Until the onset of puberty, the mammary ducts grow at the same rate as the body. However, this growth becomes exponential in the presence of high levels of hormones at puberty; a rapid proliferation and elongation of the epithelial ducts occur at the same time that the stroma is remodeled to allow those ducts to migrate and fill the entirety of the organ. These events are tightly controlled by hormones and mutual communication between the stroma and the epithelium. Disruption of any of the interactions/mechanisms that are in place in the mammary gland to maintain a perfect balance between both compartments during this very active period would result in a decreased ability of the gland to respond to potential carcinogenic challenges (e.g. exogenous hormones, radiation, environmental toxins). Thus, the abnormal reaction of the mammary gland could be manifested as a disease (such as cancer) or functional aberrations (such as reduced capacity to lactate) later in life.

Studies using transplantation of mammary tumor cells into the mammary stroma at different ages showed that prepubertal and pubertal glands support the growth of those tumor cells. In contrast, post-pubertal adult and parous glands were able to instruct those same tumor cells to become normal mammary ducts [57]. This suggests that a resting gland provides a balanced and stable environment while the extensive tissue remodeling and cell proliferation that occur during puberty increases the chances for normal development to go awry.

## Xenoestrogens exposure during puberty and breast cancer

Dichlorodiphenyltrichloroethane (DDT) is a potent and persistent xenoestrogen. It was introduced in the USA in 1945; the peak use of this pesticide was 1959 [58] and the highest dietary content of DDT has been estimated to have been in 1965 [59]. In 1972, DDT was banned in the USA.

Because of its persistency and massive release into the environment over 60 years ago, it was thought that DDT was a suitable marker of exposure for breast cancer; its presence or the presence of its metabolite dichlorodiphenyldichloroethylene (DDE) (even more persistent in the environment and biological systems) in serum may represent cumulative exposure during a lifetime. Three studies claimed a correlation between the occurrence of breast cancer and levels of xenoestrogen. Wolff *et al.* found that serum DDE levels correlated with breast cancer [60]. Another study documented that ER-positive breast cancer correlated with higher concentrations of DDE in participants' tissues [61]. Krieger *et al.* studied 150 women with breast cancer and 150 controls; each set was made up of 50 Black, 50 White and 50 Asian women. When the cases and matching controls were evaluated separately according to their ethnic group, high serum DDE levels were correlated to breast cancer incidence in White and Black women, but there was no significant correlation in Asian [62]. Although very important correlations between breast cancer incidence and xenoestrogen levels were found, these studies measure the levels of DDE long after exposure time.

A more recent study tested the hypothesis that the association between DDT and breast cancer resides in the age at the time of exposure. Cohn *et al.* measured the amount of DDT and DDE in serum collected between 1959 and 1967 from a cohort of young women (mean age: 26 years). They found that women who were 14 years of age at the time DDT was first introduced into the environment and had high levels of serum DDT had a 5-fold increased risk of breast cancer [21]. They observed similar correlations in women who were younger than 20 years of age at the time of the peak use of DDT. These findings strongly indicated that exposure to the xenoestrogen DDT during childhood and adolescence increased the risk of breast cancer. The implications of these results could be even stronger considering the large number of women exposed worldwide, the long latency of breast cancer, and the increase in women exposed at early ages entering menopause in the next decades.

Other persistent and heavily used xenoestrogens are polychlorinated biphenyls or PCBs. Evidence of a link between exposure to PCBs and breast cancer incidence is equivocal [63]. However, these studies aimed at correlating exposure to total PCBs, rather than to the levels of specific congeners. In order to clarify the relevance of these findings, epidemiological studies are now being conducted involving larger sample sizes. However, testing only for the presence of DDT metabolites or total PCBs may not clarify whether or not xenoestrogens play a role in breast cancer incidence, because (i) not all the PCB congeners are estrogenic, and (ii) many other environmental estrogens may also play a role. Methods to identify and measure new xenoestrogens in bodily fluids and tissues have yet to be developed. Nevertheless, the core of the problem remains whether or not the combined exposure to xenoestrogens correlates with breast cancer incidence. Methodology developed to measure the total xenoestrogen burden is being used to assess this hypothesis [64, 65]. For instance, Ibarluzea *et al.* have found that the total effective xenoestrogen burden (measure in body fat) of lean post-menopausal women correlates with an increased risk of breast cancer [66].

## Radiation

Ionizing radiation is another environmental agent considered a carcinogen. Gestational exposure to low doses of X-rays causes an increased incidence of several childhood cancers. In addition, the exposure of infants to radiation has been associated with the development of thyroid and breast cancer later in life [67].

Much of the information regarding correlations between breast cancer incidence and radiation exposure comes from epidemiological studies of the survivors of the Hiroshima–Nagasaki atomic bomb. A recent report analyzing a cohort from 1950–1990 atomic bomb survivors indicated that exposure to radiation before the age of 20 years was associated with an increased excess relative risk compared with exposure at older ages [19]. Interestingly, of those women exposed under the age of 20 that developed breast cancer, 4.9% developed primary cancer in both breasts. Only 2.3% of those exposed at older age developed double primary tumors. After reviewing a pool of eight different cohorts, Preston *et al.* also concluded that age at exposure correlated with increased risk [68].

These epidemiologic data strengthen the hypothesis that radiation-associated breast cancer risk is higher in women exposed during childhood and adolescence than as adults.

Multiple animal models of mammary carcinogenesis have been perfected for maximum tumor incidence based on the time of exposure. The highest incidence of tumors, i.e. 90–100%, is obtained when rats are exposed during puberty. Before or after this window of susceptibility, the incidence drops to levels below 20%, highlighting once again the relevance of animal models as surrogates for human exposures.

## Cancer as a consequence of altered tissue organization

The majority of research on cancer and carcinogenesis performed in the last 50 years has been based upon the theory that cancer arises due to the accumulation of mutations in the genome of a cell (somatic mutation theory) [69]. More recently, supporters of the novel theory of fetal origins of adult diseases have investigated how changes in epigenomic expression in a cell might play a vital and central role in carcinogenesis. One study found that neonatal exposure to BPA or estradiol benzoate increased the propensity for the development of neoplastic lesions in the prostate following subsequent exposure to a carcinogen [70]. The authors proposed that the exposure of the prostate to either BPA or estradiol may have permanently altered the methylation pattern of cell-signaling genes in the tissue, leading to neoplastic development. Both the somatic mutation theory and the epigenetic theory of carcinogenesis consider cancer a genetic disease that starts in one cell that ultimately escapes regulation of proliferation [69].

In contrast, the tissue organization field theory postulates that carcinogenesis is a problem of tissue organization and that proliferation is the default state of *all* cells [71]. When a carcinogen or teratogen disrupts the normal dynamic interaction of neighboring cells and tissues, during either development or adulthood, cancer arises. This is a process similar to "organogenesis gone awry."

Although there are hereditary cases of breast cancer with long familial histories of women affected by the disease, these cases make up less than 10% of the total incidences of breast cancer. The remaining cases (greater than 90%) are "sporadic" cases with no genetic link. The most important risk factor for developing breast cancer is lifetime exposure to estrogens. According

to a report published in 2002 by The National Cancer Institute's (NCI) Surveillance, Epidemiology and End Results (SEER) Program, a woman's lifetime risk for developing breast cancer has increased from 1 in 22 in the 1940s to 1 in 8 when the report was released. This time-span coincides with the introduction of man-made chemicals into the natural and urban environment, many of which act as xenoestrogens.

Regulation of expression of estrogen-target genes involved in tissue patterning, and tissue and cell differentiation are believed to mediate the direct effects of estrogens on target organs in the reproductive system as well as the mammary gland. Estrogens are considered morphogens that directly regulate the expression of genes important for the normal patterning of an organ. It is therefore plausible that fetal xenoestrogens may alter the expression of this set of genes, thereby affecting morphogenesis and perhaps leading to neoplastic development. Bisphenol-A is also suspected to alter the methylation patterns of genes involved in the reciprocal interactions between tissues that mediate morphogenesis. It is critical that we re-evaluate our understanding of development and carcinogenesis in light of the information that has been collected on DES, BPA, and endocrine disruptors in general. It is now clear that environmental exposure to these chemicals at levels previously thought to be irrelevant can have clear and distinct effects, especially during critical periods of development on target organs. This raises grave concern over the potentially deleterious effects these chemicals could be having on human development and subsequent disease. Extrapolating conclusions from animal studies to human beings must be done cautiously, as there can be great variation within strains of a species and certainly between species. However, rodents have proven an excellent model for the understanding of perinatal DES exposure. Given the growing evidence of the risk posed by endocrine-disrupting chemicals such as BPA, regulatory agencies should be encouraged to apply the precautionary principle and ban or substitute chemicals that may put human beings and animals at risk by interfering with normal development.

## Acknowledgments

The authors are grateful to Cheryl M. Schaeberle and Gregory A. Loomis for assistance in the preparation of the figures. The work outlined herein was supported by NIEHS grants ES08314, ES012301, and ES013884.

# References

1. Rosen PP. Anatomy and physiologic morphology. In *Rosen's Breast Pathology*. New York: Lippincott, Williams and Wilkins, 2008.

2. Anbazhagan R, Bartek J, Monaghan P. *et al.* Growth and development of the human infant breast. *Am J Anat* 1991; **192**: 407–17.

3. Cunha GR, Bigsby RM, Cooke PS. *et al.* Stromal-epithelial interactions in adult organs. *Cell Different* 1985; **17**: 137–48.

4. Robinson GW, Karpf ABC, Kratochwil K. Regulation of mammary gland development by tissue interaction. *J Mammary Gland Biol Neoplasia* 1999; **4**: 9–19.

5. Vandenberg LN, Maffini MV, Wadia PR. *et al.* Exposure to the xenoestrogen bisphenol-A alters development of the fetal mammary gland. *Endocrinology* 2007; **148**: 116–27.

6. Humphreys RC, Krajewska M, Krnacik S. *et al.* Apoptosis in the terminal end bud of the murine mammary gland: a mechanism of ductal morphogenesis. *Development* 1996; **122**: 4013–22.

7. Daniel CW, Smith GH. The mammary gland: a model for development. *J Mammary Gland Biol Neoplasia* 1999; **4**: 3–8.

8. Campbell CH, Bulayeva N, Brown DB. *et al.* Regulation of the membrane estrogen receptor-α: role of cell density, serum, cell passage number, and estradiol. *FASEB (Fed Am Soc Exp Biol ) J* 2002; **16**: 1917–27.

9. Dressing GE, Thomas P. Identification of membrane progestin receptors in human breast cancer cell lines and biopsies and their potential involvement in breast cancer. *Steroids* 2007; **72**: 111–16.

10. Keeling JW, Özer E, King G. *et al.* Oestrogen receptor alpha in female fetal, infant, and child mammary tissue. *J Pathol* 2000; **191**: 449–51.

11. Bartow SA. Use of the autopsy to study ontogeny and expression of the estrogen receptor gene in human breast. *J Mammary Gland Biol Neoplasia* 1998; **3**: 37–48.

12. Weihua Z, Saji S, Makinen S. *et al.* Estrogen receptor (ER) beta, a modulator of ER-alpha in the uterus. *Proc Natl Acad Sci USA* 2000; **97**: 5936–41.

13. Shyamala G, Chou Y-C, Louie SG. *et al.* Cellular expression of estrogen and progesterone receptors in mammary glands: regulation by hormones, development and aging. *J Steroid Biochem Molec Biol* 2002; **80**: 137–48.

14. Press MF, Greene GL. Localization of progesterone receptor with monoclonal antibodies to the human progestin receptor. *Endocrinology* 1988; **122**: 1165–75.

15. Lemmen JG, Broekhof JLM, Kuiper GGJM. *et al.* Expression of estrogen receptor alpha and beta during mouse embryogenesis. *Mech Dev* 1999; **81**: 163–67.

16. Narbaitz R, Stumpf WE, Sar M. Estrogen receptors in the mammary gland primordia of fetal mouse. *Anat Embryol* 1980; **158**: 161–66.

17. Saji S, Jensen EV, Nilsson S. *et al.* Estrogen receptors α and β in the rodent mammary gland. *Proc Natl Acad Sci USA* 2000; **97**: 337–42.

18. Palmer JR, Wise LA, Hatch EE. *et al.* Prenatal diethylstilbestrol exposure and risk of breast cancer. *Cancer Epidem Biomar* 2006; **15**: 1509–14.

19. Land CE, Tokunaga M, Koyama K. *et al.* Incidence of female breast cancer among atomic bomb survivors, Hiroshima and Nagasaki, 1950–1990. *Radiation Res* 2003; **160**: 707–17.

20. Murray TJ, Maffini MV, Ucci AA. *et al.* Induction of mammary gland ductal hyperplasias and carcinoma in situ following fetal Bisphenol A exposure. *Reprod Toxicol* 2007; **23**: 383–90.

21. Cohn BA, Wolff MS, Cirillo PM. *et al.* DDT and breast cancer in young women: new data on the significance of age at exposure. *Environ Health Perspect* 2007; **115**: 1406–14.

22. Fenton SE, Hamm JT, Birnbaum L. *et al.* Persistent abnormalities in the rat mammary gland following gestational and lactational exposure to 2,3,7,8-tetrachlorodibenzo-p-dioxin (TCDD). *Toxicol Sci* 2002; **67**: 63–74.

23. Bern HA. The fragile fetus. In Colborn T, Clement C, eds. *Chemically-Induced Alterations in Sexual and Functional Development: The Wildlife/Human Connection*. Princeton: Princeton Scientific Publishing Co., Inc., 1992; 9–15.

24. Newbold RR. Diethylstilbestrol (DES) and environmental estrogens influence the developing female reproductive system. In Naz RK, ed. *Endocrine Disruptors: Effects on the Male and Female Reproductive Sytems*. Boca Raton: CRC Press, 1999; 39–56.

25. Newbold RR, Jefferson WN, Banks EP. Developmental exposure to low doses of diethylstilbestrol (DES) results in permanent alterations in the reproductive tract. *The Endocrine Society, Annual Meeting* 1999.

26. Markey CM, Michaelson CL, Veson EC. *et al.* The mouse uterotropic assay: a re-evaluation of its validity in assessing the estrogenicity of bisphenol A. *Environ Health Perspect* 2001; **109**: 55–60.

27. Boylan ES, Calhoon RE. Mammary tumorigenesis in the rat following prenatal exposure to diethylstilbestrol and postnatal treatment with 7,12-dimethylbenz[a]anthracene. *J Toxicol Environ Health* 1979; **5**: 1059–71.

28. Boylan ES, Calhoon RE. Transplacental action of diethylstilbestrol on mammary carcinogenesis in female rats given one or two doses of 7,12-dimethylbenz(a)anthracene. *Cancer Res* 1983; **43**: 4879–84.

29. Rothschild TC, Boylan ES, Calhoon RE. *et al.* Transplacental effects of diethylstilbestrol on mammary development and tumorigenesis in female ACI rats. *Cancer Res* 1987; **47**: 4508–16.

30. Walker BE. Tumors in female offspring of control and diethylstilbestrol-exposed mice fed high-fat diets. *J Nat Cancer Inst* 1990; **82**: 50–4.

31. Markey CM, Michaelson CL, Sonnenschein C. *et al.* Alkylphenols and bisphenol A as environmental estrogens. In Metzler M, ed. *The Handbook of Environmental Chemistry Vol 3. Part L, Endocrine Disruptors – Part I*. Berlin: Springer Verlag, 2001; 129–53.

32. Dodds EC, Lawson W. Molecular structure in relation to oestrogenic activity. Compounds without a phenathrene nucleus. *Proc Roy Soc B* 1938; **125**: 222–32.

33. Brotons JA, Olea-Serrano MF, Villalobos M. *et al.* Xenoestrogens released from lacquer coating in food cans. *Environ Health Perspect* 1994; **103**: 608–12.

34. Biles JE, McNeal TP, Begley TH. *et al.* Determination of bisphenol-A in reusable polycarbonate food-contact plastics and migration to food simulating liquids. *J Agric Food Chem* 1997; **45**: 3541–4.

35. Olea N, Pulgar R, Perez P. *et al.* Estrogenicity of resin-based composites and sealants used in dentistry. *Environ Health Perspect* 1996; **104(3)**: 298–305.

36. Berkner S, Streck G, Herrmann R. Development and validation of a method for determination of trace levels of alkylphenols and bisphenol A in atmospheric samples. *Chemosphere* 2004; **54(4)**: 575–84.

37. Behnisch PA, Fujii K, Shiozaki K. *et al.* Estrogenic and dioxin-like potency in each step of a controlled landfill leachate treatment plant in Japan. *Chemosphere* 2001; **43**: 977–84.

38. Rodrigues-Mozaz S, Lopez de Alda M, Barcelo D. Analysis of bisphenol A in natural waters by means of an optical immunosensor. *Water Res* 2005; **39**: 5071–9.

39. Yoo SD, Shin BS, Lee BM. *et al.* Bioavailability and mammary excretion of bisphenol A in Sprague Dawley rats. *J Toxicol and Environ Health A* 2001; **64**: 417–26.

40. Calafat AM, Ye X, Wong LY. *et al.* Exposure of the U.S. population to bisphenol A and 4-tertiary-octylphenol: 2003–2004. *Environ Health Perspect* 2008; **116**: 39–44.

41. Schonfelder G, Wittfoht W, Hopp H. *et al.* Parent bisphenol A accumulation in the human maternal-fetal-placental unit. *Environ Health Perspect* 2002; **110**: A703–7.

42. Ikezuki Y, Tsutsumi O, Takai Y. *et al.* Determination of bisphenol A concentrations in human biological fluids reveals significant early prenatal exposure. *Hum Reprod* 2002; **17**: 2839–41.

43. Takahashi O, Oishi S. Disposition of orally administered 2,2-bis(4-hydroxyphenyl) propane (Bisphenol A) in pregnant rats and placental transfer to fetuses. *Environ Health Perspect* 2000; **108**: 931–5.

44. Munoz de Toro MM, Markey CM, Wadia PR. *et al.* Perinatal exposure to bisphenol A alters peripubertal mammary gland development in mice. *Endocrinology* 2005; **146**: 4138–47.

45. Markey CM, Luque EH, Munoz de Toro MM. *et al.* In utero exposure to bisphenol A alters the development and tissue organization of the mouse mammary gland. *Biol Reprod* 2001; **65**: 1215–23.

46. Vandenberg LN, Maffini MV, Schaeberle CM. *et al.* Perinatal exposure to the xenoestrogen bisphenol-A induces mammary intraductal hyperplasias in adult CD-1 mice. *Reprod Toxico* 2008; **26**: 210–19.

47. Prevedouros K, Cousins IT, Buck RC. *et al.* Sources, fate and transport of perfluorocarboxylates. *Environ Sci Technol* 2006; **40**: 32–44.

48. Emmett EA, Shofer FS, Zhang H. *et al.* Community exposure to perfluorooctanoate: relationships between serum concentrations and exposure sources. *J Occup Environ Med* 2006; **48**: 759–70.

49. White SS, Calafat AM, Kuklenyik Z. *et al.* Gestational PFOA exposure of mice is associated with altered mammary gland development in dams and female offspring. *Toxicol Sci* 2007; **96**: 133–44.

50. Curwin BD, Hein MJ, Sanderson WT. *et al.* Urinary and hand wipe pesticide levels among farmers and nonfarmers in Iowa. *J Expo Anal Environ Epidemiol* 2005; **15**: 500–8.

51. Norrgran J, Bravo R, Bishop AM. *et al.* Quantification of six herbicide metabolites in human urine. *J Chromatogr B Analyt Technol Biomed Life Sci* 2006; **830**: 185–95.

52. Enoch RR, Stanko JP, Greiner SN. *et al.* Mammary gland development as a sensitive end point after acute prenatal exposure to an atrazine metabolite mixture in female Long–Evans rats. *Environ Health Perspect* 2007; **115**: 541–7.

53. Warner M, Eskenazi B, Mocarelli P. *et al.* Serum dioxin concentrations and breast cancer risk in the Seveso Women's Health Study. *Environ Health Perspect* 2002; **110**: 625–8.

54. Brown NM, Manzolillo PA, Zhang JX. *et al.* Prenatal TCDD and predisposition to mammary cancer in the rat. *Carcinogenesis* 1998; **19**: 1623–9.

55. Fenton SE, Hamm JT, Birnbaum LS. *et al.* Adverse effects of TCDD on mammary gland development in Long Evans rats: a two generational study. *Organohalogen Compounds* 2000; **48**: 157–60.

56. Birnbaum L, Fenton SE. Cancer and developmental exposure to endocrine disruptors. *Environ Health Perspect* 2003; **111**: 389–94.

57. Maffini MV, Calabro JM, Soto AM. *et al.* Stromal regulation of neoplastic development: age-dependent normalization of neoplastic mammary cells by mammary stroma. *Am J Pathol* 2005; **67**: 1405–10.

58. USEPA. *DDT, a Review of Scientific and Economic Aspects of the Decision to Ban its Use as a Pesticide.*

*EPA-540/1–75–022.* Washington DC: US Environmental Protection Agency, 1975.

59. Wolff MS, Britton JA, Teitelbaum SL. *et al.* Improving organochlorine biomarker models for cancer research. *Cancer Epidem Biomar* 2005; **14**: 2224–36.

60. Wolff MS, Toniolo PG, Lee EW. *et al.* Blood levels of organochlorine residues and risk of breast cancer. *J Nat Cancer Inst* 1993; **85**: 648–52.

61. Dewailly E, Dodin S, Verreault R. *et al.* High organochlorine body burden in women with estrogen receptor positive breast cancer. *J Nat Cancer Inst* 1994; **86**: 232–4.

62. Krieger N, Wolff MS, Hiatt RA. *et al.* Breast cancer and serum organochlorines: a prospective study among white, black, and Asian women. *J Nat Cancer Inst* 1994; **86**: 589–99.

63. Wolff MS, Toniolo PG. Environmental organochlorine exposure as a potential etiologic factor in breast cancer. *Environ Health Perspect* 1995; **103**: 141–5.

64. Soto AM, Fernandez MF, Luizzi MF. *et al.* Developing a marker of exposure to xenoestrogen mixtures in human serum. *Environ Health Perspect* 1997; **105**: 647–54.

65. Pazos P, Perez P, Rivas A. *et al.* Development of a marker of estrogen exposure in breast cancer patients. *Adv Exp Med Biol* 1998; **444**: 29–40.

66. Ibarluzea JM, Fernández MF, Santa-Marina L. *et al.* Breast cancer risk in the combined effect of environmental estrogens. *Cancer Causes Contr* 2004; **15**: 591–600.

67. Boice JD, Jr., Miller RW. Childhood and adult cancer after intrauterine exposure to ionizing radiation. *Teratology* 1999; **59**: 227–33.

68. Preston DL, Mattsson A, Holmberg E. *et al.* Radiation effects on breast cancer risk: a pooled analysis of eight cohorts. *Radiat Res* 2002; **158**: 220–35.

69. Weinberg RA. *The Biology of Cancer.* New York: Taylor & Francis, 2006.

70. Ho S-M, Tang WY, Belmonte de Frausto J. *et al.* Developmental exposure to estradiol and bisphenol a increases susceptibility to prostate carcinogenesis and epigenetically regulates phosphodiesterase type 4 variant 4. *Cancer Res* 2006; **66**: 5624–32.

71. Soto AM, Sonnenschein C. The somatic mutation theory of cancer: growing problems with the paradigm? *BioEssays* 2004; **26**: 1097–107.

# Development and maturation of the normal male reproductive system

Richard M. Sharpe

## Introduction

To be fertile as an adult, a properly functioning male reproductive system has to be established. To ensure this, each component part has to work satisfactorily; this includes the testis, internal reproductive tract/accessory sex organs, the penis, and also the brain. The last controls libido but also ensures that the hormonal aspects of the male reproductive system (the hypothalamic–pituitary–testicular axis) work normally. Deficiencies in any of the component parts of the male reproductive system may impair fertility or cause other reproductive disorders. Such disorders can arise via a variety of mechanisms and at different ages. However, some ages are more important than others in terms of the impact that aberrant changes may have on development or function of the reproductive system and, as detailed below, fetal life is probably the most important period. This chapter will review current understanding about key events occurring at different stages of development in the normal human male and how this impacts reproductive function in adulthood.

## Key periods in development of the male reproductive system

Development of the normal male reproductive system can be divided into five periods (fetal, neonatal, infancy/childhood, puberty, adulthood), as illustrated in Fig. 4.1. These periods are essentially defined by changes in activity of the reproductive hormonal axis, illustrated in Fig. 4.1 by the changing levels of testosterone. Details of the events occurring within each of these periods and their functional importance are considered separately in the sections below. Here the emphasis is on providing perspective on the relative importance and contribution of each of these phases for normal reproductive function in adulthood. For example, a key event that determines the capacity of a man to produce sperm in adulthood in numbers sufficient to ensure his fertility is the number of Sertoli cells, as each of these cells can support only a finite number of germ cells; thus the number of Sertoli cells determines the ceiling of sperm production capacity in any individual [1, 2]. As shown in Fig. 4.1, Sertoli cells proliferate during fetal and neonatal periods and in the period around the start of puberty [1, 2]. Therefore, three phases of life are important in determining adult sperm-producing capacity. One implication of this (in theory anyway) is that if deficiencies in Sertoli cell number arise in fetal or neonatal life it could be compensated for around the time of puberty, so that no deficit in sperm-producing capacity results (Fig. 4.1); evidence from studies in marmosets [3] and rats [4, 5] supports this notion. In this example, it is the same process (Sertoli cell proliferation) taking place in each of the three phases and this applies also to other aspects of reproductive development, for example penile growth. The penis grows during the fetal and neonatal periods but especially during puberty [6, 7]; these periods of growth coinciding with high or rising levels of testosterone, on which this growth depends (Fig. 4.1). The relative importance of these different phases is uncertain, but a working hypothesis based on clinical experience and emerging experimental animal data suggests that in normal males androgen action at all three ages is required to ensure normal penile size, but early deficiencies in growth may be correctable during puberty [8], much as argued for correction of Sertoli cell number. Ultimate size of the penis is firstly dependent on its correct formation in fetal life during the masculinization process [9]. Details of this are covered below, but an important point to note is that masculinization of the reproductive tract (including the genitalia) occurs during an earlier time window in

*Environmental Impacts on Reproductive Health and Fertility*, ed. T. J. Woodruff, S. J. Janssen, L. J. Guillette, and L. C. Giudice. Published by Cambridge University Press. © Cambridge University Press 2010.

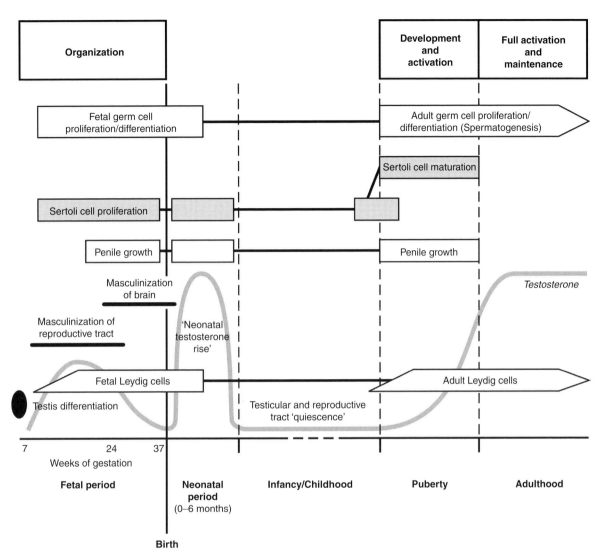

**Fig. 4.1.** Timing of the main events that shape reproductive development and function of the human male, from the time of testis differentiation through to adulthood. Fetal life is when the testis and reproductive system are organized, puberty is when the fully formed reproductive system is developed into its adult form and its functions first activated, and adulthood involves the long-term maintenance of this activation and function. The key events and the relative importance of the different life phases in relation to normal reproductive development are detailed in the text.

fetal life [9] than does masculinization of the brain [10] which is a relatively late event (Fig. 4.1). It may be that this difference is simply a reflection of the longer time necessary for the large brain to develop and grow to the stage at which it is ready for masculinization.

Although at first glance it appears that germ cell development is similar in the perinatal period and during puberty/adulthood, in that proliferation and differentiation are both occurring, what happens to the germ cells in these two periods is fundamentally different. In perinatal life, the germ cells begin differentiating from pluripotent (fetal) germ cells into semi-differentiated germ cells (pre-spermatogonia and then spermatogonia) that are committed to (later) spermatogenesis [11, 12]. During puberty, these cells proliferate and differentiate and then develop into spermatozoa via the complex process of spermatogenesis [2]. As this process is fuelled by spermatogonia and their continuous proliferation, it is ultimately dependent on the successful proliferation and differentiation of fetal germ cells. This example illustrates that a good way of viewing development of the reproductive system is through three step-wise events (Fig. 4.1), namely: (i) organization of the reproductive system, which occurs primarily in fetal life but may extend into the neonatal period; (ii) further development and activation of the reproductive system during puberty; (iii) full activation, and then maintenance, of this system throughout the remainder of adulthood. Clearly, the two later events are predicated on successful organization of the reproductive system many years earlier in fetal life. This highlights the importance of the fetal period; if things go wrong, or are incomplete in terms of organization of the reproductive system during this period, then it is likely to affect development, activation, and maintenance of the reproductive system in later life and lead to reproductive disorders.

It is worth emphasizing the inherent difficulties in acquiring detailed understanding about the processes illustrated in Fig. 4.1 and especially in elucidating what can go wrong mechanistically to result in reproductive malfunction. A major problem is there are relatively few good animal models for reproductive development in the human male. This is mainly because of the lengthy period required for full development which contrasts with reproductive development in rodents and most domestic animals in which the various phases of development shown in Fig. 4.1 are condensed and may even overlap, especially in rodents [1]. As much of our understanding about normal reproductive system development derives from studies in these species, there may be limitations in extrapolating details of these processes to the human. The most striking difference between humans and rodents is the events that occur between birth and puberty, namely the period of the neonatal testosterone rise [13, 14] and the period of reproductive quiescence during childhood [15, 16] (Fig. 4.1). The neonatal testosterone rise in rodents is literally confined to a matter of hours around the time of birth and a period of "childhood" is barely perceptible, as puberty occurs rapidly and there is never an obvious period of testicular or reproductive tract quiescence, and this is only slightly more visible in domestic species such as bulls and rams. In contrast, most primates exhibit similar phases of development to the human [13, 16], and this has been well established in particular for the macaque family and for marmosets [13, 16, 17]. However, even in these species the comparability is not absolute because the period of childhood quiescence is still relatively short when compared with the ~10-year period in the human.

# The fetal period

This is the most important period for determining how normal or otherwise the development and function of the reproductive system will be in the human male. This is when the whole of the reproductive system is organized/stabilized and is therefore the period when the most fundamental errors can occur, which cannot then be corrected [18]. There are three separate aspects to reproductive development during this period, defined as: (i) differentiation of the testis from an indifferent genital ridge; this is termed sexual differentiation because it is the pivotal moment when "maleness" is determined at the molecular level; (ii) masculinization of the fetus. This is essentially putting into practice for the whole of the body what has already been determined for the gonad itself, and this body-wide masculinization is achieved via the production of hormones by the recently differentiated testis; (iii) the start of events that will continue in one form or another throughout fetal, neonatal, and later life and fully develop the reproductive system. This involves Sertoli cell proliferation, penis formation and then growth, germ cell proliferation and differentiation. These three events are sequential as a testis has to normally differentiate (i) if masculinization (ii) is then to ensue and development of the processes in (iii) are to take place. Each of these events will therefore be considered in more detail and their relevance to disorders of reproduction in the human male considered.

## Testicular differentiation (sexual differentiation)

A recognizable testis first forms at around 7 weeks of gestation in the human male [19]. Prior to this, males and females are indistinguishable based on the size or morphology of the genital ridge, from which the testis and ovary form [19, 20]. At this age, males and females cannot be distinguished on the basis of their reproductive systems as both possess müllerian ducts, wolffian ducts, and a genital tubercle from which a penis or clitoris will develop [20]. Current understanding of gonadal differentiation suggests that the "set-up" is for the fetus to develop as a female, whereas becoming a male requires modification of this "set-up" program [18, 21]. It used to be stated that female development was "by default," but it is now clear that a sequence of molecular events occurs to ensure successful female development in the same way that development along the male pathway involves a (different) sequence of molecular changes [22, 23]. (See Chapter 3 for more detail on female development.)

So the fetus will activate a female sequence of events unless there is intervention to switch to the male pathway. This switch initially involves activation of the *Sry* gene on the Y chromosome which then triggers a cascade of other molecular changes [21–23]. The current view is that a cascade of "snowball" events occurs which reinforce each other and reinforce development along the male pathway whereas a different sequence of "snowball" changes occur in the female [22, 23]. A key reinforcing event in the male is switching on expression of the gene *Sox9* [21–23]. According to studies in the mouse, *Sox9* is expressed initially in both ovary and testis but its expression is rapidly lost in the ovary because of the lack of a reinforcing stimulatory signal as occurs in the male, namely *Sry* [24]. Additionally in the male, expression of *Fgf9* also reinforces *Sox9* expression [22] whereas, in the female, expression of *Wnt4* is thought to down-regulate *Sox9* expression as well as inhibiting development of steroidogenic (Leydig) cells [23]. Progressive reinforcement of *Sox9* expression is thus the hallmark of testis differentiation and is the pivotal point of separation from further development along the female pathway [23]. Other genes are also involved in reinforcing development at this early stage, down either male or female pathways, and details can be found elsewhere [21–23]. As increasing numbers of genes are being identified as playing reinforcing roles in early gonad development, it is likely the relative importance of individual genes may vary between species. Nevertheless, it is clear in the human that individuals with inactivating/activating mutations of *Sox9* or *Wnt4* have abnormal sexual development [25–27], similar to that in mice. As only ~35% of sex reversal cases in the human (i.e. in which phenotype does not match genotype) can be explained by mutations in key genes (*Sry*, *Sox9*, *Wnt4*), other genes may be important in this process in the human [28] and our understanding will grow progressively as new genes are identified via studies in the mouse. However, care should be taken in assuming that exactly the same sequence of events occurs during human gonad differentiation as in the mouse, until direct evidence is available.

The differentiation of Sertoli cells is what defines that a testis has formed and is the pivotal step in male development [21–23] as all subsequent steps along the male pathway follow from this. One such effect is on the fetal germ cells (gonocytes), which earlier migrated into the indifferent genital ridge [29]. They can develop along male or female pathways, involving either their arrest at a step prior to meiosis (male pathway) or their entry into meiosis (female pathway). Sertoli cell differentiation is the key event ensuring that the germ cells do not enter meiosis in males [30], and studies in mice point to a potential mechanism. Thus, retinoic acid (RA), produced by cells in the mesonephros lying adjacent to the gonad, diffuses into the gonad and induces the germ cells to enter meiosis; this should only happen in the ovary [31]. Retinoic acid also diffuses into the developing male gonad but, when Sertoli cells differentiate they switch on an enzyme (CYP26B1) which inactivates RA and thus prevents the gonocytes from entering meiosis [31, 32]. It remains to be shown if a similar mechanism occurs in the human testis, because there are some fundamentally important differences between germ cell development during fetal and early postnatal life in rodents and humans (see below).

## Masculinization

Following *Sry*-induced differentiation of the testis, a male phenotype does not automatically develop [18]. For this to occur the differentiated testis must produce three hormones, the actions of which then bring about masculinization of the internal and external reproductive organs as well as masculinization of the brain and the rest of the body. Normal hormonal functioning of the fetal testis is therefore essential for masculinization and thus for development of a male reproductive system [18]. The three hormones are anti-müllerian hormone (AMH), insulin-like factor 3 (Insl3), and testosterone.

Anti-müllerian hormone synthesis/secretion is switched on in Sertoli cells almost immediately after their differentiation and it is then transported to the müllerian ducts where it induces their regression [18, 33]. Anti-müllerian hormone-induced degeneration of the müllerian ducts is an early event in masculinization [33]. Based on studies in rodents, AMH may have other roles to play in the development of the male reproductive system. For example, continued production of AMH suppresses development of the adult generation of Leydig cells and thus could participate in regulating differentiation of these cells during the early stages of puberty [34, 35]. Whether this occurs in humans and whether there may be other effects of AMH are currently unclear. The primary known role of Insl3 (based mainly on studies in rodents) is to regulate transabdominal testicular descent [36] (see below) but there

51

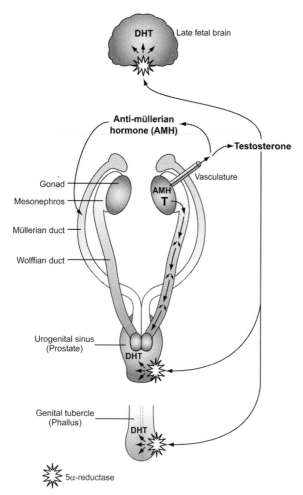

**Fig. 4.2.** The main hormonal events that bring about masculinization of the human male. Note that the diagram is not strictly accurate as masculinization of the brain is a late fetal event, at which time testis differentiation and masculinization of the reproductive tract and genital tubercle (and disappearance of the müllerian ducts) have long occurred. Note also that Insl3, which plays a role in masculinization via regulation of testis descent (Fig. 4.4), is not depicted.

is evidence that it may also play some role in germ cell development postnatally [37].

By far and away the most important of the hormones produced by the fetal testis is testosterone, as it is the actions of this hormone and its metabolites throughout the body that leads to body-wide masculinization (Fig. 4.2). Testosterone itself probably has effects only within the testis and the adjacent wolffian duct [18], as it is somehow transported out of the testis and delivered locally down the wolffian duct lumen where it acts to stabilize and differentiate it so that it will develop into the epididymis, vas deferens, and seminal vesicles

[9, 38]. In these organs, testosterone induces its effects via directly binding to the androgen receptor (AR), but for its actions in the rest of the body it is metabolized within target tissues to the more potent androgen dihydrotestosterone (DHT) which then acts via androgen receptors [39, 40]. Otherwise, the dilution of testosterone in the peripheral circulation would mean that its concentration was insufficient to ensure "masculinizing" effects via ARs in its target reproductive tissues. The conversion of testosterone to DHT occurs via the enzyme 5α-reductase, of which there are types 1 and 2. Type 2 is the form expressed in the urogenital sinus and genital tubercle (Fig. 4.2) whereas type 1 is the form expressed predominantly in the brain and skin [41]. Individuals with inactivating mutations in the type 2 enzyme usually present at birth with ambiguous genitalia [39, 40]. An alternative possibility is for testosterone to be converted via the enzyme aromatase to estradiol which can then exert effects via estrogen receptors (ERs). In rodents, some of the masculinizing effects of androgens on the brain are mediated via their local conversion to estradiol, including regulation of male sexual behavior [42]. In contrast, in the human the predominant masculinizing effect on the brain occurs via androgens themselves, presumably DHT [43, 44] (Fig. 4.2). However, ERs are expressed in many of the developing reproductive tissues of the fetal male, including the genital tubercle, and some evidence from both rodents and humans suggest that estrogens could play a role in some aspects of penile development [45]. Whatever this role is, it is of minor significance in comparison to the role of androgens [46].

Disorders of masculinization resulting in frank sex reversal or intersex in humans are rare and are usually explained by mutations in AR, 5α-reductase or in genes involved in earlier testis differentiation, such as *Sry* or *Sox9* [47]. In contrast, milder disorders of masculinization in humans are amongst the commonest congenital disorders, namely the failure of testis descent into the scrotum (cryptorchidism, see details below) and hypospadias; the latter condition is when the urethral meatus does not open in the middle of the tip of the penis but is displaced to the edge or the shaft of the penis or, in severe cases, to the perineal region [48]. At birth, hypospadias affects 0.3–1.0% of boys, depending on the country [49], whereas cryptorchidism affects 2–9% of boys [50, 51]. As testicular descent is regulated by androgens and Insl3 and androgens play a key role in penile development, the high prevalence of these disorders suggests that mild impairment of masculinization is common [9, 18, 52]. Cryptorchidism and hypospadias are considered to be potential manifestations of a broader "testicular dysgenesis syndrome" (TDS) which also includes adult onset disorders such as some cases of low sperm counts and testicular germ cell cancer [52, 53]. These disorders are all thought to have a common origin in fetal life, resulting one way or another from abnormal testis differentiation or function, leading to downstream disorders that manifest either at birth or after puberty [52, 53]. Details on TDS can be found in other chapters. However, the fetal origin of TDS disorders provides a focus for understanding the details of the masculinization process, and how it might malfunction. An important recent development has been the discovery in rodents of a "male programming window" [9].

## 'Male (masculinization) programming window'

Once the testis differentiates and starts to produce hormones, masculinization of the reproductive system ensues but it is not instantaneous [9]. The fetal ages at which the various reproductive structures emerge in recognizable form varies according to the organ (Fig. 4.3). For example, a recognizable penis is not evident until ~14 weeks of gestation and a recognizable prostate and differentiation of the wolffian duct does not occur until this time or later (Fig. 4.3). From studies in the rat, it has been shown that differentiation of these reproductive structures is driven by androgen action during an earlier fetal time window than when they actually differentiate, referred to as the male programming window [9]. By analogy, it is predicted that this programming window occurs at ~8–12 weeks of gestation in humans, possibly extending to 14 weeks (Fig. 4.3). In the corresponding time window in the rat, androgen action is essential for the later normal development of each of the component reproductive tract structures including the penis, but within the programming window itself there is little sign of morphological change in these structures so they appear broadly comparable in males and females [9].

An important implication of the male programming window is that, in rats, cryptorchidism and hypospadias can only arise due to deficient androgen action within this programming window [9]. Impaired androgen action at any later age, including at the time at which a morphologically recognizable penis manifests and testes descent is completed, fails to have

effects. Similarly, other aspects of reproductive development (final penile length, size of prostate and seminal vesicles) are also determined by androgen action within this programming window [9]. The available evidence suggests that this information can be transcribed from the rat to the human (Fig. 4.3). Therefore, the size of accessory sex organs in adulthood in human males, as well as penile length, may also be affected by the normality of androgen action during the male programming window, early in gestation. Another clinically relevant observation from these animal studies is that ano-genital distance (AGD), which is normally ~1.7 times as long in males as in females, is also programmed by androgen action within the male programming window, and provides a lifelong read-out of androgen levels/action at this time [9]. Smaller AGD predicts cryptorchidism, hypospadias (and its severity), penile length, prostate and testis size in rats [5, 9].

In contrast to masculinization of the reproductive tract, masculinization of the brain is not programmed within the male programming window but is determined by androgen action later in gestation [44] (Fig. 4.3). This suggests that masculinization of the body and the brain are separate and, therefore, there could be disorders of one without disorders of the other, for example gender dysphoria [54].

## Testicular development

After its differentiation, the testis undergoes important developmental changes in fetal life. The three most important changes are: (i) increase in Sertoli cell numbers; (ii) expansion and differentiation of the germ cell population; (iii) testis descent through the abdomen and pelvis to reach its final location in the base of the scrotum prior to birth. Each of these events is important for fertility and normal testis function in adulthood. Proliferation of Sertoli [1] and germ cells [11, 12] commence soon after testicular differentiation and both of these processes continue into the neonatal period (Fig. 4.1). For germ cells, important differentiation changes also occur in the same period. This involves loss of expression of pluripotency factors, associated with embryonic stem cell-like activity, and switching on of germ cell-specific genes associated with more mature germ cells (i.e. spermatogonia-like changes) [11, 12]. This differentiation is an important step along the pathway towards later spermatogenesis, and in relation to the possibility of developing testicular germ cell cancer (TGCT). This arises from premalignant, precursor cells termed carcinoma *in situ* (CIS),

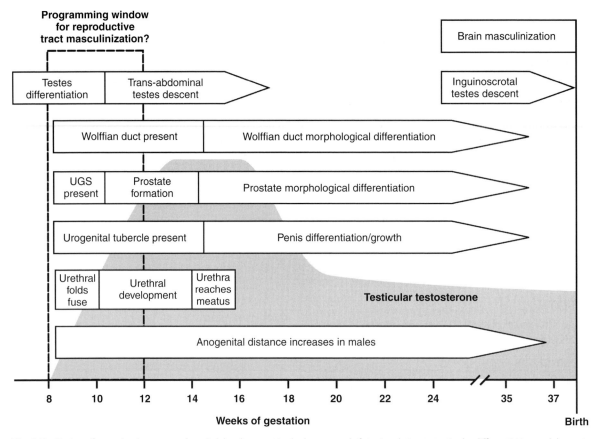

**Fig. 4.3.** Timing of reproductive tract and genital development in the human male fetus in relation to testicular differentiation and descent, the testicular levels of testosterone and brain masculinization. The postulated timing of the "male programming window" [9] is also shown. Timings are based on numerous published studies [9] UGS: urogenital sinus.

and the CIS cells share many features with fetal germ cells, including expression of pluripotency genes and lack of expression of more differentiated germ cell genes (which would normally be expressed) [55]. Details on the origins of CIS cells and TGCT and the associated risk factors can be found elsewhere (see Chapter 11).

Androgen action is also thought to be important for Sertoli cell proliferation in fetal and neonatal life, based on studies in rodents which have examined the impacts of inactivation of the AR or by lowering fetal intratesticular testosterone levels [1, 5, 56]. At least in theory, subnormal androgen production by the human fetal testis could lead to reduced numbers of Sertoli cells and, if this was not compensated for by extra Sertoli cell proliferation in the postnatal period (Fig. 4.1), it would lead to reduced Sertoli cell numbers in adulthood which would translate into a lower sperm count [1, 52]. Thus, subnormal testosterone production by the fetal testis could lead to this change as well as to the other changes associated with TDS [52].

Testicular descent is a key fetal event which places the testis in the scrotum, which is necessary for full, normal spermatogenesis to take place subsequently from mid-puberty onwards (Fig. 4.1). Descent of the testis occurs in two phases [57, 58], the first occurring early in gestation and involving movement of the testes from their point of origin by the kidney into the inguinal region (Fig. 4.4). Here the testes remain until the second phase of testes descent through the pelvis and into the bottom of the scrotum, which occurs late in gestation [58] (Fig. 4.4). The trans-abdominal phase of descent is thought to be regulated by Insl3, based on studies in mice [36, 57, 58], but androgens may also play some role, whereas the trans-inguinal phase of testes descent is regulated by androgens alone [57, 58]. It is this second phase of testis descent which goes wrong most commonly in human crytorchidism [58], suggestive of impaired androgen production/action as the cause [9]. Moreover, it is now established for the rat that this second phase of testicular descent is

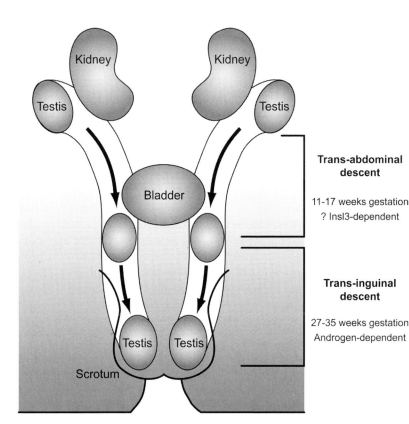

**Fig. 4.4.** The two phases of testicular descent in the human male fetus and their hormone dependence. Note that failure of testis descent (cryptorchidism) in boys at birth is due mainly to incompletion of the second phase of descent.

programmed by androgens in the "male programming window" [9] (see above) even though the lapse of time between this programing window and the timing of the second phase of testis descent is quite considerable (Fig. 4.1).

## The neonatal period (0–6 months)

In neonatal male and female babies there is activation of the hypothalamic–pituitary axis and consequent increase in circulating levels of luteinizing hormone (LH) and follicle-stimulating hormone (FSH) [13, 16]. In the female this is not accompanied by gonadal steroidogenesis whereas in the male it is associated with stimulation of the Leydig cells and elevation of testosterone levels into the low adult range [13, 14](Fig. 4.1). The role of this increase in testosterone continues to be debated. During this neonatal period, Sertoli cells continue to proliferate [1] and this is arguably the most important period in life in terms of the magnitude of increase in Sertoli cell numbers; however, there is a paucity of data for the human and this is inferred from what is seen in other animals [1]. It had been presumed that the neonatal increase in Sertoli cell number was a consequence of stimulation by the elevated levels of FSH, but rodent studies showing the importance of

androgens in driving increased Sertoli cell proliferation in fetal and neonatal periods [1, 52, 56], suggest that testosterone may also be important in this context in the human. Another effect of androgens during the neonatal period in the human is to increase penile length [59], although the data are limited. In rodents, the masculinizing effects of androgens on the brain occur primarily during the immediate postnatal period [42, 43]. Whether masculinizing effects of androgens on the brain occur during neonatal life in human males is unknown [44]. However, studies in non-human primates in which blockade of the neonatal testosterone rise has been induced experimentally have shown that in general there are no consequences for later fertility or sexual behavior [13, 60]. Nevertheless, it seems likely that there will be some effect of testosterone on androgen target tissues during this period, and high on this list might be organs such as the developing prostate. Our unpublished studies in the marmoset suggest that the prostate may grow during the period of the neonatal testosterone rise and that this growth is diminished if the neonatal testosterone rise is blocked. As androgens in the male have effects on nearly all of the main tissues and organs of the body, and the time windows within which these organs are affected are largely if not completely unknown, it remains possible that some of these effects could occur during the neonatal period.

# Infancy and childhood (6 months – ~12 years)

After the neonatal period, there is a protracted period of testicular and reproductive quiescence, typified by low circulating levels of gonadotropins and testosterone [15]. However, it has been suggested that it is perhaps more accurate to consider the testis as "quietly active" rather than completely quiescent [15]. This is because studies have shown, for example, that germ cell proliferation and development occur during this period but at a low level; germ cell numbers increase by ~three-fold during childhood and testis weight also increases [61], as occurs also in marmosets [16]. Together with these changes, testosterone secretion from the testis may be somewhat increased in later childhood, especially during the nighttime when there is activation of pulsatile LH secretion [62]. These developmental changes are relatively minor in comparison to the dramatic changes that occur subsequently during puberty and it seems most likely that their purpose is to "prepare the ground" for these later changes. A particular reason for interest in these changes is that in boys who are unfortunate enough to develop cancer during infancy/childhood and who require therapy, this can result in complete loss of germ cells for some therapies and consequent sterility in adulthood [63].

A further period of Sertoli cell proliferation is known to occur at some stage during the childhood/early puberty period but for the human there is insufficient information to establish precisely when this occurs [1]. As it is presumed that this will involve stimulation by FSH and/or testosterone, this most likely occurs in the period leading into puberty and direct studies in the marmoset and other animals support this interpretation [1].

# Puberty and adulthood

The onset of puberty is characterized by increased activity of the hypothalamic–pituitary (HP) axis and consequent increased frequency of pulsatile LH secretion, especially at night [62]. Activation of the HP axis at the start of puberty is more accurately viewed as a re-awakening, and it is suggested that the correct question to ask is "what actually puts the brake on the HP axis in childhood between the neonatal period when it is active and puberty when it is active?" [64]. This question is currently undergoing revision with the discovery of important new players that regulate this activity, namely kisspeptin and its cognate receptor (GPR54). This is beyond the scope of the present chapter but the latest thinking can be found elsewhere [65, 66]. Testosterone levels rise progressively during puberty as the adult Leydig cell population differentiates and increases in number and as the LH drive to these cells increases. Testosterone has effects on many of the androgen-dependent reproductive organs, in particular it stimulates further penile growth so that it attains its full adult size and it also acts on the internal organs of the reproductive tract to induce their growth to adult size and to switch on their various androgen-driven secretory functions. This applies in particular to the prostate and seminal vesicles but also to some extent to the epididymis and vas deferens. Based on studies in the rat, the final size of the accessory sex organs may be determined not by the level of androgen stimulation during puberty and into adulthood but by the level of androgen action that occurred during the male programming window in fetal life [9] (Fig. 4.1). In addition to their effects on the reproductive tract, the rising androgen levels have effects throughout the body, especially on the brain to fully activate sexual behavior and libido [10, 44, 54]. Arguably, the most important new effects that androgens have during puberty and through into adulthood is their effects on the Sertoli cell to support spermatogenesis [2].

The Sertoli cell is not a direct androgen target prior to puberty in the human as it does not express the AR [1, 67]. However, as already outlined, androgens have important effects on Sertoli cells to regulate their proliferation in perinatal life, but these effects are thought to be mediated indirectly via the AR-positive peritubular myoid cells [1, 56]. Sertoli cells start expressing AR at the onset of puberty and this is considered one sign of maturation of these cells, as they terminally differentiate and cease proliferating [1]. This is a prerequisite for onset and expansion of spermatogenesis, as adjacent Sertoli cells must develop interlocking tight junctions to form an occluding barrier that is largely impenetrable and which creates a new "adluminal compartment" within the seminiferous tubules [2]. Formation of the tight junctions enables formation of a lumen which is continuous along the length of the seminiferous tubules and which provides the conduit via which spermatozoa can be transported out of the testis to the epididymis. Formation of a tubule lumen is an indirect indicator of tight junction formation and is one of the earliest hallmarks of the onset of spermatogenesis [2]. The secretion of seminiferous tubule fluid (STF) is driven by androgens and is a feature of the adult testis [2]. Creation of the adluminal compartment provides a unique environment in which meiotic and post-meiotic germ cells can differentiate into sperm and be fully supported by the secretions of the Sertoli cells but be protected from immune surveillance and attack. Maintenance of intact tight junctions between Sertoli cells (sometimes referred to as the blood–testis barrier) is therefore essential for maintenance of full normal spermatogenesis and for protection of the germ cell components of spermatogenesis from immune attack [2].

The process of spermatogenesis is hormonally regulated by the combined effects of FSH from the pituitary gland and by testosterone produced locally within the testis by the adult generation of Leydig cells [2]. Testosterone levels in the testis are ~200-fold higher than levels in peripheral blood [2] and this is necessary to drive spermatogenesis, as suppression of intra-testicular testosterone to levels found in blood results in incomplete spermatogenesis and loss of fertility [2, 68]. Androgen-receptor knock-out studies in mice have established that androgen action via the AR in Sertoli cells is essential for maintenance of full spermatogenesis and for the development of germ cells through meiosis [69]. In addition to switching on of the AR, formation of tight junctions and commencement of STF secretion, there are numerous other functional changes that occur to the Sertoli cell as part of its "maturation" [1, 70]. Essentially, this involves the switching off of functions that predominated during early life (such as proliferation) and the switching on of a wide range of new functions, the purpose of which is to provide physical and metabolic support for germ cells during spermatogenesis [1]. Details of these events are beyond the scope of this chapter and the reader is referred to other reviews [1, 2]. Importantly, for normal spermatogenesis to occur, the testes must be descended into the bottom of the scrotum. Therefore, failure of this process in fetal life (Fig. 4.4), without subsequent correction, will result in failure of sperm production in the affected testis.

Once puberty has ended, adulthood has effectively been attained and all that is important now is to maintain both steroidogenic and spermatogenic activity of the testis and the supporting functions of other reproductive organs to ensure constant fertility and normal reproductive behavior for the rest of adulthood. This is dependent upon a normally functioning HP axis as this provides FSH and, more importantly, LH as essential drives to the testis to maintain steroidogenesis and spermatogenesis. Disorders of spermatogenesis, and in particular low sperm counts, are extremely common in humans [52, 53, 71] and little is understood about the causes and origins of these problems [2]. Consequently, there is little effective treatment for such disorders. As outlined above, it is thought that some cases of low sperm counts in young men may have their origins in fetal life, but whether this results from effects on Sertoli cell number or function or on germ cell number and function or even on Leydig cell number and function, or a combination of these, is unknown. Connecting together events separated by 20–30 or more years, as with adult-onset reproductive disorders with fetal origins, such as low sperm counts, is problematic and therefore information derived from animal models is probably going to be the quickest way to obtain the understanding necessary to enable prevention or treatment of the disorders in human males.

# References

1. Sharpe RM, McKinnell C, Kivlin C. *et al.* Proliferation and functional maturation of Sertoli cells, and their relevance to disorders of testis function in adulthood. *Reproduction* 2003; **125**: 769–84.

2. Sharpe RM. Regulation of spermatogenesis. In Knobil E, Neill JD, eds. *The Physiology of Reproduction*, 2nd Edition New York: Raven Press, 1994; 1363–434.

3. Sharpe RM, Walker M, Millar MR. *et al.* Effect of neonatal gonadotropin-releasing hormone antagonist administration on Sertoli cell number and testicular development in the marmoset: comparison with the rat. *Biol Reprod* 2000; **62**: 1685–93.

4. Hutchison G, Scott HM, Walker M. *et al.* Sertoli cell development and function in an animal model of testicular dysgenesis syndrome. *Biol Reprod* 2008; **78**: 352–60.

5. Scott HM, Hutchison GR, Jobling MS. *et al.* Relationship between androgen action in the 'male programming window', fetal Sertoli cell number and adult testis size in the rat. *Endocrinology* 2008; **149**: 5280–7.

6. George FW, Wilson J. Gonads and ducts in mammals. In Knobil E, Neill JD, eds. *The Physiology of Reproduction*. 2nd Edition. New York: Raven Press, 1994; 3–28.

7. Brown GR, Nevison CM, Fraser HM. Manipulation of postnatal testosterone levels affects phallic and clitoral development in infant rhesus monkeys. *Int J Androl* 1999; **22**: 119–28.

8. Bin-Abbas B, Conte FA, Grumbach MM. *et al.* Congenital hypogonadotropic hypogonadism and micropenis: effect of testosterone treatment on adult penis size, why sex reversal is not indicated. *J Pediatr* 1999; **134**: 579–83.

9. Welsh M, Saunders PTK, Fisken M. *et al.* Identification in rats of a programming window for reproductive tract masculinization, disruption of which leads to hypospadias and cryptorchidism. *J Clin Invest* 2008; **118**: 1479–90.

10. Cohen-Bendahan CC, van de Beek C, Berenbaum SA. Prenatal sex hormone effects on child and adult sex-typed behavior: methods and findings. *Neurosci Biobehav Rev* 2005; **29**: 353–84.

11. Gaskell TL, Esnal A, Robinson LL. *et al.* Immunohistochemical profiling of germ cells within the human fetal testis: identification of three subpopulations. *Biol Reprod* 2004; **71**: 2012–21.

12. Mitchell R, Cowan G, Morris KD. *et al.* Germ cell differentiation in the marmoset (*Callithrix jacchus*) during fetal and neonatal life closely parallels that in the human. *Hum Reprod* 2008; **23**: 2755–65.

13. Mann DR, Fraser HM. The neonatal period: a critical interval in male primate development. *J Endocrinol* 1996; **149**: 191–7.

14. Andersson AM, Toppari J, Haavisto AM. Longitudinal reproductive hormone profiles in infants: peak of inhibin B levels in infant boys exceeds levels in adult men. *J Clin Endocrinol Metab* 1998; **83**: 675–81.

15. Chemes HE. Infancy is not a quiescent period of testicular development. *Int J Androl* 2001; **24**: 2–7.

16. Kelnar CJ, McKinnell C, Walker M. *et al.* Testicular changes during infantile 'quiescence' in the marmoset and their gonadotrophin dependence: a model for investigating susceptibility of the prepubertal human testis to cancer therapy? *Hum Reprod* 2002; **17**: 1367–78.

17. Plant TM, Ramaswamy S, Simorangkir D. *et al.* Postnatal and pubertal development of the rhesus monkey (*Macaca mulatta*) testis. *Ann NY Acad Sci USA* 2005; **1061**: 149–162.

18. Sharpe RM. Pathways of endocrine disruption during male sexual differentiation and masculinization. *Best Pract Res Clin Endocrinol Metab* 2006; **20**: 91–110.

19. Krone N, Hanley NA, Arlt W. Age-specific changes in sex steroid biosynthesis and sex development. *Best Pract Res Clin Endocrinol Metab* 2007; **21**: 393–401.

20. Jirasek JE. Morphogenesis of the genital system in the human. *Birth Defects Orig Artic Ser* 1977; **13**: 13–39.

21. Brennan J, Capel B. One tissue, two fates: molecular genetic events that underlie testis versus ovary development. *Nature Rev Gen* 2004; **7**: 509–21.

22. Wilhelm D, Palmer S, Koopman P. Sex determination and gonadal development in mammals. *Physiol Rev* 2007; **8**: 1–28.

23. DiNapoli L, Capel B. SRY and the standoff in sex determination. *Mol Endocrinol* 2008; **22**: 1–9.

24. Kim Y, Capel B. Balancing the bipotential gonad between alternative organ fates: a new perspective on an old problem. *Dev Dyn* 2006; **235**: 2292–300.

25. Sim H, Argentaro A, Harley VR. Boys, girls and shuttling of SRY and SOX9. *Trends Endocrinol Metab* 2008; **19**: 213–22.

26. Biason-Lauber A, Konrad D, Navratil F, *et al.* A WNT4 mutation associated with Müllerian duct regression and virilization in a 46,XX woman. *New Engl J Med* 2004; **351**: 792–8.

27. Bernard P, Harley VR. Wnt4 action in gonadal development and sex determination. *Int J Biochem Cell Biol* 2007; **39**: 31–43.

28. McElreavey K, Fellous M. Sex-determining genes. *Trends Endocrinol Metab* 1997; **8**: 342–6.

29. Molyneaux K, Wylie C. Primordial germ cell migration. *Int J Dev Biol* 2004; **48**: 537–44.

30. McLaren A, Buehr M. Development of mouse germ cells in cultures of fetal gonads. *Cell Differ Dev* 1990; **31**: 185–95.

31. Bowles J, Koopman P. Retinoic acid, meiosis and germ cell fate in mammals. *Development* 2007; **134**: 3401–11.

32. Bowles J, Knight D, Smith C. *et al.* Sex-specific regulation of retinoic acid levels in developing mouse gonads determines germ cell fate. *Science* 2006; **312**: 596–600.

33. Klattig J, Englert C. The Müllerian duct: recent insights into its development and regression. *Sex Dev* 2007; **1**: 271–8.

34. Wu X, Arumugam R, Baker SP. *et al.* Pubertal and adult Leydig cell function in Müllerian inhibiting substance-deficient mice. *Endocrinology* 2005; **146**: 589–95.

35. Salva A, Hardy MP, Wu XF. *et al.* Müllerian-inhibiting substance inhibits rat Leydig cell regeneration after ethylene dimethanesulphonate ablation. *Biol Reprod* 2004; **70**: 600–7.

36. Adhami IM, Agoulnik AI. Insulin-like 3 signalling in testicular descent. *Int J Androl*; 2004; **27**: 257–65.

37. Kawamura K, Kumagai J, Sudo S. *et al.* Paracrine regulation of mammalian oocyte maturation and male germ cell survival. *Proc Natl Acad Sci USA* 2004; **101**: 7323–8.

38. Welsh, M, Saunders PT, Sharpe RM. The critical time window for androgen-dependent development of the Wolffian duct in the rat. *Endocrinology* 2007; **148**: 3185–95.

39. Hughes IA. Minireview: sex differentiation. *Endocrinology* 2001; **142**: 3281–7.

40. Sultan C, Paris F, Terouanne B. *et al.* Disorders linked to insufficient androgen action in male children. *Hum Reprod Update* 2001; **7**: 314–22.

41. Ellsworth K, Harris G. Expression of the type 1 and 2 steroid 5 alpha-reductases in human fetal tissues. *Biochem Biophys Res Commun* 1995; **215**: 774–80.

42. Schwarz JM, McCarthy MM. Cellular mechanisms of estradiol-mediated masculinization of the brain. *J Steroid Biochem Mol Biol* 2008; **109**: 300–6.

43. Swaab DF. Sexual differentiation of the human brain: relevance for gender identity, trans-sexualism and sexual orientation. *Gynecol Endocrinol.* 2004; **19**: 301–12.

44. Goy RW, Bercovitch FB, McBrair MC. Behavioral masculinization is independent of genital masculinization in prenatally androgenized female rhesus macaques. *Horm Behav* 1988; **22**: 552–71.

45. Agras K, Willingham E, Shiroyanagi Y. *et al.* Estrogen receptor-alpha and beta are differentially distributed, expressed and activated in the fetal genital tubercle. *J Urol* 2007; **177**: 2386–92.

46. Agras K, Willingham E, Liu B. *et al.* Ontogeny of androgen receptor and disruption of its mRNA expression by exogenous estrogens during morphogenesis of the genital tubercle. *J Urol* 2006; **176**: 1883–8.

47. Hughes IA. Disorders of sex development: a new definition and classification. *Best Pract Res Clin Endocrinol Metab* 2008; **22**: 119–34.

48. Wang MH, Baskin LS. Endocrine disruptors, genital development and hypospadias. *J Androl* 2008; **29**: 499–505.

49. Boisen, KA, Chellakooty M, Schmidt IM. *et al.* Hypospadias in a cohort of 1072 Danish newborn boys: prevalence and relationship to placental weight, anthropometrical measurements at birth, and reproductive hormone levels at three months of age. *J Clin Endocrinol Metab* 2005; **90**: 4041–6.

50. Toppari J, Kaleva M, Virtanen HE. Trends in the incidence of cryptorchidism and hypospadias, and methodological limitations of registry-based data. *Human Reprod* 2001; **7**: 282–6.

51. Boisen KA, Kaleva M, Main KM. *et al.* Difference in prevalence of congenital cryptorchidism in infants between two Nordic countries. *Lancet* 2004; **363**: 1264–9.

52. Sharpe RM, Skakkebaek NE. Testicular dysgenesis syndrome: mechanistic insights and potential new downstream effects. *Fertil Steril*; 2008; **89** Suppl 1: e33–8.

53. Skakkebaek NE, Rajpert-De Meyts E, Main, KM. Testicular dysgenesis syndrome: an increasingly common developmental disorder with environmental aspects. *Hum Reprod* 2001; **16**: 972–8.

54. Gooren LJ, Kruijver FP. Androgens and male behaviour. *Mol Cell Endocrinol* 2002; **198**: 31–40.

55. Rajpert-De Meyts E. Developmental model for the pathogenesis of testicular carcinoma in situ: genetic and environmental aspects. *Hum Reprod Update* 2006; **12**: 303–23.

56. Scott HM, Hutchison GR, Mahood IK. *et al.* Role of androgens in fetal testis development and dysgenesis. *Endocrinology* 2007; **148**: 2027–36.

57. Klonisch T, Fowler PA, Hombach-Klonisch S. Molecular and genetic regulation of testis descent and external genitalia development. *Dev Biol* 2004; **270**: 1–18.

58. Amann RP, Veeramachaneni DN. Cryptorchidism in common eutherian mammals. *Reproduction* 2007; **133**: 541–61.

59. Boas M, Boisen KA, Virtanen HE. *et al.* Postnatal penile length and growth rate correlate to serum testosterone levels: a longitudinal study of 1962 normal boys. *Eur J Endocrinol* 2006; **154**: 125–9.

60. Tan KAL, Walker M, Morris K. *et al.* Infant feeding with soy formula milk: effects on puberty progression, reproductive function and testicular cell numbers in marmoset monkeys in adulthood. *Hum Reprod* 2006; **21**: 896–904.

61. Müller J, Skakkebaek NE. Fluctuations in the number of germ cells during the late foetal and early postnatal periods in boys. *Acta Endocrinol* 1984; **105**: 271–4.

62. Grumbach MM. The neuroendocrinology of human puberty revisited. *Horm Res* 2002; **57** Suppl 2: 2–14.

63. Brougham MF, Kelnar CJ, Sharpe RM. *et al.* Male fertility following childhood cancer: current concepts and future therapies. *Asian J Androl* 2003; **5**: 325–37.

64. Plant TM, Barker-Gibb ML. Neurobiological mechanisms of puberty in higher primates. *Hum Reprod Update* 2004; **10**: 67–77.

65. Chan YM, Broder-Fingert S, Seminara SB. Reproductive functions of kisspeptin and Gpr54 across the life cycle of mice and men. *Peptides* 2009; **30**: 42–8.

66. Castellano JM, Roa J, Lucque RM. *et al.* KISS-1/kisspeptins and the metabolic control of reproduction: physiologic roles and putative physiopathological implications. *Peptides* 2009; **30**: 139–45.

67. Sharpe RM. Sertoli cell endocrinology and signal transduction: androgen regulation. In: Skinner MK, Griswold MD, eds. *Sertoli Cell Biology.* London: Elsevier Academic Press, 2005: 199–216.

68. Page ST, Amory JK, Bremner WJ. Advances in male contraception. *Endocr Rev* 2008; **29**: 465–93.

69. De Gendt K, Swinnen JV, Saunders Ptk. *et al.* A Sertoli cell-selective knockout of the androgen receptor causes spermatogenic arrest in meiosis. *Proc Natl Acad Sci USA* 2004; **101**: 1327–32.

70. Tan KA, De Gendt K, Atanassova N. *et al.* The role of androgens in Sertoli cell proliferation and functional maturation: studies in mice with total or Sertoli cell-selective ablation of the androgen receptor. *Endocrinology* 2005; **146**: 2674–83.

71. Jørgensen N, Asklund C, Carlsen E. *et al.* Coordinated European investigations of semen quality: results from studies of Scandinavian young men is a matter of concern. *Int J Androl* 2006; **29**: 54–61.

# Modern genetics of reproductive biology

Taisen Iguchi, Shinichi Miyagawa, and Tamotsu Sudo

## Introduction

"Epigenetics" has been described as the study of changes in gene expression that occur not due to changes in DNA sequence, but rather due to remodeling of the chromatin or modifications in DNA such as methylation, a process by which methyl groups are added to the base cytosine in DNA [1]. Waddington [2] defined "epigenetics" as "… the interactions of genes with their environment which bring the phenotype into being." In those days, the gene as the unit of heritable material was a theoretical concept without a physical identity. Holliday and Pugh [3] proposed that covalent chemical DNA modifications, including methylation of cytosine–guanine (CpG) dinucleotides, were the molecular mechanisms behind Waddington's hypothesis. Developmental processes are regulated largely by epigenetics, because different cell types maintain their fate during cell division even though their DNA sequences are essentially the same. The further revelations that X chromosome inactivation in mammals and genomic imprinting are regulated by epigenetic mechanisms highlighted the heritable nature of epigenetic gene-regulation mechanisms [4]. The genomics revolution inspired the investigation of global, rather than local, gene analyses, and the term "epigenomics" was coined as the study of the "… effects of chromatin structure, including the higher order of chromatin folding and attachment to the nuclear matrix, packaging of DNA around nucleosomes, covalent modifications of histone tails (acetylation, methylation, phosphorylation, ubiquitination), and DNA methylation" [5]. The resistance of some gene loci to methylation reprogramming during embryogenesis revealed the possibility that epigenetic modifications are inherited not only during somatic-cell division, but also in subsequent generations [6].

Transcription factors play roles in regulating gene expression levels, however, DNA methylation and structural changes in chromatin involve switching "on/off" of gene expression. In most studies, increased methylation is associated with gene silencing and decreased methylation is associated with gene activation. These events occur in cells during the normal development of mammals [7].

## Epigenetics and disease

Epigenetic changes are involved in disease processes, including cessation of embryonic development and malformation of embryos as well as during normal development. A unifying theme of disease epigenetics is the occurrence of defects in phenotypic plasticity – the cells' ability to change their behavior in response to internal or external environmental cues. Several defects in the epigenome are known to lead to disease, including changes in the localization or global density of DNA methylation, and incorrect histone modification, altered distribution or function of chromatin-modifying proteins that in turn leads to aberrant gene expression, or the disruption of higher-order loop structure in disease. For example, Rett syndrome, an X-linked dominant neurodevelopmental disorder affecting 1/10 000–15 000 girls, involves mutations of the methyl CpG-binding protein 2 (*MeCP2*) gene, which encodes a protein that binds to methylated DNA sequences [8]. Several examples of DNA methylation changes in diseases have been summarized [9]. Beckwith–Wiedemann syndrome patients, characterized by prenatal overgrowth, a midline abdominal wall and other malformations and cancer, show disrupted imprinting of either or both of two neighboring imprinted subdomains on 11p15. In Prader–Willi syndrome and Angelman syndrome, disorders of a pair of imprinted genes are associated with mental retardation [10]. In cancer cells, changes in DNA methylation and histone modification have been reported in the

*Environmental Impacts on Reproductive Health and Fertility*, ed. T. J. Woodruff, S. J. Janssen, L. J. Guillette, and L. C. Giudice. Published by Cambridge University Press. © Cambridge University Press 2010.

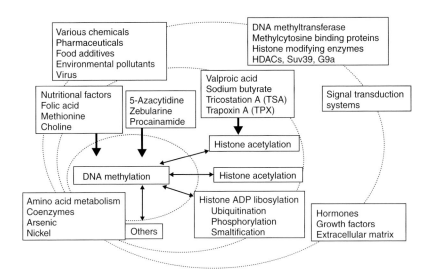

**Fig. 5.1.** Various factors affecting DNA methylation. DNA methylation and histone modification are major mechanisms of epigenetic changes.

promoter regions of oncogenes or tumor suppressor genes [11]. DNA methylation is affected by various factors (Fig. 5.1).

Epidemiologic studies and animal studies increasingly suggest that exposures to environmental chemicals, nutrition, physical factors, and other factors early in development have a role in susceptibility to disease in later life [12]. In addition, some of these environmental effects seem to be passed on to subsequent generations. Epigenetic modifications provide a plausible link between the environment and alterations in gene expression that might lead to disease phenotypes [6].

## Morphogenesis genes in female reproductive tracts

The mammalian female reproductive system arises from the uniform paramesonephric duct, the müllerian duct. The embryonic müllerian duct derives from the intermediate mesoderm and gives rise to the oviduct, uterus, cervix, and upper third of the vagina during mammalian embryonic development. The initial formation of the müllerian duct requires Lim-1 expression because female mice lacking this homeodomain protein have no uterus [13]. Subsequently, expressions of *Abdominal B HOX* genes are required to establish the segmental boundaries between these structures along the developing müllerian duct, as mutations in these genes result in region-specific developmental defects in the female reproductive tract [14, 15]. *HOXA10* knock-out mice, for example, show defective implantation and decidualization in uterine

stromal cells that result in infertility. Stromal cell proliferation in *HOXA10* knock-out mice in response to progesterone (P4) and 17β-estradiol (E2) was significantly reduced, while epithelial cell proliferation was normal in response to E2, suggesting that stromal cell responsiveness to P4 with respect to cell proliferation is impaired in *HOXA10*(-/-) mice, and that *HOXA10* is involved in mediating stromal cell proliferation [16]. *HOXA* genes have crucial roles for patterning of the developing müllerian duct. *HOXA9* is expressed in the oviduct, *HOXA10* in the uterus, *HOXA11* in the uterus and uterine cervix, and *HOXA13* in the upper vagina. These genes continue to be expressed in the adult mouse and are expressed in the same pattern in the human. The female reproductive system undergoes dramatic structural and functional changes during the estrous cycle and in pregnancy, retaining a high degree of developmental plasticity [17]. *HOXA10* is expressed in the adult human uterus and its expression is dramatically increased during the midsecretory phase of the menstrual cycle, corresponding to the time of implantation and an increase in circulating P4 [18].

*Wnt7a-/-* mice are sterile and develop an abnormal stratified uterine epithelium [19]. In particular, the oviducts are not coiled, and are reduced in size or absent. However, the uterine horns are normal in length but have a markedly reduced diameter. The size of the cervix and vagina appear to be normal but in many cases, the midline fails to fuse appropriately. The oviducts acquire a uterus-like appearance (simple columnar epithelium with gland-like inclusions). The uterus completely lacks glands and the normal simple columnar epithelium of the uterus is replaced by a stratified epithelium resembling the cytoarchitecture of the vagina. In addition, the myometrium is disorganized and larger than in the wild-type female.

During embryonic development, members of the *Wnt* gene family are mostly expressed in complementary patterns. *Wnt5a* is expressed at high levels in the adult female reproductive tract, but during gestation, *Wnt5a* is down-regulated [20]. *Wnt4* and *Wnt7a* are detected at high levels in the female reproductive tract. In the adult, *Wnt4*, *Wnt5a*, and *Wnt7a* are expressed in specific mesenchymal–epithelial patterns in the uterus and vagina. *Wnt4* is expressed strongly in the stroma adjacent to the luminal epithelium of the uterus, but *Wnt5a* is also expressed in the stroma of the uterus and is restricted from the epithelium and the uterine myometrium. *Wnt7a* is expressed only within the luminal epithelium of the uterus and not within the glandular epithelium. In the vagina, *Wnt4* expression is detected in the vaginal epithelium but expression of *Wnt5a* and *Wnt7a* are not detectable. In the adult female reproductive tract, levels of *Wnt4*, *Wnt5a*, and *Wnt7a* fluctuate during the estrous cycle, as determined by the varying intensity of signals from *in situ* expression analysis [21]. Estrogenic hormones directly or indirectly repress *Wnt7a*, expression similar to the situation observed for *HOXA* genes in the uterus. Cross-talk of *Wnt* genes and *HOX* genes has been summarized by Kitajewski and Sassoon [22].

The uterine luminal and glandular columnar epithelia are derived from the anterior müllerian epithelium, whereas the vaginal stratified squamous epithelium is derived from the posterior müllerian epithelium. Tissue recombination experiments demonstrated that this cell fate determination event involves reciprocal interactions between the epithelium and the underlying stroma [23]. The determination of uterine epithelium occurs between postnatal days 5 and 7 and is thought to be mediated by signals from the stroma. Before this time, the fate of the uterine epithelium can be changed to that of vaginal epithelium when combined with vaginal mesenchyme, whereas the converse recombination results in uterine epithelial differentiation [23]. After postnatal day 7, the fate of uterine epithelium is determined and cannot be changed by mesenchymal cues from the vagina. Epithelial p63 expression is induced by signals from the cervical or vaginal mesenchyme and is thought to be an "identity switch" that controls stratified epithelial differentiation in the female reproductive tract [24]. Although the nature of these stromal signals is not clear at present, swapping the homeodomain of *HOXA11* with that of *HOXA13* resulted in the expression of a hybrid *HOX* protein in the uterine stroma and subsequent stratification of uterine epithelium, suggesting that the stromal signal is likely controlled by *Hox* proteins [25].

# Disordered expression of HOX genes in female reproductive diseases

Epithelial ovarian cancer (EOC) is the leading cause of death from gynecological malignancies in the great majority of developed countries. Most investigators believe that EOC develops within a single layer of ovarian surface epithelium (OSE) that covers the ovary or that lines inclusion cysts immediately beneath the ovarian surface. The "incessant ovulation" hypothesis argues that repeated cycles of ovulation-induced trauma and repair of the OSE at the site of ovulation contributes to ovarian cancer development. However, it has proved difficult to fully understand the underlying mechanisms of the tumorigenic process. The major subtypes of EOCs show morphologic features that resemble those of the müllerian duct-derived epithelia of the reproductive tract. Cheng *et al.* [26] reported that ectopic expression of *HOXA9* in tumorigenic mouse OSE cells gave rise to papillary tumors resembling serous EOCs. In contrast, *HOXA10* and *HOXA11* induced morphogenesis of endometrioid-like and mucinous-like EOCs, respectively. Yoshida *et al.* [27] reported that *HOXA10* expression is down-regulated in endometrial carcinomas and is associated with methylation of the *HOXA10* promoter. They also found that *Hoxa10* induced expression of the epithelial cell adhesion molecule E-cadherin by down-regulating expression of Snail, a repressor of *E-cadherin* gene transcription, resulting in a novel role for *HOXA10* deregulation by promoting epithelial–mesenchymal transition. Endometriosis is a common gynecological disorder that is characterized by the presence of uterine endometrial tissue outside of the uterine cavity and is mainly associated with severe pelvic pain and/or infertility. Taylor *et al.* [28] showed that patients with endometriosis failed to show the expected mid-luteal rise in *HOXA10* and *HOXA11* gene expressions suggesting that aberrant *HOX* gene expression also may contribute to the etiology of infertility in patients with endometriosis.

# Estrogen-receptor signaling and estrogen-responsive genes in female reproductive tracts

Estrogens exert profound effects on cell proliferation, development, differentiation, and homeostasis. Estrogenic effects are mediated through specific intracellular receptors that act via multiple mechanisms. The mechanism of action of estrogen begins upon 17β-estradiol (E2) binding to its receptors (ER-α and ER-β). Ligand-activated ER dimerizes and translocates to the nucleus where it recognizes estrogen response elements (ERE) located in or near promoter DNA regions of target organs. Estrogen (17β-estradiol, E2) also modulates gene expression by a second indirect mechanism that involves the interaction of ER with other transcription factors which, in turn, bind their cognate DNA elements. Estrogen receptor modulates the activities of transcription factors such as the activation protein-1 (AP-1), nuclear factor-κB (NF-κB) and stimulating protein-1 (Sp-1), by stabilizing DNA-protein complexes and/or recruiting co-activators. The E2 binding to ER may also exert rapid actions that start with the activation of a variety of signal transduction pathways (e.g. ERK/MAPK, p38/MAPK, PI3K/AKT, PLC/PKC) [29]. In addition to the nuclear ERs, plasma membrane-associated ERs mediate the non-genomic signaling pathway, which can lead both to cytoplasmic alterations and to regulation of "rapid or non-genomic" gene expression [29] (Fig. 5.2).

Estrogen-receptor-alpha is predominantly expressed in the reproductive tracts of mammals. In the ovary, both ER-α and ER-β are expressed in interstitial cells and granulosa cells, respectively. Estrogen receptor protein (possibly ER-α) begins to be expressed at 5 days of age in the mouse uterine epithelial cells, but ER-α

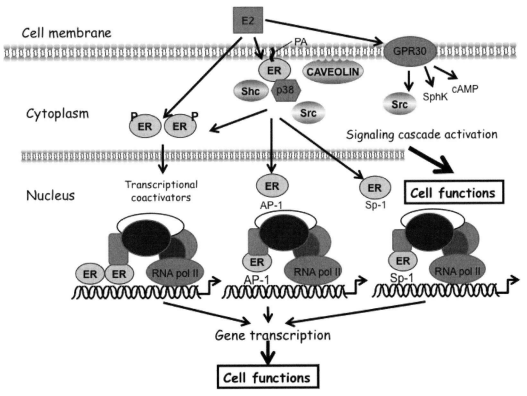

**Fig. 5.2.** Models of the relationship between rapid, intermediate, and long-term actions of estrogen (17β-estradiol, E2) on target cells. Palmitoylation (palmitic acid, PA) allows the estrogen receptor (ER) localization at the cell membrane. E2 binding induces ER relocalization, association to signaling proteins, and triggers the activation of signaling cascades. The kinase activations phosphorylate ER, modulate transcriptional coactivator recruitment, enhance activation protein-1 (AP-1) and stimulate protein-1 (Sp-1) activation. After dimerization, ERs directly interact with ERE on DNA. ERs-DNA indirect association occurs through protein–protein interactions with the Sp-1 and AP-1 transcription factors. Newly identified membrane ER is G-protein coupled receptor 30 (GPR30) located in the plasma membrane and induces rapid intracellular signaling. MNAR: modulator of non-genomic activity of ER-α; SphK: sphingosine kinase. (Partly modified from a figure in Marino *et al.* [29]).

is already expressed in the uterine stromal cells and vaginal epithelial and stromal cells at the day of birth. Recombination studies of the epithelium and the stroma from ER-α knock-out mice and wild-type mice revealed that wild-type mouse stroma can induce proliferation of epithelial cells from ER-α knock-out mice, but the stroma from ER-α knock-out mice could not induce proliferation of epithelium from knock-out mice, suggesting that stromal cells induce epithelial cell proliferation through paracrine factors induced by estrogen stimulation [30]. ER-α is dominant in the female reproductive tracts. ER-α knock-out mice are infertile and ER-β knock-out mice are fertile but produce less offspring than the wild-type mice [31]. Estrogen-responsive genes in the mouse uterus [32] and mouse vagina [33] have been identified using microarray techniques. We

demonstrated that 299 genes are up-regulated and 317 genes are down-regulated in mouse uterus after 6 h of estrogen stimulation [32]. Physiological (E2) and non-physiological (DES) estrogens, nonylphenol (NP) as well as dioxin have different patterns of gene expression in the mouse uterus [34, 35] (Fig. 5.3). In the liver, NP and dioxin activate a set of genes that are distinct from estrogen-responsive genes [35, 36]. Nonylphenol has very similar effects to E2 on gene expression in the uterus but not in hepatic tissue. Organ-specific effects, therefore, should be considered in order to elucidate the distinct effects of various EDCs. Also, 1234 genes having an ERE in the promoter region of estrogen target genes have been identified [37, 38]. This information is useful for the understanding of the molecular mechanism of the physiological response to estrogen as well

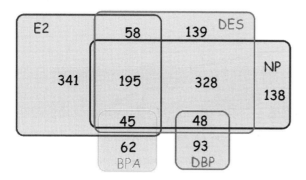

**Fig. 5.3.** Genes showed expression change in ovariectomized adult mouse uterus after 6 h exposure of various estrogenic chemicals. E2 17β-estradiol; DES diethylstilbestrol; NP nonylphenol; BPA: bisphenol-A; DBP, dibutyl phthalate. Total genes examined were 12 588.

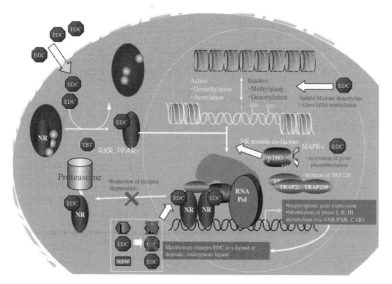

**Fig. 5.4.** Endocrine-disrupting chemicals (EDCs) may operate by a variety of mechanisms. When EDCs arrive at a cell membrane (top left) they may bind to a membrane estrogen receptor (mER), or pass through the membrane and bind to a nuclear estrogen receptor (ER) in the nucleus. When the complex of EDC and ER binds to a gene containing an estrogen-responsive element it recruits molecules that help to cause gene expression by boosting gene transcription by the RNA polymerase complex (large ovals), and so may cause gene expression at inappropriate times. EDC/ER complexes can also bind to proteasomes, which can lead to a reduction of the normal process of degradation of ER.

as the abnormalities induced by perinatal exposure to estrogens and estrogenic chemicals.

Estrogens are a critical class of steroids in vertebrate physiology, exerting effects both at the transcriptional level as well as at the level of rapid intracellular signaling through second messengers. Many of estrogen's transcriptional effects are mediated through classical nuclear ERs but recent studies also demonstrate the existence of a 7-transmembrane G protein-coupled receptor, GPR30 (membrane ER) that responds to estrogen with rapid cellular signaling [39]. There is controversy over the ability of classical ERs to recapitulate GPR30-mediated signaling mechanisms and vice versa. Further studies are needed to clarify the detailed function of the membrane ER.

Receptor-mediated mechanisms have received the most attention, but other mechanisms (e.g. hormone synthesis, transport and metabolism, nuclear receptors, gene methylation) have been shown to be equally important [40] (Fig. 5.4). For most associations reported between exposure to chemicals such as endocrine disrupting chemicals and a variety of biological outcomes including effects on human health, the mechanism(s) of action are poorly understood.

## Diethylstilbestrol syndrome and epigenetics

Perinatal exposure to an estrogen, including a synthetic estrogen such as diethylstilbestrol (DES), induces anovulation through alterations of the hypothalamo–hypophyseal–ovarian axis, polyovular follicles, uterine hypoplasia, and persistent epithelial cell proliferation and superficial keratinization in the vagina, even after ovariectomy in mice. This results in uterine lesions later in life, as well as smooth muscle disorganization and epithelial squamous metaplasia in the uterus [41, 42]. In humans, treatment with DES during pregnancy because it was believed to prevent miscarriage, resulted in uterine hypoplasia and vaginal adenocarcinoma in female offspring, and prostate cancer and reduction of sperm count in male offspring [43]. Vaginal adenocarcinoma was also experimentally induced in mice by prenatal exposure to DES [44]. The mechanisms underlying these developmentally induced lesions have not been clarified yet. However, DES altered the normal differentiation of the epithelial cells of the fetal vagina and cervix such that they responded abnormally to estrogen stimulation at puberty, as evidenced by the postpubertal appearance of cancers, as no cancers had

been seen in prepubescent girls or prepubertal female mice. Ovariectomy of developmentally DES-treated mice prevented the subsequent expression of uterine and vaginal adenocarcinomas.

The effects of DES in humans and/or mice are predominantly (1) malformation of the oviducts; (2) paucity of uterine glands; (3) increase of disorganized smooth muscle compartment; (4) adenosis of the cervix and vagina; and (5) stratified epithelium (vagina-like) in the uterus [43]. These phenotypes resemble those in HOXA10 knock-out mice, suggesting that HOXA10 gene expression might be repressed by DES treatment during reproductive tract morphogenesis. Exposure of the developing female reproductive tract to DES, either in vivo or in organ culture, repressed the expression of HOXA10 in the uterus and resulted in uterine metaplasia [45]. Msx2, a homeodomain transcription factor, has been shown to function downstream of DES and is required for the proper expression of several genes in the uterine epithelium including Wnt7a, PLAP, and K2.16 in the mouse uterus [46]. Msx2-/- mice exhibited abnormal water trafficking after DES exposure [46]. Prenatal DES exposure produced posterior shifts in Hox gene expression and homeotic anterior transformations of the mouse reproductive tracts [47]. Diethylstilbestrol-treated mice and Wnt7a-mutant mice also displayed similar malformations in female reproductive tracts [22]. Perinatal DES exposure down-regulated the Wnt7a gene and resulted in uterine metaplasia [48]. Diethylstilbestrol treatment significantly decreased uterine expression of HOXA10, HOXA11, and Wnt7a genes in wild-type mice but had no effect in the ER-α knock-out mice. In contrast, the DES effect on uterine expression of Wnt4 and Wnt5a was observed in both genotypes, suggesting a developmental role for ER-β. Adult ER-α knock-out mice exhibited complete resistance to the chronic effects of neonatal DES exposure, including atrophy, decreased weight, smooth muscle disorganization, and epithelial squamous metaplasia in the uterus, proliferative lesions of the oviduct; and persistent vaginal cornification exhibited in treated wild-type animals. Therefore, the lack of DES effects on gene expression and tissue differentiation in the ER-α knock-out mice provides unequivocal evidence of an obligatory role for ER-α in mediating the detrimental actions of neonatal DES exposure in the mouse reproductive tract [49].

Methoxychlor (MXC), a pesticide having weak estrogenic activity, has adverse effects on reproductive

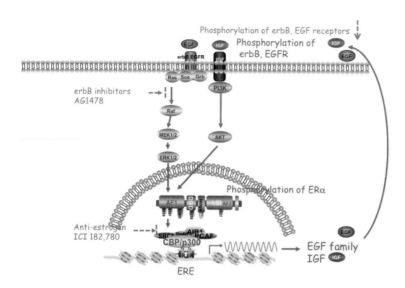

**Fig. 5.5.** Possible mechanism of persistent proliferation of mouse vaginal epithelial cells induced by perinatal exposure to diethylstilbestrol (DES). Auto-stimulation cascade has been established in the mouse vaginal epithelial cells exposed perinatally to DES: persistently expressed EGF-related growth factors and IGF-1 induced persistent phosphorylation of estrogen receptor-α, erbB, EGF receptor and IGF-1 receptor.

capability in mice. Methoxychlor (1 mg/kg/bw per day) treatment of mice produced a mild uterotropic response as measured by increased uterine weight and epithelial cell height. In vivo, MXC blocked the effect of E2 on *HOXA10* expression. Neonatal MXC treatment (2 μg/kg/bw per day from day 1 to 14 of age) resulted in an immediate suppression of *HOXA10* expression as well as a permanent generalized decrease in expression that persisted in the adult [50]. Neonatal treatment of female mice with a PCB mixture (Arachlor 1254) (500 μg/g/bw per day) and low levels of DES (10 ng/g/bw per day) resulted in the down-regulation of *Wnt7a* expression and also induced changes in uterine myometrium and gland formation and morphologic changes became more pronounced during postnatal and adult life, suggesting that the female reproductive tract is permanently reprogrammed after exposure even to weak estrogenic compounds. *Wnt7a* heterozygous mice were more sensitive to PCB exposure and *Wnt7a* expression in the mouse uterus can be used as biomarker for detecting the estrogenic activity of chemicals.

Persistent expression of *fos* and *jun* genes [51, 52, 53] and persistent phosphorylation of ER-α, erbB receptors and JNK1 and sustained expression of EGF-like growth factors, interleukin-1 (IL-1)-related genes and IGF-1 mRNA [54, 55] contributed to persistent activity of these signaling pathways in the perinatally DES-exposed mouse vagina (Fig. 5.5). Persistent expression of other genes such as *retinol binding protein 2* [56] and *trefoil factor 1*, a mucin-associated gastrointestinal growth factor [57] were reported in

the neonatally E2-exposed mouse vagina. Neonatal treatment of female rats with E2 and bisphenol-A (BPA), a high-production-volume chemical used in the manufacture of polycarbonate plastics, induces anovulation and persistent vaginal keratinization as a consequence of insufficient phasic secretion of gonadotropins from the hypothalamic–pituitary axis [58].

Most activities of estrogenic chemicals, described to date, are mediated through ER-α and/or ER-β. However, little is known about the relative contribution of the individual ER subtypes in induction of abnormalities. Nakamura *et al.* [59] tested the effects of neonatal exposure to ER selective ligands, ER-α agonist (propyl pyrazole triol, PPT) and the ER-β agonist (diarylpropionitrile, DPN), and DES. Persistent estrous smears and anovulation were induced in all mice by DES and PPT, but not by DPN, suggesting that the observed anovulation was primarily mediated through ER-α. Disorganization of uterine musculature and ovary-independent vaginal epithelial cell proliferation accompanied by persistent expression of EGF-related genes and interleukin-1-related genes were also mediated through ER-α. In contrast, polyovular follicles were induced by neonatal treatment with both ER-α and ER-β ligands, suggesting that ovarian abnormalities are mediated through both ER subtypes.

## Transgenerational effect of DES

Prenatal or neonatal treatment with DES led to cancers in the female and male genital tract, and in addition, the susceptibility to cancers was transmitted to the descendants through the maternal germ cell lineage [60]. Mice were treated with DES prenatally (2.5, 5, or 10 µg/kg/bw per day) on days 9–16 of gestation, or neonatally (0.002 µg/pup per day) on days 1–5; the highest doses were used that did not drastically interfere with fertility later in life. When female mice reached sexual maturity, they were bred to control untreated males. In DES-lineage females, an increased incidence of uterine adenocarcinoma was observed. An increased incidence of proliferative lesions of the rete testis (an estrogen target tissue in the male) and cancers of the reproductive tract were observed in DES-lineage males at 17–24 months of age. Transgenerational occurrence of cancers in mice treated with DES prenatally was also reported [61, 62]. Tomatis [63] reviewed the evidence for transgenerational carcinogenesis in epidemiological studies and experimental studies. These data suggested that alterations occurred in germ cells and were passed to subsequent generations. The high risk of reproductive dysfunction seen in women exposed to DES in utero was not observed in their daughters. However, menstrual irregularity and possible infertility were reported in the third generation of DES-exposed women [64], suggesting transgenerational transmission of DES-related epigenetic alterations in humans.

Epigenetic change in the molecular program of cell differentiation in the affected tissues may be a common mechanism. The clear cell adenocarcinoma in the vagina in DES-exposed women displayed genetic instability consistent with epigenetic imprints in the absence of any expected mutation in classical oncogenes or tumor suppressor genes. Using a mouse model for DES syndrome, Li *et al.* [65] demonstrated that one of the estrogen-inducible genes in the mouse uterus, *lactotransferrin* gene, that had been shown earlier to be persistently up-regulated by developmental DES exposure, had an altered pattern of CpG methylation in the promoter region of the gene upstream from the ERE. Li *et al.* [53] have also shown that neonatal exposure to DES in mice induces a persistent increase in *c-fos* mRNA expression and hypomethylation of specific enhancer-binding sites. Altered DNA methylation by DES is probably a gene-specific phenomenon because the CpG methylation of the promoters of the *HOXA10* and *HOXA11* genes is not altered by neonatal exposure to DES, even though DES dramatically downregulates expression of these genes [66]. Increase in 18S and 45S ribosomal DNA methylation in uterine

samples exposed prenatally to low (0.1 µg/kg/bw per day) and high (100 µg/kg/bw per day) doses of DES was reported [67]. Ruden *et al.* [68] proposed the hypothesis that CpG methylation alterations in many of the key uterine cancer genes are stabilized by WNT signaling during gametogenesis and that this might explain the trans-generational effects of DES exposure on uterine development.

As mentioned above, persistently expressed genes were identified in the mouse reproductive tracts exposed perinatally to DES. Thus, DES and other environmental estrogens alter the program of differentiation of estrogen target cells in the reproductive tract through an epigenetic mechanism, as suggested by Crews and McLachlan [69]. The transmission of uniquely specific changes in the program of development in mice has implications for similarly exposed humans as well as for the biology of hormonally induced diseases.

It is likely that the trans generational epigenetic effects seen with environmental estrogens and DES also occur with other endocrine-disrupting chemicals (EDCs). Rats treated with the estrogenic pesticide MXC or the anti-androgenic fungicide vinclozolin during pregnancy produced male offspring that have decreased sperm capacity and fertility [70]. Remarkably, compromised fertility was passed through the adult male germ line for four generations with high penetrance. The authors demonstrated altered patterns of DNA methylation in the germ cells of generations two and three. Interestingly, individuals initially were fertile, but with age, fertility was reduced. This study is an elegant demonstration of epigenetic alterations in genes apparently important to reproductive function by two kinds of EDCs in an age-dependent manner. However, Kawabe *et al.* [71] reported that they were unable to confirm the results of this experiment. Further studies are needed to clarify this inconsistency.

## Other examples of DNA methylation changes by environmental factors

There is now significant evidence that the risk of many chronic adult diseases and disorders results from exposure to environmental factors early in development [72, 73]. Moreover, there is a link between what we are exposed to in utero and disease formation in adulthood that involves epigenetic modifications such as DNA methylation of transposable elements and cis-acting, imprinting regulatory elements [6]. Many xenobiotics, ubiquitously present in the environment, have estrogenic properties and function as endocrine disruptors [40]; however, their potential to modify the epigenome remains largely unexplored [69]. The epigenome is particularly susceptible to deregulation during gestation, neonatal development, puberty, and old age. Nevertheless, it is most vulnerable to environmental exposures during embryogenesis because the elaborate DNA methylation and chromatin patterning required for normal tissue development is programmed during early development.

Most regions of the mammalian genome exhibit little variability among individuals in tissue-specific DNA methylation levels. In contrast, DNA methylation is determined stochastically at some transposable element insertion sites. This potentially can affect the expression of neighboring genes, resulting in the formation of loci with metastable epialleles [6]. Cellular epigenetic mosaicism and individual phenotypic variability then can occur even in genetically identical individuals. These sites are also particularly vulnerable to environmentally induced epigenetic alterations [74, 75].

The hypothesis of fetal origins of adult disease posits that early developmental exposures involve epigenetic modifications, such as DNA methylation, that influence adult disease susceptibility. In utero exposure to genistein (250 mg/kg diet), a phytoestrogen, at levels comparable to that of humans consuming high-soy diets, shifted the coat color of heterozygous viable yellow agouti ($A^{vy}$/a) offspring toward pseudoagouti. This phenotypic change was significantly associated with increased methylation of six CpG sites in a retrotransposon upstream of the transcription start site of the *Agouti* gene. This genistein-induced hypermethylation persisted into adulthood, decreasing ectopic Agouti expression and protecting offspring from obesity. This is the first evidence that in utero dietary genistein affects gene expression and alters susceptibility to obesity in adulthood by permanently altering the epigenome [75]. In utero or neonatal exposure to BPA is associated with higher body weight, increased risk for breast and prostate cancer, and altered reproductive function. Dolinoy *et al.* [76] showed that maternal exposure to BPA shifted the coat color distribution of viable yellow agouti ($A^{vy}$) mouse offspring toward yellow by decreasing CpG methylation in an intracisternal A particle retrotransposon upstream of the *Agouti* gene. CpG methylation also was decreased at another metastable locus, the CDK5 activator-binding protein (*Cabp^{IAP}*). DNA methylation at the $A^{vy}$ locus was similar

in tissues from the three germ layers, providing evidence that epigenetic patterning during early stem cell development is sensitive to BPA exposure. Moreover, maternal dietary supplementation, with either methyl donors like folic acid or the phytoestrogen genistein, negated the DNA hypomethylating effect of BPA. Thus, early developmental exposure to BPA can change offspring phenotype by stably altering the epigenome, an effect that can be counteracted by maternal dietary supplements. The metabolic phenotype of adult rats, including the propensity to obesity, hyperinsulinemia, and hyperphagia, showed plasticity in response to prenatal nutrition and to neonatal administration of the adipokine leptin. Effects of neonatal leptin on hepatic gene expression and epigenetic status in adulthood are directionally dependent on the animals' nutritional status in utero [77].

Environmentally relevant doses of BPA or E2 increase prostate gland susceptibility to adult-onset precancerous lesions and hormonal carcinogenesis [78]. To identify a molecular basis for estrogen imprinting, DNA methylation changes were screened over time in the prostate glands exposed to BPA (10 µg/kg bw/day, neonatal days 1, 3, and 5) and E2 (0.1 µg/kg bw/day). For phosphodiesterase type 4 variant 4 (PDE4D4), an enzyme responsible for intracellular cyclic adenosine monophosphate breakdown, a specific methylation cluster was identified in the 5′-flanking CpG island that gradually hypermethylated with aging in normal prostates resulting in loss of gene expression. In prostates exposed to neonatal E2 or BPA, this region became hypomethylated with aging resulting in persistent and elevated PDE4D4 expression [79].

The fetuses exposed to 2,3,7,8-tetrachlorodibenzo-*p*-dioxin (TCDD) during the preimplantation stage (from 1-cell stage to blastocyst stage) weighed less on embryonic day 14 than the fetuses in the unexposed control group. Also the expression levels of imprinted genes *H19* and *Igf2* (insulin-like growth factor 2) genes were less in the TCDD-exposed fetuses than in the controls. Use of the bisulfate genomic sequencing demonstrated that the methylation level of the 430-base pair *H19/Igf2* imprint control region was higher in TCDD-exposed embryos and fetuses than in the controls, and methyltransferase activity was also higher in the TCDD-exposed embryos than in the controls [80].

## Conclusions

We are beginning to understand the mechanisms by which estrogens, and environmental chemicals with estrogenic activity, can alter the genetic program of target cells during development, without altering the sequence of DNA itself. It is important to determine the epigenetic imprints associated with hormones in normal cells and organs, and compare these with the same patterns in affected or dysfunctional ones. Patterns of imprints are the result of a network of signaling pathways that are often developmentally active. Endocrine changes underline all major life-history transitions such as birth, puberty, reproduction, and aging. In the context of epigenetic programming and gene imprinting, irreversible changes in cell function that lead to disease as a result of exogenous hormone/chemical exposures can be explained in detail in the near future. During mammalian development, the direction of the response to one cue can be determined by previous exposure to another, indicating the potential for a discontinuous distribution of environmentally induced phenotypes. Future analyses of epigenetic imprints of genes will explain the developmental origins of disease.

## Acknowledgments

These studies are supported in part by Grants-in-Aid for Scientific Research from the Ministry of Education, Culture, Sports, Science and Technology (T.I., T.S.) and grants from the Ministry of Health Labor and Welfare, Japan (T.I.).

## References

1. Wolffe AP, Matzke MA. Epigenetics: regulation through repression. *Science* 1999; **286**: 481–6.

2. Waddington CH. *Organisers and Genes.* Cambridge: Cambridge University Press, 1940.

3. Holliday R, Pugh JE. DNA modification mechanisms and gene activity during development. *Science* 1975; **187**: 226–32.

4. Willard HF, Brown CJ, Carrel L, Hendrich B, Miller AP. Epigenetic and chromosomal control of gene expression: molecular and genetic analysis of X chromosome inactivation. *Cold Spring Harbor Symp Quant Biol* 1993; **58**: 315–22.

5. Murrell A, Rakyan VK, Beck S. From genome to epigenome. *Human Mol Genet* 2005; **14**: R3–10.

6. Jirtle RL, Skinner MK. Environmental epigenomics and disease susceptibility. *Nature Rev Genet* 2007; **8**: 253–62.

7. Reik W. Stability and flexibility of epigenetic gene regulation in mammalian development. *Nature* 2007; **447**: 425–32.

8. Amir RE, Van den Veyver IB, Wan M. *et al.* Rett syndrome is caused by mutations in X-linked MECP2, encoding methyl-CpG-binding protein 2. *Nature Genet* 1999; **23**: 185–8.

9. Feinberg AP. Phenotypic plasticity and the epigenetics of human disease. *Nature* 2007; **447**: 433–40.

10. Horsthemke B, Buiting K. Imprinting defects on human chromosome 15. *Cytogenet Genome Res* 2006; **113**: 292–9.

11. Esteller M. Epigenetics in cancer. *New Engl J Med* 2008; **358**: 1148–59.

12. Heindel JJ. Animal models for probing the developmental basis of disease and dysfunction paradigm. *J Compil* 2008; **102**: 76–81.

13. Kobayashi A, Shawlot W, Kania A, Behringer RR. Requirement of Lim1 for female reproductive tract development. *Development* 2004; **131**: 539–49.

14. Satokata I, Benson G, Maas R. Sexually dimorphic sterility phenotypes in Hoxa-10 deficient mice. *Nature* 1995; **374**: 460–3.

15. Mortlock DP, Innis JW. Mutation of HOXA13 in hand-foot-genital syndrome. *Nature Genet* 1997; **15**: 179–80.

16. Lim H, Ma L, Ma WG, Maas RL, Dey SK. Hoxa-10 regulates uterine stromal cell responsiveness to progesterone during implantation and decidualization in the mouse. *Mol Endocrinol* 1999; **13**: 1005–17.

17. Taylor HS, Vanden Heuvel GB, Igarashi P. A conserved Hox axis in the mouse and human female reproductive system: late establishment and persistent adult expression of the Hoxa cluster genes. *Biol Reprod* 1997; **57**: 1338–45.

18. Taylor HS, Arici A, Olive D, Igarashi P. HOXA 10 is expressed in response to sex steroids at the time of implantation in the human endometrium. *J Clin Invest* 1998; **101**: 1379–84.

19. Miller C, Sassoon DA. Wnt-7a maintains appropriate uterine patterning during the development of the mouse female reproductive tract. *Development* 1998; **125**: 3201–11.

20. Pavlova A, Boutin E, Cunha G, Sassoon D. Msx1 (Hox-7.1) in the adult mouse uterus: cellular interactions underlying regulation of expression. *Development* 1994; **120**: 335–46.

21. Miller C, Pavlova A, Sassoon D. Differential expression patterns of Wnt genes in the murine female reproductive tract during development and the estrous cycle. *Mech Dev* 1998; **76**: 91–9.

22. Kitajewski J, Sassoon D. The emergence of molecular gynecology: homeobox and Wnt genes in the female reproductive tract. *BioEssays* 2000; **22**: 902–10.

23. Cunha GR. Stromal induction and specification of morphogenesis and cytodifferentiation of the epithelia of the Müllerian ducts and urogenital sinus during development of the uterus and vagina in mice. *J Exp Zool* 1976; **196**: 361–70.

24. Kurita T, Mills AA, Cunha GR. Roles of p63 in the diethylstilbestrol-induced cervicovaginal adenosis. *Development* 2004; **131**: 1639–49.

25. Zhao Y, Potter SS. Functional specificity of the Hoxa13 homeobox. *Development* 2001; **128**: 3197–207.

26. Cheng W, Liu J, Yoshida H, Rosen D, Naora H. Lineage infidelity of epithelial ovarian cancers is controlled by HOX genes that specify regional identity in the reproductive tract. *Nature Med* 2005; **11**:531–7.

27. Yoshida H, Broaddus R, Cheng W, Xie S, Naora H. Deregulation of the HOXA10 homeobox gene in endometrial carcinoma: role in epithelial-mesenchymal transition. *Cancer Res* 2006; **15**:889–97.

28. Taylor HS, Bagot C, Kardana A, Olive D, Arici A. HOX gene expression is altered in the endometrium of women with endometriosis. *Human Reprod* 1999; **14**: 1328–31.

29. Marino M, Galluzzo P, Ascenzi P. Estrogen signaling multiple pathways to impact gene transcription. *Curr Genomics* 2006; **7**: 497–508.

30. Bigsby RM, Caperell-Grant A, Berry N, Nephew K, Lubahn D. Estrogen induces a systemic growth factor through an estrogen receptor-alpha-dependent mechanism. *Biol Reprod* 2004; **70**: 178–83.

31. Couse JF, Korach KS. Estrogen receptor null mice: what have we learned and where will they lead us? *Endocr Rev* 1999; **20**: 358–417.

32. Watanabe H, Suzuki A, Mizutani T. *et al*. Genome-wide analysis of changes in early gene expression induced by estrogen. *Genes Cells* 2002; **7**: 497–507.

33. Suzuki A, Watanabe H, Mizutani T. *et al*. Global gene expression in mouse vaginae exposed to diethylstilbestrol at different ages. *Exp Biol Med* 2006; **231**: 632–40.

34. Watanabe H, Suzuki A, Kobayashi M. *et al*. Similarities and differences in uterine gene expression patterns caused by treatment with physiological and non-physiological estrogen. *J Mol Endocrinol* 2003; **31**: 487–97.

35. Watanabe H, Suzuki A, Goto M. *et al*. Tissue-specific estrogenic and non-estrogenic effects of a xenoestrogen, nonylphenol. *J Mol Endocrinol* 2004; **33**: 243–52.

36. Watanabe H, Suzuki A, Goto M. *et al*. Comparative uterine gene expression analysis after dioxin and estradiol administration. *J Mol Endocrinol* 2004; **33**: 763–71.

37. Kobayashi M, Takahashi E, Miyagawa S, Watanabe H, Iguchi, T. Chromatin immunoprecipitation-mediated identification of aquaporin 5 as a regulatory target of estrogen in the uterus. *Genes Cells* 2006; **11**: 1133–43.

38. Lin CY, Vega VB, Thomsen JS. *et al*. Whole-genome cartography of estrogen receptor alpha binding sites. *PLoS Genet* 2007; **3**: e87.

39. Prossnitz ER, Arterburn JB, Sklar LA. GPR30: a G protein-coupled receptor for estrogen. *Mol Cell Endocrinol* 2007; **265–266**: 138–42.

40. Damstra T, Barlow S, Bergman A, Kavlock R, Van Der Kraak G (eds.) *Global Assessment of the State-of-the-Science of Endocrine Disruptors*. WHO/IPCS, 2002.

41. Takasugi N, Bern HA, DeOme KB. Persistent vaginal cornification in mice. *Science* 1962; **138**: 438–9.

42. Iguchi T. Cellular effects of early exposure to sex hormones and antihormones. *Int Rev Cytol* 1992; **139**: 1–57.

43. Herbst AL, Bern HA (eds.) *Developmental Effects of Diethylstilbestrol (DES) in Pregnancy*. New York: Thieme Stratton Inc., 1981.

44. McLachlan JA, Newbold RR, Bullock BC. Long-term effects on the female mouse genital tract associated with prenatal exposure to diethylstilbestrol. *Cancer Res* 1980; **40**: 3988–99.

45. Ma L, Benson G, Lim H, Dey SK, Maas RL. Abdominal B (AbdB) hoax genes: regulation in adult uterus by estrogen and progesterone and repression in Müllerian duct by the synthetic estrogen diethylstilbestrol (DES). *Dev Biol* 1998; **197**: 141–54.

46. Huang WW, Yin Y, Bi Q. *et al*.Developmental diethylstilbestrol exposure alters genetic pathways of uterine cytodifferentiation. *Mol Endocrinol* 2005; **19**: 669–82.

47. Block K, Kardana A, Igarashi P, Taylor HS. In utero diethylstilbestrol (DES) exposure alters Hox gene expression in the developing Müllerian system. *FASEB J* 2000; **14**: 1101–8.

48. Miller C, Degenhardt K, Sassoon DA. Fetal exposure to DES results in de-regulation of Wnt7a during uterine morphogenesis. *Nature Genet* 1998; **20**: 228–30.

49. Couse JF, Dixon D, Yates M. *et al*. Estrogen receptor-α knockout mice exhibit resistance to the developmental effects of neonatal diethylstilbestrol exposure on the female reproductive tract. *Dev Biol* 2001; **238**: 224–38.

50. Fei X, Chung H, Taylor HS. Methoxychlor disrupts uterine Hoxa10 gene expression. *Endocrinology* 2005; **146**: 3445–51.

51. Iguchi T, Fukazawa Y, Bern HA. Effects of sex hormones on oncogene expression in the vagina and on the development of sexual dimorphism of the pelvis and anococcygeous muscle in the mouse. *Environ Health Perspect* 1995; **103**: 79–82.

52. Kamiya K, Sato T, Nishimura N. *et al*. Expression of estrogen receptor and proto-oncogene messenger ribonucleic acids in reproductive tracts of neonatally diethylstilbestrol-exposed female mice with or without postpubertal estrogen administration. *Exp Clin Endocrinol Diabetes* 1996; **104**: 111–22.

53. Li S, Hansman R, Newbold RR. *et al*. Neonatal diethylstilbestrol exposure induces persistent elevation of c-fos expression and hypomethylation in its exon-4 in mouse uterus. *Mol Carcinog* 2003; **38**: 78–84.

54. Miyagawa S, Katsu Y, Watanabe H, Iguchi T. Estrogen-independent activation of ErbBs signaling and estrogen receptor α in the mouse vagina exposed neonatally to diethylstilbestrol. *Oncogene* 2004; **23**: 340–9.

55. Miyagawa S, Suzuki A, Katsu Y. *et al.* Persistent gene expression in mouse vagina exposed neonatally to diethylstilbestrol. *J Mol Endocrinol* 2004; **32**: 663–77.

56. Matsuda M, Masui F, Mori T. Neonatal estrogenization leads to increased expression of cellular retinol binding protein 2 in the mouse reproductive tract. *Cell Tissue Res* 2004; **316**: 131–9.

57. Masui F, Kuraosaki K, Mori T, Matsuda M. Persistent trefoil factor 1 expression imprinted on mouse vaginal epithelium by neonatal estrogenization. *Cell Tissue Res* 2006; **323**: 167–75.

58. Kato H, Furuhashi T, Tanaka M. *et al.* Effects of bisphenol A given neonatally on reproductive functions of male rats. *Reprod Toxicol* 2006; **22**: 20–9.

59. Nakamura T, Katsu Y, Watanabe H, Iguchi T. Estrogen receptor subtypes selectively mediate female mouse reproductive abnormalities induced by neonatal exposure to estrogenic chemicals. *Toxicology* 2008; **253**; 117–24.

60. Newbold RR, Padilla-Banks E, Jefferson WN. Adverse effects of the model environmental estrogen diethylstilbestrol are transmitted to subsequent generations. *Endocrinology* 2006; 147: S11–17.

61. Turusov VS, Trukhanova LS, Parfenov Yu D, Tomatis L. Occurrence of tumours in the descendants of CBA male mice prenatally treated with diethylstilbestrol. *Int J Cancer* 1992; **50**: 131–5.

62. Walker BE, Haven MI. Intensity of multigenerational carcinogenesis from diethylstilbestrol in mice. *Carcinogenesis* 1997; **18**: 791–3.

63. Tomatis L. Transgeneration carcinogenesis: a review of the experimental and epidemiological evidence. *Jpn J Cancer Res* 1994; **85**: 443–54.

64. Titus-Ernstoff L, Troisi R, Hatch EE. *et al.* Menstrual and reproductive characteristics of women whose mothers were exposed in utero to diethylstilbestrol (DES). *Int J Epidemiol* 2006; **35**: 862–8.

65. Li S, Washburn KA, Moore R. *et al.* Developmental exposure to diethylstilbestrol elicits demethylation of estrogen-responsive lactotransferrin gene in the mouse uterus. *Cancer Res* 1997; **57**: 4356–9.

66. Li S, Ma L, Chiang T. *et al.* Promoter CpG methylation of Hox-a10 and Hox-a11 in mouse uterus not altered upon neonatal diethylstilbestrol exposure. *Mol Carcinog* 2001; **32**: 213–19.

67. Alworth LC, Howdeshell KL, Ruhlen RL. *et al.* Uterine responsiveness to estradiol and DNA methylation are altered by fetal exposure to diethylstilbestrol and methoxychlor in CD-1 mice: effects of low versus high doses. *Toxicol Appl Pharmacol* 2002; **183**: 10–22.

68. Ruden DM, Xia L, Garfinkel MD, Lu X. Hsp90 and environmental impacts on epigenetic stages: a model for the trans-generational effects of diethylstilbestrol

on uterine development and cancer. *Human Mol Genet* 2005; **14**: R149–55.

69. Crews D, McLachlan JA. Epigenetics, evolution, endocrine disruption, health, and disease. *Endocrinology* 2006; **147**: S4–10.

70. Anway MD, Cupp AS, Uzumcu M, Skinner MK. Epigenetic transgenerational actions of endocrine disruptors and male fertility. *Science* 2005; **308**: 1466–9.

71. Kawabe M, Takahashi S, Doi Y. *et al.* Maternal exposure to anti-androgenic compounds has no effects on spermatogenesis and DNA methylation in male rats of subsequent generation. Abstract 264, *Int Congress Toxicol* 2007.

72. McMillen IC, Robinson JS. Developmental origins of the metabolic syndrome: prediction, plasticity, and programming. *Physiol Rev* 2005; **85**: 571–633.

73. Crain DA, Janssen SJ, Edwards TM. *et al.* Female reproductive disruption: the roles of endocrine disrupting compounds and developmental timing. *Fertil Steril* 2008; **90**: 911–40.

74. Waterland R, Jirtle R. Transposable elements: targets for early nutritional effects on epigenetic gene regulation. *Mol Cell Biol* 2003; **23**: 5293–300.

75. Dolinoy DC, Wiedman J, Waterland R, Jirtle RL. Maternal genistein alters coat color and protects Avy mouse offspring from obesity by modifying the fetal epigenome. *Environ Health Perspect* 2006; **114**: 567–72.

76. Dolinoy DC, Huang D, Jirtle RL. Maternal nutrient supplementation counteracts bisphenol A-induced DNA hypomethylation in early development. *Proc Natl Acad Sci USA* 2007; **104**: 13 056–61.

77. Gluckman PD, Lillycrop KA, Vickers MH. *et al.* Metabolic plasticity during mammalian development is directionally dependent on early nutritional status. *Proc Natl Acad Sci USA* 2007; **104**: 12 796–800.

78. Prins GS, Tang W-Y, Belmonte J, Ho S-M. Perinatal exposure to oestradiol and bisphenol A alters the prostate epigenome and increases susceptibility to carcinogenesis. *J Comp* 2008; **102**: 134–8.

79. Ho S-M, Tang W-Y, Belmonte de Frausto J, Prins GS. Developmental exposure to estradiol and bisphenol A increases susceptibility to prostate carcinogenesis and epigenetically regulates phosphodiesterase type 4 variant 4. *Cancer Res* 2006; **66**: 5624–32.

80. Wu Q, Ohsako S, Ishimura R, Suzuki JS, Tohyama C. Exposure of mouse preimplantation embryos to 2,3,7,8-tetrachlorodibenzo-p-dioxin (TCDD) alters the methylation status of imprinted genes H19 and Igf2. *Biol Reprod* 2004; **70**: 1790–7.

# Mechanisms of endocrine disruption

K. Leigh Greathouse and Cheryl L. Walker

## Introduction

As described in Chapter 1, chemicals that disrupt the endocrine system do so via several mechanisms, including interfering with hormone synthesis, metabolism, ligand binding, and gene expression. Importantly, Chapter 1 highlights the fact that organogenesis is one of the most critical periods of susceptibility to developmental reprogramming by endocrine-disrupting chemicals (EDCs). The term developmental reprogramming was coined by Barker *et al.* in 1989 [1] to explain the observed correlation between birthweight and cardiovascular disease in adulthood. Barker observed that individuals with low birthweight (lowest quartile) and low weight at one year had significantly higher mortality rates from cardiovascular disease and significantly higher rates of diabetes than individuals in the higher quartiles of birthweight. From these data he hypothesized that low birthweight, secondary to in utero growth restriction (IUGR), developmentally reprogrammed the response of tissues to normal physiological signals to promote the onset of disease in adulthood.

This chapter will focus on the mechanisms by which environmental exposures can induce endocrine disruption and highlights the mechanisms that play important roles in developmental programming.

## Targets for endocrine disruption: understanding the endocrine system

### Target systems of endocrine-disrupting chemicals

#### (a) The hypothalamic–pituitary–gonadal (HPG) axis

The endocrine system is the master regulator for metabolic homeostasis. It functions as a series of feedback loops designed to maintain a balance between the activity of the major endocrine organs which are the adrenals, hypothalamus, pituitary, thyroid, and gonads. While the endocrine system is extensive and complex, this chapter will focus on the HPG axis (including the thyroid, adrenals, and mammary glands) as it relates to the reproductive system.

The classical description of the function of the endocrine system is the secretion of hormone(s) by an endocrine organ, which then travel through the blood to a distant effector organ. Contact of hormone with cells expressing receptors for that hormone elicits a response in the target tissue. One of the responses of the target organ may be to produce another hormone, which feeds back to the original secretory organ to inhibit further hormone secretion, creating a negative feedback loop and maintaining homeostasis of the system.

The HPG axis is made up of three organ systems: (1) the hypothalamic neurons that release gonadotropin-releasing hormone (GnRH); (2) the anterior pituitary, which produces luteinizing and follicle-stimulating hormone, LH and FSH (gonadotropes); and (3) the gonads, which consist of the ovary and testis, that produce steroid hormones (e.g. estrogen and testosterone) in response to LH and FSH. The initial signal is triggered within the hypothalamus by GnRH neurons, which release GnRH in a pulsatile fashion into the blood. GnRH receptors located on the gonadotrope cells of the anterior pituitary bind GnRH and respond by releasing LH and FSH into the blood. In the gonads, Sertoli and Leydig (testis) and theca and granulosa (ovary) cells with receptors for LH or FSH, produce steroid hormones including estrogen and testosterone, as well as other factors (such as inhibin B) that induce direct effects on hormone-responsive tissues. These hormones also feed back to the hypothalamus,

*Environmental Impacts on Reproductive Health and Fertility*, ed. T. J. Woodruff, S. J. Janssen, L. J. Guillette, and L. C. Giudice. Published by Cambridge University Press. ©Cambridge University Press 2010.

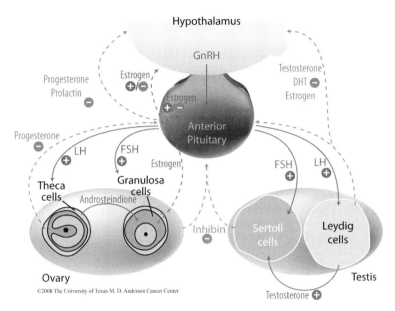

Hypothalamus

GnRH

Progesterone
Prolactin

Estrogen
⊕/⊖

Testosterone
DHT ⊖
Estrogen

Estrogen
⊕/⊖

Anterior
Pituitary

Progesterone ⊖

LH ⊕   FSH ⊕

Estrogen

FSH ⊕   LH ⊕

Theca
cells

Granulosa
cells

Androsteindione

Inhibin ⊖

Sertoli
cells

Leydig
cells

Ovary

©2008 The University of Texas M. D. Anderson Cancer Center

Testis

Testosterone ⊕

**Fig. 6.1.** Illustrative representation of the mammalian hypothalamic–pituitary–gonadal (HPG) axis. In the hypothalamus gonadotropin releasing hormone (GnRH) is secreted from GnRH neurons into the portal blood system. GnRH receptors in the pituitary bind GnRH, which induces the production and secretion of the gonadotropins luteinizing hormone (LH) and follicle stimulating hormone (FSH). LH and FSH then travel systemically to the ovary (females) or testis (males) to induce production of steroid hormones. In the ovary, LH binds LH receptors in the theca cells to produce progesterone and androsteindione. Androsteindione is secreted in a paracrine manner to the granulosa cells while progesterone feeds back negatively to the pituitary and hypothalamus to reduce secretion of GnRH, LH and prolactin. Prolactin secreted from the pituitary also feeds back negatively to the hypothalamus to reduce corticotrophin releasing hormone. FSH binds FSH receptors in granulosa cells to produce estradiol, which feeds back positively to the hypothalamus to increase GnRH secretion and negatively to the hypothalamus and pituitary to reduce FSH secretion. In the testis, LH binds receptors on the Leydig cells, which secrete testosterone in a paracrine manner to the Sertoli cells. Testosterone, dihydrotestosterone (DHT) and/or estradiol negatively feed back from the testis to the hypothalamus and pituitary to reduce secretion of GnRH and LH. FSH binds to receptors on the Sertoli cells stimulating them to produce inhibin B, which is also secreted from the granulosa cells, and feeds back negatively to the pituitary to reduce secretion of FSH. This illustration is representative of the HPG axis, and it should be noted that testosterone and estradiol also have other target tissues within the body, for example bone and muscle. (© 2008 University of Texas M. D. Anderson Cancer Center.)

to inhibit GnRH release, and to the pituitary, to inhibit LH and FSH release (Fig. 6.1).

Hormones can also have paracrine and autocrine activity. Paracrine activity is defined by communication between cells of different cell types (e.g. stromal to epithelial signaling). Paracrine signaling plays an important role in hormone-responsive tissues such as the prostate and uterus where estrogen and testosterone are mitogenic. For example, testosterone secreted from testicular Leydig cells stimulates spermatogenesis in the seminiferous tubules and supports stability of the prostatic epithelium. Similarly, mammary epithelium in response to estrogen utilizes paracrine signaling via ER positive epithelial cells signaling to ER negative cells to induce proliferation and morphogenesis [2].

In contrast, autocrine signaling is defined by the secretion of a factor (hormone or growth factor) from a cell that acts on itself. Autocrine signaling mainly applies to cytokines of the immune system that regulate inflammatory responses as well as growth factors that control proliferation. As it relates to reproductive function, autocrine signaling has been shown to function in hypothalamic neurons, granulosa cells, and mammary epithelial cells. In the hypothalamus, GnRH secretion occurs in a pulsatile fashion through positive and negative autocrine feedback loops in GnRH neurons. Additionally, granulosa cells utilize autocrine signaling to regulate progesterone secretion [3]. In the mammary epithelium during puberty, growth hormone (GH) also works in an autocrine manner to prevent mammary differentiation [4]. Tumor-associated autocrine signaling, a key component of transformation of breast and prostate cells into tumor cells, involves a transition from normal regulation via endocrine or paracrine hormone signaling to autocrine signaling in

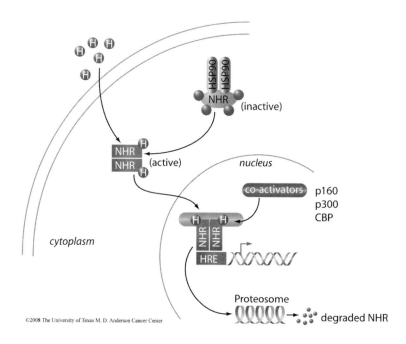

**Fig. 6.2.** Diagram of genomic nuclear hormone receptor signaling and transcriptional activation. Hormone (H) and certain endocrine disrupting chemicals (EDCs) can enter the cell where nuclear hormone receptors (NHR) are kept inactive by chaperone proteins including heat shock protein-90 (HSP90) until liganded by hormones (or EDCs). Liganded NHRs form dimers and translocate to the nucleus where they interact with co-activators (e.g. p160, p300, or CBP) and bind to hormone responsive elements (HRE) in the DNA. After gene transactivation, NHRs are degraded by the proteosome or recycled back to the cytoplasm. (© 2008 University of Texas M. D. Anderson Cancer Center.)

order to supplant dependence on exogenous mitogenic signals[5, 6].

## Target mechanisms of EDCs: genomic modulation

One of the important mechanisms by which hormones and EDCs act is via nuclear hormone receptors, directly activating or inhibiting these receptors or indirectly modulating hormone metabolism. Determined generally by whether they are hydrophilic or lipophilic, hormones can activate cellular membrane receptors (i.e. hydrophilic) and initiate rapid signaling to affect cellular function, or freely enter cells (i.e. lipophilic) to activate nuclear hormone receptors (NHRs) and regulate gene expression [7].

### Nuclear hormone receptors

One of the first mechanisms by which EDCs were identified to act was via their interaction with NHRs. Nuclear hormone receptors are a class of ligand-activated proteins that enter the nucleus and function as transcription factors to transactivate or repress gene expression. This ligand-induced gene expression facilitates changes in cellular function, a process that can be modulated by EDCs. There are three classes of NHRs: Type I NHRs, which are receptors for steroid hormones, e.g. estrogen receptor (ER), androgen receptor (AR), progesterone receptor (PR); Type II,

which are receptors for non-steroid hormones, e.g. thyroid receptor (TR), retinoic acid receptor (RAR), retinoid X receptor (RXR); and Type III, which are receptors with no known ligand or *orphan* receptors, e.g. G-protein coupled receptor (GPCR), farnesoid X receptor (FXR), liver X receptor (LXR). The activation domain of the NHR binds the hormone, which induces a conformational change in the protein, to activate or inhibit its ability to function as a transcription factor, often via binding of co-activator or co-repressor accessory proteins. The activity of NHRs is best illustrated by the ER. The ER has two classical forms, ER-α and ER-β, which can act in an antagonistic manner towards one another, for example with ER-β antagonizing the proliferative effects of ER-α. When unbound by ligand, ER is maintained in an inactive state in the cytosol bound to large complexes of proteins including heat shock protein-90 (HSP90). Upon ligand binding, ER monomers dimerize, and the liganded ER dimer then binds to the DNA of specific genes that have a recognition sequence termed a hormone responsive element (HRE) (Fig. 6.2). In addition to promoter binding, co-activator or co-repressor recruitment facilitates initiation or repression of transcription (respectively).

Endocrine-disrupting chemicals, which mimic the activity of endogenous hormones and activate receptors are termed agonists, whereas those that inhibit receptor activity are termed antagonists. For, example, ER-α liganded by DES can dimerize and transactivate

**Table 6.1.** Compilation of references that exemplify molecular mechanisms utilized by endocrine disruptors to interfere with endocrine signaling, reproduction or fertility.

| Classification | Xenocompound | Associated Mechanism | Refs |
|---|---|---|---|
| *Anti-androgens* | DDT | Anti-androgen, Ca++ mobilization alteration, phosphorylation of c-ERB2/c-met, inhibition of p450scc | 25, 87, 116, 123 |
| | DDE | Anti-androgen, activates MAPK pathway, activates PI3K, interacts with GPR30 | 25, 88, 93, 111 |
| | Methoxychlor | Activates ER, induce CYP2B, CYP23A and CAR, alters germline DNA methlylation, anti-androgen and transgenerational effects | 36, 40–42, 171, 184 |
| | Vinclozolin | Anti-androgen, alters DNA methylation, transgenerational effects | 14, 171, 184–185 |
| | Atrazine | Anti-androgen, PKC/cAMP modulation | 27, 108–109 |
| *Xenoestrogens* | Genistein | ER agonist/antagonist (dose-dependent), Ca++ mobilization alteration, interacts with GPR30, inhibition of sulfotransferases, DNA methylation alteration | 9–13, 87, 112, 144, 171 |
| | Octylphenol | Ca++ mobilization alteration | 87 |
| | Nonylphenol | MAPK pathway activation, PKC/cAMP modulation, reduces CYP1A1 expression | 28, 88, 112 |
| | Bisphenol A | ER agonist/antagonist, increased ARHH expression, increased expression of ERβ/TRAPP220, Ca++ mobilization alteration, PKC/cAMP modulation, aromatase inhibition, inhibition of sulfotransferases, DNA methylation alteration | 28, 34–37, 51, 70, 87, 108–109, 144, 170 |
| | Diethylstilbestrol (DES) | ER agonist, reduced AR expression, alteration of Ca++ mobilization, MAPK pathway activation, PI3K pathway activation, PKA/cAMP modulation, DNA methylation alterations | 8, 30, 87, 88, 93–94, 108–109, 169 |

estrogen-responsive gene promoters containing an estrogen responsive element (ERE) such as *Hoxa9* and *Hoxa10* [8]. However, agonism and antagonism can sometimes be difficult to discern. An example of an EDC hormone mimetic is the phytoestrogen genistein, found in soybeans. At low doses, genistein acts as an estrogen receptor agonist, to promote cell growth, while at high doses in vitro (9–100 μM) genistein can inhibit signaling molecules (receptor tyrosine kinases, RTKs) [9, 10] to inhibit cell proliferation. Similarly, genistein binding to ER-β can antagonize ER-α activity, as ligand-bound ER-β can suppress the transcriptional activation of ER-α. Given that genistein binds with higher affinity to ER-β (8.4 nM vs. 145 nM) than ER-α[11], genistein-bound ER-β could suppress the activity of ER-α, even though it is an ER-β agonist [12, 13]. Endocrine-disrupting chemicals can also act as receptor antagonists, such as the antiandrogens, which act to inhibit the effects of androgens by interfering with ligand-AR binding. Two

such antiandrogens are vinclozolin and DDE, which have both been shown to be inhibitors of AR-mediated gene expression (Table 6.1) [14].

# Androgen receptor-mediated endocrine disruption

During the perinatal period programming of the endocrine axis occurs, making this a vulnerable period of exposure to endogenous and exogenous stimuli. Of importance during this programming is the initial feedback of hormones from the gonads to the hypothalamus and pituitary. For males, testosterone produced mainly by the testis around gestational day 65 (humans) [15] is critical in establishing sexual behaviors, male reproductive tract development, and masculinization of other organs. Like steroid hormones produced by other organs, the secretion of LH from the pituitary controls synthesis of testosterone. The NHR for testosterone and its metabolite dihydrotestosterone (DHT) is the AR, which is expressed in multiple organs, including the hypothalamus [16], pituitary, kidney, prostate, and adrenals (and ovary) [17, 18]. Aromatization of testosterone to 17β-estradiol by an aromatase, CYP19, is also critical for proper brain development [19]. If testosterone fails to be produced in the male fetus (for example due to exposure to antiandrogens, a genetic mutation in AR or blocked metabolism of testosterone) the fetus will develop as a phenotypic female with testes. This extreme sensitivity to EDC exposure is not as pronounced in the adult once the HPG axis is established, however, exposure of adult males to antiandrogens can result in alteration in sperm production and reduced libido [20, 21]. Therefore, exposure to EDCs during male reproductive tract development that disturbs the binding of testosterone to AR or its metabolism can permanently reprogram the male reproductive tract and its coordination with the HPG axis.

Endocrine-disrupting chemicals disrupt androgen homeostasis via several different mechanisms, including decreasing levels of AR [22], by altering LH stimulation [23] or when binding of the EDC to the AR alters proper folding of the ligand-binding domain (LBD) of the AR. Misfolding of the LBD blocks the recruitment of co-activators, prevents transcriptional initiation, and leads to abrogation of AR activity. Antiandrogenic EDCs acting via this mechanism include vinclozolin (in the presence of testosterone) [24], DDT [25], tris-(4-chlorophenyl)-methanol, procymidone [26], linuron, atrazine, lindane, dieldrin [27], methoxychlor [15], nonylphenol, octylphenol, and bisphenol-A [28]. Another mechanism by which EDCs affect AR activity is reducing the expression of AR. Reduction in AR levels is a mechanism shared by multiple EDCs including PCBs [29], DES [30], cyproterone acetate (CPA), and hydroxyflutamide (OHF) [22]. Ultimately, EDCs that disrupt AR ligand binding, dimerization, DNA binding, or receptor levels reduce or eliminate expression of AR target genes, which affects downstream cellular responses, such as differentiation and cell communication.

## Estrogen receptor-mediated endocrine disruption

Among the EDCs, xenoestrogens have garnered a significant amount of attention due to the well-known effects of the xenoestrogen DES in humans, and the identification of many other estrogenic anthropogenic chemicals [31, 32]. Analogous to testosterone, estrogen (E2) is a key hormone involved in development and maintenance of the female reproductive tract, brain, bone and cardiovascular system, and as mentioned earlier, a key component in male development. In the adult female, E2 plays important roles in metabolism and in coordinating the morphological alterations that occur during the menstrual cycle and pregnancy, and for differentiation and proliferation of hormone-responsive tissues.

Estrogens work in part by binding to the ER to transactivate the expression of estrogen-responsive genes. Xenoestrogens that function as agonists lead to the expression of estrogen-responsive genes by binding to the ER, as has been demonstrated for DES, 7-methyl-benz[a]anthracene-3,9-diol (MBA), coumestrol, and genistein (GEN) [33] among others. In contrast, in some cases xenoestrogens can act as antagonists by preventing the binding of ER to DNA (e.g. BPA) [34] or by inhibiting the binding of ER co-activators [35] to prevent transactivation of gene expression. Estrogen-responsive genes contain an estrogen-responsive element (ERE) or recognition sequences for other transcription factors such as those for transcription factors, SP1 and AP1, to which the ER binds. Until liganded by E2, or a xenoestrogen, ER remains bound in an inactive state by HSP90. In response to binding by ERs, an agonist/ER complex binds to DNA and coordinates transcription with the aid of co-activators. Important target genes of E2/ER include the progesterone receptor (nuclear hormone receptors), vascular endothelial growth factor (growth factors), c-fos/c-jun (proto-oncogenes) and cyclin D1 (cell cycle regulators). Several EDCs show ER-mediated effects on gene expression including DES, BPA, methoxychlor [36], and genistein. While all of these compounds act as xenoestrogens, their affinity for ER-α or ER-β, however, differ substantially. For example, DES and methoxychlor have a higher affinity for ER-α, while genistein and BPA bind ER-β with higher affinity [35]. Differential ER-α or ER-β mediated effects may partially account for the differential effects of EDCs on different target tissues. This is exemplified in the reproductive tract where studies have shown that the deleterious effects of EDCs are xenoestrogen-specific [37].

In conclusion, xenoestrogens disrupt the endocrine system by acting as ER agonists or antagonists due to differential effects on ER-α or ER-β or via differential binding affinity.

# Xenobiotic nuclear receptor-mediated endocrine disruption

In order to defend against xenobiotics, some of which act as EDCs, a unique system of xenobiotic sensors have evolved that can activate metabolic pathways to aid in the detoxification and elimination of these potentially toxic compounds. These sensors include several NHRs, such as steroid and xenobiotic receptor/pregnane X receptor (SXR/PXR), constitutive androstane receptor (CAR), peroxisome proliferator-activated receptor (PPAR), liver X receptor (LXR), farnesol X receptor (FXR), and the aryl hydrocarbon receptor (AhR). These receptors facilitate the metabolism of xenobiotics by binding to a battery of genes whose expression initiates Phase I (activation) and Phase II (conjugation) metabolism. These xenobiotic receptors, expressed in the brain, ovaries, testes, liver, and intestines can be rather promiscuous in their ligand-binding affinity, being activated by pesticides, pharmaceuticals, xenoestrogens, and steroid hormones [38, 39].

Xenobiotics can also perturb steroid hormone homeostasis by activating xenobiotic receptors or inducing the expression of CYP p450 enzymes that modulate production of steroidogenic metabolites. This mechanism was illustrated by several in vitro studies in rat hepatocytes [40–42] showing that both methoxychlor, and its estrogenic metabolites bis-OH-methoxychlor [1,1,1-trichloro-2,2-bis(p-hydroxyphenyl)ethane] (HPTE), can induce the cytochrome p450 enzymes CYP2B and CYP23A as well as the orphan nuclear receptor CAR. An alternative mechanism by which xenobiotics can disrupt endocrine signaling is via modulating the availability of co-regulators that are shared between xenobiotic receptors and NHRs (i.e. ER). Specifically, the CAR agonist 1,4-bis-(2-(3,5-dichloropyridoxyl)) benzene can inhibit the expression of estrogen-responsive genes through competitive binding of p160 (GRIP1), a co-activator for ER [43], decreasing p160 availability and attenuating ER activity.

Aryl hydrocarbon receptor is one of the most extensively researched xenobiotic receptors, due to its important role in detoxification of the anthropogenic chemicals polycyclic aromatic hydrocarbons (PAHs), dioxins, alkylphenols, and polychlorinated biphenyls (PCBs) [44]. The AhR is a nuclear receptor bound by cytoplasmic chaperones such as HSP90 [45], which disassociate once AhR is bound by a ligand, allowing the liganded receptor to be translocated to the nucleus. Inside the nucleus AhR heterodimerizes with aryl hydrocarbon nuclear translocator (ARNT), and binds to dioxin response elements (DRE) to induce the expression of genes involved in xenobiotic metabolism (e.g. CYP1A1 and glutathione S transferase) [46], [47] and to induce AhR feedback inhibition via the aryl hydrocarbon receptor repressor (AHRR) [48].

Xenobiotics are also modulators of the regulatory cross-talk between AhR and ER-α. While AhR is crucial for female reproductive function via its cooperation with other transcription factors in ovarian granulosa cells to induce CYP19 expression, a key aromatase enzyme in estrogen synthesis [49], activated AhR can bind ER-α and be recruited to estrogen-responsive genes to induce transcription. Ohtake *et al.* [50] showed that in response to AhR agonist such as TCDD and 3-MC, activated AhR dimerizes with ARNT allowing its association with unliganded-ER and recruitment co-activators, such as p300, that transactivate estrogen-responsive genes [50]. Conversely, xenoestrogens can inhibit the activation of AhR via increasing the expression of the negative-feedback gene AHRR, as was demonstrated after in utero exposure to BPA [51]. These examples illustrate the importance of xenobiotic receptors in mediating not only metabolism of anthropogenic chemicals, but also via inappropriate activation and cross-talk with other steroid hormone receptor systems.

# Nuclear receptor co-regulator-mediated endocrine disruption

An exquisite ballet is performed around chromatin to coordinate the process of gene transcription. In order for the transcription machinery to access DNA, the chromatin structure of genes to be transcribed must be de-compacted. Heterochromatin (transcriptionally silent) is transformed into euchromatin (transcriptionally competent) through histone modifications, including acetylation (and additional modifications to be described later), which is accomplished by histone acetyltransferases (HATs). An agonist binding to NHRs induces a conformational change in the NHR to recruit co-activator proteins, many of which are HATs. In contrast, when acted upon by an antagonist, NHR either fail to recruit co-activators or recruit co-repressors, which are usually histone deacetylases (HDACs). Thus far all of the NHRs, and many xenobiotic receptors, have been found to participate with co-regulators to initiate gene transcription (Table 6.2), [52, 53, 54–67].

**Table 6.2.** List of nuclear receptor co-regulators and nuclear receptors reported to interact with one another. Nuclear co-regulators are classified as histone acetyl transferases (HATs) (co-activators) or as histone deactylases (HDACs) (co-repressors), which regulate nuclear receptor activity.

| Co-regulators | Receptors |
|---|---|
| HATs | |
| CARM1 | ER [52], AR [53] |
| CBP/p300 | ER [54], PR [55], RAR/RXR [56], TR [58],AR [57] |
| GRIP1/p160s | ER [60], GR [59], AR [62], RAR [62], TR [61] |
| GCN5/TRAPP | ER [63], TR [64] |
| pCAF/AIB1 | RAR/RXR [65] |
| HDACs | |
| NCoR/SMRT | TR [66], ER [67], RAR/RXR [66] |

Like the NHRs themselves, the expression of co-regulators is also often tissue-specific, and this tissue- and cell-type specificity contributes to differential effects of steroid hormones and xenobiotics in different tissues. The widely used selective estrogen receptor modulators (SERMs), the prototype of which is tamoxifen, exhibit tissue-specific agonist and antagonist activity in the breast (antagonist) and uterus (agonist) due to the differential expression of co-regulators in the breast and uterus. Tamoxifen inhibits ER activity in the breast where it functions as an antagonist, but not in the uterus, where it functions as an agonist, due in part to the higher concentration of steroid receptor co-activator (SRC-1) in the uterus compared with the breast [68].

Given the importance of co-regulators as modulators for NHRs, these accessory proteins have also been a focus of endocrine disruptor research. Currently, three mechanisms for co-regulator modulation by EDCs have been identified. First is xenobiotic-induced NHR co-regulator competition. As mentioned above, CAR can suppress ER transcriptional activation by competing with ER for its shared co-activator GRIP-1 (p160) [43]. This was one of the first examples of xenobiotic regulation of hormone activity via co-regulator squelching. Second is xenobiotic modulation of co-regulator protein levels, which occurs via regulation of target gene expression. An example is modulation of the co-activator thyroid hormone receptor activator protein (TRAP220) in vivo. After exposure of uterine tissue to BPA, TRAP220 interaction with ER-β was enhanced due to increased expression of both ER-β and TRAP220 [69] which functions as an ER-β co-activator,

indicating that xenoestrogens can increase the expression of both NHRs and their co-regulators. Finally, EDC-mediated co-regulator modulation via post-translational modifications (PTMs) of co-regulators is a third mechanism. Endocrine-disrupting chemicals can modulate cell signaling pathways that induce rapid cellular changes termed non-genomic signaling (see below). One of the signaling pathways modulated by EDCs is mitogen-activated protein-kinase (MAPK). Font de Mora and Brown [70] demonstrated that activation of MAPK could induce phosphorylation of the ER co-activators, amplified in breast cancer 1 (AIB1) and p300, to enhance transcription mediated by interaction of these co-activators with the ER.

# Target mechanisms of EDCs: non-genomic signaling

Steroid hormones activate NHRs via two distinct pathways: genomic signaling, which as described above occurs in the nucleus via NHR-DNA binding to regulate expression of target genes, or via non-genomic signaling, which occurs in the cytoplasm, and does not require NHR-DNA binding. While several steroid hormone receptors participate in non-genomic signaling, including GR, TR, MR, PR, RXR, and AR, the majority of the data on activation of non-genomic signaling by EDCs has been obtained for the ER [71–80], which will be used as an example of both potential and established pathways of hormone- and EDC-mediated non-genomic signaling.

Losel and Wehling [73] provided the first evidence, suggesting a non-genomic function for hormones was obtained in cells lacking a "normal" nucleus (e.g. spermatozoa) where genomic signaling is not possible. In nucleated cells, several criteria that define non-genomic signaling can be used to discern genomic from non-genomic signaling as it relates to the classical steroid receptors or EDCs. First, non-genomic signaling is rapid (seconds → minutes) compared with the slower genomic signaling (hours → days). Second, since transcription and protein synthesis result from genomic signaling, hormone-induced events that occur in the presence of inhibitors of either (e.g. actinomycin D or cycloheximide, respectively) is consistent with non-genomic signaling. And third, the effects of hormones or xenoestrogens that cannot traverse the cell membrane can also be inferred not to be the result of genomic signaling, such as those elicited by E2 bound to BSA.

Several pathways for non-genomic signaling have been identified including induction of ion channels

(Ca++), activation of protein kinase signal transduction pathways leading to generation of second messengers (IP$_3$) and activation of growth factor receptors (GFRs) (Fig. 6.3). In the reproductive tract non-genomic responses to E2 include Ca++ mobilization [81] and increased intracellular Ca++ concentrations [82–85], which have multiple biological consequences including altered gene expression, apoptosis, cell division, synaptic transmission, and muscle contraction. Endocrine-disrupting chemicals that have been demonstrated to perturb Ca++ mobilization or concentration include xenoestrogens BPA, genistein, DES, DDT, and octyphenol [86], indicating that like estrogen, xenoestrogens can induce non-genomic changes in Ca++ modulation.

In response to estrogens, increased levels of intracellular Ca++ can activate kinases that participate in signal transduction of mitogenic, stress, and inflammatory signaling [81]. However, these same pathways can be activated by steroid hormone receptors and their endogenous ligands, including PR, AR, GR, and MR [72] as well as by xenoestrogens (e.g. BPA, DES, nonylphenol, and genistein). An ER liganded by E2, for example, can activate the Ras-Raf1-MEK-ERK/MAPK pathway in vitro independently of Ca++ [87], a mechanism also utilized by several xenoestrogens (DES, coumestrol, nonylphenol, DDE, endosulfan, and dieldrin). Downstream effects of non-genomic kinase activation are numerous, and include phosphorylation of effector proteins, including co-regulators such as SRC-1, that can modulate gene transcription (i.e. Elk-1, STAT3), and proteins that regulate cell cycle (i.e. cyclin D) and apoptosis (i.e. BAD). Importantly, the activation of kinases such as MAPKs and protein kinase C (PKC) by E2, growth factors [88] or xenoestrogens can induce phosphorylation of ER (Ser118), which has been shown to recruit ER co-activators to enhance ER-mediated transcription of estrogen-responsive genes [89–91]. Additionally, ER can directly bind p85, a subunit of phosphoinositol-3-kinase (PI3K), to enhance the activation of PI3K signaling, which induces (via its second messenger PIP3) phosphorylation and activation of AKT, resulting in pleotropic biologic effects, which culminate in cell survival. Activation of the PI3K pathway has been demonstrated by Bulayeva and Watson [92] as a mechanism by which the xenoestrogens endosulfan, DDE, coumestrol, and DES act to regulate estrogen-responsive gene expression [93].

Membrane-associated receptor signaling is a specific type of receptor-mediated non-genomic signaling utilized by hormones to activate cellular responses. For ER, both ER-α and ER-β have been found to reside in the nuclear, plasma, and mitochondrial membranes, as well as the cystosol [94–96]. Reports indicate that E2-induced signaling via a membrane-bound receptor can occur via G protein-coupled receptors (GPCRs) in several cell types including nuclear estrogen-receptor negative breast cancer epithelium [97, 98], hypothalamic neurons [99, 100], osteoblasts [101], vascular endothelium [102], and renal cells [103]. Specifically, Razandi et al. [94] demonstrated that E2-liganded ER stimulates G-proteins in the membrane, resulting in activation of the enzyme adenylate cyclase, which uses ATP to produce the second messenger cyclic adenosine 3', 5'-monophosphate (cAMP) [94, 104]. In turn, cAMP binds to protein kinase A (PKA), which phosphorylates proteins that modulate steroidogenesis, apoptosis, differentiation, proliferation, and neuronal conductivity. The cAMP-bound R subunit of PKA also phosphorylates cAMP response-element-binding protein (CREB), which is a common mediator of non-genomic steroid hormone signaling [105]. CREB, a transcription factor, initiates transcription of stress-response and estrogen-responsive target genes including c-fos/c-jun and lactate dehydrogenase [106]. Another target of cAMP is protein kinase C (PKC), which also regulates Ca++ flux and feeds back to enhance PKC activity. Xenoestrogens that have been implicated in modulation of cAMP and PKC in vitro include BPA, DES, atrazine, and nonylphenol [107, 108]. The identification of a potential G-protein coupled membrane estrogen receptor GPR30 has been reported to mediate the estrogenic effects of E2 [109, 110] and xenoestrogens, DDE [110, 111], BPA, genistein, nonylphenol, and kepone [111], however, it remains a controversial issue as to whether this receptor functions as a true mediator of estrogen signaling [112, 113].

Another mechanism by which ER-mediated non-genomic signaling modulates the activity of GFRs, including EGFR and the insulin-like growth factor 1-receptor (IGF-1R), is via the association of E2/ER with scaffolding proteins such as Shc, which induces autophosphorylation and activation of EGFR [114]. Activated EGFR can then induce activation of signal transduction pathways including MAPK. Additionally, E2/ER has been shown to induced autophosphorylation of IGF-1R, which also activates the MAPK pathway. This has been shown to occur in response to DDT, which increases tyrosine phosphorylation of growth factor receptors c-erB2 and c-met after in vitro

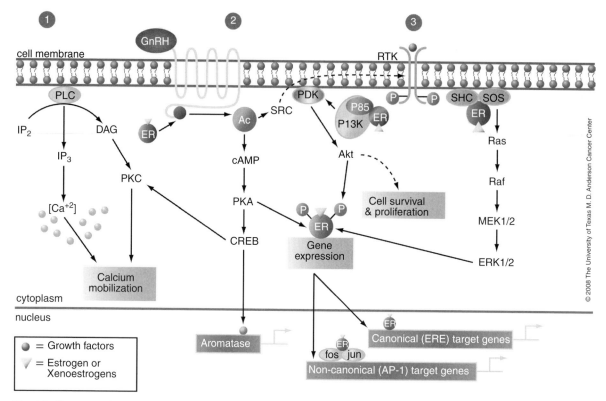

**Fig. 6.3.** Illustration of non-genomic NHR signaling. (1) Calcium mobilization, as the result of non-genomic signaling through protein kinase C (PKC) via activation of GPCRs and CREB by liganded ER, is one of the consequences of estrogen or xenoestrogen exposure. (2) Activation of GPCRs by estrogen or xenoestrogens also induces non-genomic signaling and expression of estrogen-responsive (canonical and non-canonical) genes via protein kinase A (PKA) activation of ER. Estrogen-induced GPCR activation also signals via CREB to induce aromatase expression. (3) In addition to GFs, estrogens and xenoestrogens can promote cell survival, proliferation and estrogen-responsive gene expression via activation of the PI3K/Akt and MAPK pathways. Activation of GFRs can also induce PI3K and MAPK signaling, which can both phosphorylate the ER. Alternatively, liganded-ER can bind directly to the p85 subunit of PI3K to activate Akt or bind SHC to activate the ERK1/2, which can also phosphorylate ER. (© 2008 University of Texas M. D. Anderson Cancer Center.)

exposure [115], indicating that EDCs have the ability to modulate GFR activation via rapid non-genomic signaling. Importantly, MAPK and PI3K signaling can in turn result in phosphorylation of ER, providing a positive feedback mechanism between GFR and ER signaling [116].

In conclusion the ability of EDCs to modulate non-genomic signaling or activation of second messengers or co-factors provides another avenue by which endocrine function can be disrupted.

## Target mechanisms of EDCs: modulation of hormone activity

Metabolism plays a key role in maintaining hormone homeostasis. As such, proteins that maintain steroid hormone balance are potential targets for endocrine disruption. As mentioned previously, xenobiotics activate receptors that induce the expression of enzymes that participate in activation, conjugation, and elimination of endogenous hormones and xenobiotics. These enzymes are classified as Phase I enzymes (hydrolases, reductases, and oxidases) or Phase II enzymes (conjugation enzymes). Phase I enzymes, including cytochrome P450, are primarily responsible for activating xenobiotics, and many of these enzymes are up-regulated in response to ligand binding to xenobiotic receptors. The P450s can also participate in elimination of xenobiotics via hydroxylation [117]. Importantly, P450s also participate in steroid hormone metabolism, for example via aromatization of testosterone to 17β-estradiol, and in the conversion of progesterone to testosterone [118]. Other Phase I enzymes participate in inactivation and elimination of steroid hormones including steroid reductases and hydroxysteroid dehydrogenases. Through alteration of the activity of enzymes that participate in hormone synthesis and metabolism, xenobiotics can become endocrine disruptors.

In addition, the availability of circulation hormones is regulated by hormone binding proteins. Production of sex hormone binding globulins (SHBGs), which bind both E2 and testosterone, by the liver is regulated by testosterone, (which decreases SHBG levels) and estrogen (which increases SHBG levels) [119]. However, while SHBGs can bind endogenous hormones, xenoestrogens are not recognized by these proteins. During development, for example, the critical estrogen-binding protein in the blood of the developing fetus is alpha-feto protein (AFP), which is produced by the liver at high levels until ~postnatal day 16 (in rodents) or soon after birth in humans [120]. Alpha-feto protein scavenges maternal and fetal E2, which protects developing tissues from this hormone and allows the reproductive tract, for example, to differentiate in an estrogen-independent manner. Alpha-feto protein, however, does not bind most xenoestrogens. Hence, exposure to xenoestrogens during fetal or neonatal development can result in endocrine disruption in a setting where the organism is protected from endogenous hormones, illustrating another possible mechanism of actions for EDCs.

While the liver produces proteins that regulate hormone activity (e.g. SHBG and AFP), it is the adrenals, ovary, and testes that produce steroid hormones de novo from cholesterol. In the gonads, a series of reactions take place in response to signals from the hypothalamus and pituitary that regulates the production of steroid hormone-metabolizing enzymes. As discussed earlier, cAMP is a key signal in gonads that activates the cholesterol side-chain cleavage enzyme P450scc (CYP11A) [121] to induce the production of steroid hormones from cholesterol in response to LH and FSH. This reaction produces pregnenolone, which is converted by 3β-hydroxysteroid dehydrogenase (3β-HSD) to progesterone. Both pregnenolone and progesterone are precursors for other steroid hormones, for example in the adrenals, where aldosterone and cortisol are produced from these two hormones via CYP11B2. Xenobiotics can interfere with steroid synthesis by interfering with this enzymatic pathway, or P450scc. An example of a xenobiotic that acts via this mechanism is the chemical p,p'-DDT, which when metabolized to o,p'-DDD, can specifically inhibit the production of glucocorticoids in the adrenals by inhibiting these enzymes, leading to severe adrenal dysfunction and death [122, 123].

There are also population-based studies suggesting that EDCs can interfere with steroid hormone synthesis in exposed human populations. In a large epidemiologic study of several thousand individuals who apply pesticides as part of their profession, levels of six pesticides were found to correlate with prostate cancer risk in men [124, 125]. These thiophosphate pesticides can inhibit the activity of CYP1A2 and CYP3A4, which metabolize estradiol and testosterone in the liver [126, 127] and participate in metabolism of xenobiotics in the prostate [128, 129, 130], suggesting that xenobiotics such as thiophosphate pesticides can perturb steroid hormone metabolism and potentially increase susceptibility of the prostate to cancer [131]. Another potent xenobiotic, the antifungal ketoconazole, has also been shown to modulate multiple CYP450 enzymes including P450scc, 11β-HSD, 17α-hydroxylase, and 17,20 lyase, all of which participate in the metabolism of steroid hormones [132, 133]. Concordant with this activity, ketoconazole exerts numerous effects associated with endocrine disruption including infertility, secondary to reduction or inhibition of hormone synthesis in the ovaries, uterus, and testes[134–137].

Aromatase is another P450 enzyme that is responsible for conversion of androgens to estrogens. Inhibition of aromatization in females leads to reproductive dysfunction, for example anovulation due to insufficient E2 production to trigger the LH surge needed for ovulation. Several xenoestrogens, including BPA, phytoestrogens, nonylphenol, octylphenol [28], and several isoflavones [137] effectively inhibit aromatization. For example, Akingbemi et al. [138] demonstrated that postnatal treatment (PND 21–35) of male mice with BPA (2.4 µg/kg/bw per day) resulted in the reduction of circulating and local 17ß-estradiol levels, which correlated with the ability of BPA to inhibit aromatase enzyme gene expression in Leydig cells in vitro. The dietary fatty acids linoleic and linolenic acids also inhibit aromatases. Interestingly, treatment of nude mice injected with estrogen receptor-positive, aromatase-positive MCF7 breast cancer cells with mushroom extract containing these fatty acids resulted in a reduction in tumor-cell proliferation and tumor weight [139].

Phthalates can also inhibit aromatization of testosterone to estrogen in females, and in males they can inhibit another important enzyme, 5α-reductase. 5α-reductase converts testosterone to 5α-dihydrotestosterone (5α- DHT), which has a higher binding affinity for the AR than testosterone, and is a more potent androgen. 5α-DHT is required for masculinization and is indispensable for normal prostate development and patterning of adult reproductive behavior [140]. A number of pesticides including the organotins, dibutyltin, tributyltin, and triphenyltin also demonstrate 5α-DHT inhibition in vitro in prostate epithelial cells [141], suggesting the possibility that developmental exposure to these pesticides could potentially disrupt prostate development.

The activity of sulfotransferases, phase II enzymes responsible for converting estradiol to the inactive estradiol sulfate, and steroid sulfatases, which reverse this process to produce more free active estradiol, and hence stabilize hormone balance [117], may also be disrupted by endocrine active compounds. Several different EDCs including PCBs, dioxins, dibenzofurans, BPA [142], as well as phytoestrogens, genistein, and equol [143] can inhibit sulfotransferases. Reduced enzymatic activity as a consequence of exposure to EDCs could cause an increase in estradiol availability in tissues such as the testis and endometrium, which express the estrogen sulfotransferases SULT1E1 and SULT1A1 [144], with the potential to disrupt hormone homeostasis, which has been hypothesized to increase the susceptibility to hormone-driven tumors.

In conclusion, the enzymes responsible for metabolizing xenobiotics, as well as the enzymes involved in synthesis and elimination of steroid hormones, are points at which EDCs disturb the balance of circulating and local tissue concentration of hormones with the potential to disrupt developmental and adult reproductive-tract functions.

## Target mechanisms of EDCs: epigenetic modulation

It has long been known that information beyond that encoded in DNA was responsible for the immense variations in phenotype seen in eukaryotes. One of the originators of the idea that differences in gene expression, and subsequently phenotype, were established by "canalization" of the genome in the undifferentiated cell was Conrad Waddington, a phenomenon he later termed epigenetics [145]. Epigenetics is a term used to describe heritable changes in gene expression and phenotype that are not a result of alterations in DNA sequence. The importance of epigenetics is most evident during development, where all cells of an organism start out with the same DNA, yet differentiate into a multitude of specialized cell types in the body. Accordingly, the fetal epigenome is particularly susceptible to environmental influence, as evidenced by studies of monozygotic twins, which demonstrate that even given identical DNA, two developing fetuses can present with non-identical epigenomes [146].

While we are still in the beginning stages of understanding the molecular mechanisms that regulate the epigenome, many studies already support the importance of the cellular environment in faithfully copying and transmitting epigenetic information, an environment that can be perturbed by EDCs. It is the purpose of this section to introduce the epigenetic processes of DNA methylation and histone modification, and the effects of endocrine disruptors on these processes.

### DNA methylation

DNA methylation was the first identified epigenetic alteration [147, 148]. It occurs at the 5' carbon of cytosine bases adjacent to guanine (CpG dinucleotides) in DNA. Clusters of CpG dinucleotides (DNA with > 60% CG content) are termed CpG islands (CGIs), which are located mainly in the 5' promoter region of genes [149]. While 70% of mammalian CpG sites are methylated, CGIs are usually unmethylated. Methylation of CGIs controls gene transcription, with promoter CGI methylation inhibiting gene expression, and this methylation is associated with gene silencing. This mechanism of gene silencing occurs normally in specific genes, such as those located in the X chromosome, and can also be associated with pathologies, such as tumor suppressor gene silencing in cancer cells [150].

The enzymes responsible for methylating cytosines at CpG sites are called DNA methyltransferases (DNMTs). Four DNMTs exist in mammals, DNMT1, DNMT2, DNMT3a, and DNMT3b, all of which are embryonic lethal when knocked out in mice except DNMT2 [151–156], indicating the critical role these enzymes play in normal development. Specifically, DNMT1 is considered a maintenance methylase because it has an affinity for hemimethylated DNA, and participates in faithful copying of cytosine methylation after normal cell division [150]. Conversely, DNMT3a and 3b are de novo DNA methylases, and are critical for establishing patterns of methylation during embryonic development [157].

Methylated DNA is recognized by specific proteins, methyl-CpG-binding proteins (MBDs), which bind methylated CpGs and recruit other factors that regulate transcription, including HDACs and histone methyltransferases (HMTs), to induce the compaction of chromatin into a transcriptionally silent or inactive unit.

## Histone modification

Histone proteins bind to DNA to form the nucleosome, which binds to DNA to compact it and form chromatin. There are four core histone proteins, H2A, H2B, H3, and H4, and a linker histone protein, H1. In addition to formation of chromatin, one of the other functions of histone proteins is to receive signals from the environment via post-translational modifications (PTM) of the histone "tails." The histone proteins assembled in the nucleosome have tail-like extensions protruding outward that can undergo multiple modifications including methylation, phosphorylation, sumoylation, ubiquitination, and acetylation, and the enzymes responsible for these PTMs of histones are themselves regulated by upstream signaling pathways [158]. The combination of PTMs or "marks" acquired by histones creates specific binding motifs that are recognized by other proteins, for example those containing bromo- and chromodomains, which then recognize and bind to the modified chromatin, to regulate chromatin structure and gene transcription [159]. In general, acetylation of histones is characteristic of active chromatin. Methylation of histones (H3 and H4) can be associated with either activation or repression of gene expression, which differs from DNA methylation, which is always associated with repression or silencing [160].

Histone methylation is stable and participates in epigenetic inheritance [161]. Enzymes responsible for histone methylation are called histone methyltransferases (HMTs). Currently, two classes of HMTs are known to exist, protein arginine histone methyltransferases (PRMTs) and histone lysine methyltransferases (HKMTs), both of which, similar to DNMTs, utilize S-adenosyl-methionine (SAM) as the methyl donor [162] Conversely, another family of enzymes exists to induce demethylation of methylated histones, called demethylases. An example of a histone demethylase is lysine specific demethylase 1 (LSD1), which participates in expression of hormone-responsive genes when associated with either AR or ER [163].

## Endocrine disruptor-induced epigenetic modulation

Perturbation of epigenetic regulation is beginning to emerge as an important mode of endocrine disruption, especially as a result of exposure to EDCs during development. Given that environmental cues trigger epigenetic changes during normal development and sexual reproduction, as illustrated in *Arabidopsis thaliana* which responds to temperature and time cues to regulate flowering [164], and honeybees which develop into queens from royal jelly feeding [165], it is perhaps not surprising that exposure to EDCs during development can induce aberrant epigenetic modifications.

Several windows of susceptibility exist during development when the epigenome is susceptible to reprogramming by EDCs. The earliest window of susceptibility to be identified is prior to conception, during gamete maturation. A period of de novo methylation occurs during oogenesis in females and during spermatogenesis in males [166]. The second window is the time that spans the period between fertilization and implantation, during which the zygote undergoes active demethylation of the paternal genome followed by a more gradual demethylation of the maternal genome and de novo methylation during implantation [157] . The third window includes the stage of lineage-specific cellular differentiation of pluripotent cells, which harbor bivalent chromatin awaiting signals from developmentally expressed proteins that control tissue-specific imprinting [167]. Importantly, it is thought that epigenetic alterations that occur in gametes can be inherited in the germline, with the resulting phenotypic alterations transmitted to subsequent generations. However, if epigenetic alterations occur in somatic cells, deleterious effects associated with these alterations of the epigenetic changes would not be passed to subsequent generations.

There are several lines of evidence that exposure to EDCs can reprogram the epigenome. Endocrine-disrupting chemicals, such as DES [168] , BPA, genistein [169], methoxychlor, vinclozolin [170], and arsenic [171] have all been shown to alter patterns of DNA methylation. The initial demonstration that EDCs can reprogram the epigenome came from studies [172, 173] that showed that developmental exposure to DES could induce hypomethylation of the uterine-specific genes *lactoferrin* and *c-fos,* which correlated with elevated expression of these genes in the mature uterus. However, alterations in DNA methylation were not identified that correlated with changes in expression of *HOX* family genes (i.e. *HOXA10* and *HOXA11*), essential in proper uterine development, which also occurred after exposure to DES or BPA [174, 175]. More recently, Ho *et al.* [176] demonstrated in the prostate that the gene phosphodiesterase type 4 variant 4 (PDE4D4) was differentially methylated after neonatal exposure to BPA. Increased phosphodiesterase activity leads to persistent elevation of cAMP, and was associated with increased incidence of prostate intraepithelial neoplasia (PIN) lesions in exposed animals, suggesting that

DNA methylation changes associated with BPA exposure contributed to the development of PIN lesions in the prostate. Additionally, inorganic arsenic exposure in utero was shown by Waalkes et al. [171] to significantly decrease promoter methylation of ER in the liver, resulting in increased ER expression, which correlated with increased incidence of hepatocellular carcinoma in exposed animals.

Recently, collaborative work between the laboratories of Newbold [177, 178] and Tang [179] has explored DNA methylation changes induced by developmental exposure to EDCs, specifically DES. Initial studies in CD-1 mice indicated that in addition to neonatal exposure to DES, steroid hormones were required to induce uterine neoplasias in post-pubertal animals (DES-exposed ovariectomized mice did not develop uterine neoplasias). Tang et al. demonstrated that promoter DNA methylation of nucleosomal binding protein 1 (Nsbp1) occurred after neonatal exposure to either DES or genistein. After puberty, in control animals Nsbp1 became hypermethylated (silenced), however, in neonatally DES- or genistein-exposed mice, Nsbp1 remained hypomethylated, resulting in persistent elevated expression that correlated with increased incidence of uterine neoplasias in adulthood [179].

### EDC-induced transgenerational inheritance
Phenotypic alterations inherited over multiple generations (i.e. transgenerational) can be induced by both chemical and behavioral exposures [180, 181], and are postulated to be transmissible via germline alterations. In addition to the transgenerational effects of DES (see above), other EDCs including PCBs, vinclozolin and methoxychlor have also been shown to induce phenotypic alterations in rodents through multiple generations [182, 183].

One of the first examples of transgenerational, epigenetic inheritance was described by Anway et al. [184], who demonstrated the transgenerational effects of vinclozolin and methoxychlor on spermatogenesis and fertility in males after gestational exposure to these EDCs. They showed that gestational exposure to vinclozolin or methoxychlor could alter DNA methylation patterns and affect spermatogenesis of offspring from $F_1$ through $F_4$ generations. Subsequent studies from this group have identified transgenerational effects of vinclozolin in both males [183] and females[185], though no epigenetic analyses were incorporated into these studies. For females gestationally exposed to vinclozolin, $F_1$–$F_3$ offspring

demonstrated pregnancy abnormalities in addition to increased tumor incidence as compared with control offspring (6.5% vs. 2%). Other studies have not yet corroborated the transgenerational effects observed with vinclozolin or methoxychlor, however they provide an intriguing theory whereby changes in DNA methylation contribute to transgenerational inheritance of EDC-induced phenotypic alterations associated with exposure to EDCs.

## Conclusions and future directions
Endocrine-disrupting chemicals can disturb normal hormone homeostasis, which can have both direct and indirect effects on the reproductive function of both wildlife and human populations. The molecular mechanisms by which EDCs exert their effects are varied. Primary pathways of endocrine disruption are associated with: (1) nuclear hormone receptor activity, (2) non-genomic hormone receptor signaling, (3) xenobiotic and hormone metabolism, and (4) epigenetic modifications. Perturbation of any of these pathways can induce endocrine disruption, leading to disease and impaired reproductive function, and perhaps most importantly, can induce lasting effects in adults and heritable alterations in subsequent generations following even brief developmental exposures. Continued elucidation of these mechanisms is key to the understanding of how to manage and prevent the deleterious effects of EDCs on exposed individuals and populations.

## References
1. Barker DJ, Osmond C, Golding J, Kuh D, Wadsworth ME. Growth in utero, blood pressure in childhood and adult life, and mortality from cardiovascular disease. Br Med J 1989; 298(6673): 564–7.
2. Mallepell S, Krust A, Chambon P, Brisken C. Paracrine signaling through the epithelial estrogen receptor alpha is required for proliferation and morphogenesis in the mammary gland. Proc Natl Acad Sci USA 2006; 103(7): 2196–201.
3. Rodway MR, Swan CL, Crellin NK, Gillio-Meina C, Chedrese PJ. Steroid regulation of progesterone synthesis in a stable porcine granulosa cell line: a role for progestins. J Steroid Biochem Mol Biol 1999; 68(5–6): 173–80.
4. Mukhina S, Liu D, Guo K. et al. Autocrine growth hormone prevents lactogenic differentiation of mouse mammary epithelial cells. Endocrinology 2006; 147(4): 1819–29.
5. Isaacs JT, Isaacs WB. Androgen receptor outwits prostate cancer drugs. Nat Med 2004; 10(1): 26–7.

6. Weigand M, Hantel P, Kreienberg R, Waltenberger J. Autocrine vascular endothelial growth factor signalling in breast cancer. Evidence from cell lines and primary breast cancer cultures in vitro. *Angiogenesis* 2005; **8**(3): 197–204.

7. Victor L. Davidson DBS. *Biochemistry*. Lippincott Williams & Wilkins, 1999.

8. Miki Y, Suzuki T, Tazawa C. *et al*. Analysis of gene expression induced by diethylstilbestrol (DES) in human primitive Müllerian duct cells using microarray. *Cancer Lett* 2005; **220**(2): 197–210.

9. Akiyama T, Ishida J, Nakagawa S. *et al*. Genistein, a specific inhibitor of tyrosine-specific protein kinases. *J Biol Chem* 1987; **262**(12): 5592–5.

10. Jia Z, Jia Y, Liu B. *et al*. Genistein inhibits voltage-gated sodium currents in SCG neurons through protein tyrosine kinase-dependent and kinase-independent mechanisms. *Pflugers Archiv Eur J Physiol* 2008; **456**(5): 857–66.

11. Kuiper GG, Lemmen JG, Carlsson B. *et al*. Interaction of estrogenic chemicals and phytoestrogens with estrogen receptor. *Endocrinology* 1998; **139**(10): 4252–63.

12. Paech K, Webb P, Kuiper GG. *et al*. Differential ligand activation of estrogen receptors ERα and ERβ at AP1 sites. *Science* 1997; **277**(5331): 1508–10.

13. Maruyama S, Fujimoto N, Asano K, Ito A. Suppression by estrogen receptor beta of AP-1 mediated transactivation through estrogen receptor alpha. *J Steroid Biochem Mol Biol* 2001; **78**(2): 177–84.

14. Kelce WR, Lambright CR, Gray LE, Jr., Roberts KP. Vinclozolin and p,p'-DDE alter androgen-dependent gene expression: in vivo confirmation of an androgen receptor-mediated mechanism. *Toxicol Appl Pharmacol* 1997; **142**(1): 192–200.

15. Wilson WR. In Metzler M, ed. *Endocrine Disruptors: Pt. 1 (The Handbook of Environmental Chemistry)*. Berlin: Springer-Verlag, 2001.

16. Beyer C, Green SJ, Hutchison JB. Androgens influence sexual differentiation of embryonic mouse hypothalamic aromatase neurons in vitro. *Endocrinology* 1994; **135**(3): 1220–6.

17. Burek M, Duda M, Knapczyk K, Koziorowski M, Slomczynska M. Tissue-specific distribution of the androgen receptor (AR) in the porcine fetus. *Acta Histochem* 2007; **109**(5): 358–65.

18. Davison SL, Davis SR. Androgens in women. *J Steroid Biochem Mol Biol* 2003; **85**(2–5): 363–6.

19. Holloway CC, Clayton DF. Estrogen synthesis in the male brain triggers development of the avian song control pathway in vitro. *Nat Neurosci* 2001; **4**(2): 170–5.

20. Chapin RE, Stevens JT, Hughes CL. *et al*. Endocrine modulation of reproduction. *Fundament Appl Toxicol* 1996; **29**(1): 1–17.

21. Welsch F. How can chemical compounds alter human fertility? *Eur J Obst Gynecol Reprod Biol* 2003; **106**(1): 88–91.

22. List HJ, Smith CL, Martinez E. *et al*. Effects of antiandrogens on chromatin remodeling and transcription of the integrated mouse mammary tumor virus promoter. *Exp Cell Res* 2000; **260**: 160–5.

23. Massaad C, Entezami F, Massade L. *et al*. How can chemical compounds alter human fertility? *Eur J Obst Gynecol Reprod Biol* 2002; **100**(2): 127–37.

24. Wong C, Kelce WR, Sar M, Wilson EM. Androgen receptor antagonist versus agonist activities of the fungicide vinclozolin relative to hydroxyflutamide. *J Biol Chem* 1995; **270**(34): 19 998–20 003.

25. Kelce WR, Stone CR, Laws SC. *et al*. Persistent DDT metabolite p,p'-DDE is a potent androgen receptor antagonist. *Nature* 1995; **375**(6532): 581–5.

26. Ostby J, Kelce WR, Lambright C. *et al*. The fungicide procymidone alters sexual differentiation in the male rat by acting as an androgen-receptor antagonist in vivo and in vitro. *Toxicol Ind Health* 1999; **15**(1–2): 80–93.

27. Daxenburger A. Pollutants with androgen-disrupting potency. *Eur J Lipid Sci Technol* 2002; **104**: 124–30.

28. Bonefeld-Jorgensen EC, Long M, Hofmeister MV, Vinggaard AM. Endocrine-disrupting potential of bisphenol A, bisphenol A dimethacrylate, 4-n-nonylphenol, and 4-n-octylphenol in vitro: new data and a brief review. *Environ Health Perspect* 2007; **115** (Suppl. 1): 69–76.

29. Portigal CL, Cowell SP, Fedoruk MN. *et al*. Polychlorinated biphenyls interfere with androgen-induced transcriptional activation and hormone binding. *Toxicol Appl Pharmacol* 2002; **179**: 185–94.

30. McKinnell C, Atanassova N, Williams K. *et al*. Suppression of androgen action and the induction of gross abnormalities of the reproductive tract in male rats treated neonatally with diethylstilbestrol. *J Androl* 2001; **22**(2): 323–38.

31. Vondracek J, Kozubik A, Machala M. Modulation of estrogen receptor-dependent reporter construct activation and G0/G1-S-phase transition by polycyclic aromatic hydrocarbons in human breast carcinoma MCF-7 cells. *Toxicol Sci* 2002; **70**(2): 193–201.

32. Coldham NG, Dave M, Sivapathasundaram S. *et al*. Evaluation of a recombinant yeast cell estrogen screening assay. *Environ Health Perspect* 1997; **105**(7): 734–42.

33. Oostenbrink C, van Gunsteren WF. Free energies of ligand binding for structurally diverse compounds. *Proc Natl Acad Sci USA* 2005; **102**(19): 6750–4.

34. Gould JC, Leonard LS, Maness SC. *et al*. Bisphenol A interacts with the estrogen receptor alpha in a distinct manner from estradiol. *Mol Cell Endocrinol* 1998; **142**(1–2): 203–14.

35. Routledge EJ, White R, Parker MG, Sumpter JP. Differential effects of xenoestrogens on coactivator recruitment by estrogen receptor (ER) alpha and ERbeta. *J Biol Chem* 2000; **275**(46): 35 986–93.

36. Eroschenko VP, Rourke AW, Sims WF. Estradiol or methoxychlor stimulates estrogen receptor (ER) expression in uteri. *Reprod Toxicol* 1996; **10**(4): 265–71.

37. Judy BM, Nagel SC, Thayer KA, Saal FSV, Welshons WV. Low-dose bioactivity of xenoestrogens in animals: fetal exposure to low doses of methoxychlor and other xenoestrogens increases adult prostate size in mice. *Toxicol Indust Health* 1999; **15**(1–2): 12–25.

38. Dussault I, Forman BM. The nuclear receptor PXR: a master regulator of "homeland" defense. *Crit Rev Eukaryot Gene Expr* 2002; **12**(1): 53–64.

39. Willson TM, Kliewer SA. PXR, CAR and drug metabolism. *Nat Rev Drug Discov* 2002; **1**(4): 259–66.

40. Bulger WH, Feil VJ, Kupfer D. Role of hepatic monooxygenases in generating estrogenic metabolites from methoxychlor and from its identified contaminants. *Mol Pharmacol* 1985; **27**(1): 115–24.

41. Sueyoshi T, Kawamoto T, Zelko I, Honkakoski P, Negishi M. The repressed nuclear receptor CAR responds to phenobarbital in activating the human CYP2B6 gene. *J Biol Chem* 1999; **274**(10): 6043–6.

42. Blizard D, Sueyoshi T, Negishi M, Dehal SS, Kupfer D. Mechanism of induction of cytochrome P450 enzymes by the proestrogenic endocrine disruptor pesticide methoxychlor: interactions of methoxychlor metabolites with the constitutive androstane receptor system. *Drug Metab Dispos* 2001; **29**(6): 781–5.

43. Min G, Kim H, Bae Y, Petz L, Kemper JK. Inhibitory cross-talk between estrogen receptor (ER) and constitutively activated androstane receptor (CAR). CAR inhibits ER-mediated signaling pathway by squelching p160 coactivators. *J Biol Chem* 2002; **277**(37): 34 626–33.

44. Fujii-Kuriyama Y, Mimura J. Molecular mechanisms of AhR functions in the regulation of cytochrome P450 genes. *Biochem Biophys Res Commun* 2005; **338**(1): 311–17.

45. Ma Q, Whitlock JP, Jr. A novel cytoplasmic protein that interacts with the Ah receptor, contains tetratricopeptide repeat motifs, and augments the transcriptional response to 2,3,7,8-tetrachlorodibenzo-p-dioxin. *J Biol Chem* 1997; **272**(14): 8878–84.

46. Jones KW, Whitlock JP Jr. Functional analysis of the transcriptional promoter for the CYP1A1 gene. *Mol Cell Biol* 1990; **10**(10): 5098–105.

47. Rushmore TH, Pickett CB. Transcriptional regulation of the rat glutathione S-transferase Ya subunit gene. Characterization of a xenobiotic-responsive element controlling inducible expression by phenolic antioxidants. *J Biol Chem* 1990; **265**(24): 14 648–53.

48. Mimura J, Ema M, Sogawa K, Fujii-Kuriyama Y. Identification of a novel mechanism of regulation of Ah (dioxin) receptor function. *Genes Dev* 1999; **13**(1): 20–5.

49. Baba T, Mimura J, Nakamura N. *et al.* Intrinsic function of the aryl hydrocarbon (dioxin) receptor as a key factor in female reproduction. *Mol Cell Biol* 2005; **25**(22): 10 040–51.

50. Ohtake F, Takeyama K, Matsumoto T. *et al.* Modulation of oestrogen receptor signalling by association with the activated dioxin receptor. *Nature* 2003; **423**(6939): 545–50.

51. Nishizawa H, Imanishi S, Manabe N. Effects of exposure in utero to bisphenol a on the expression of aryl hydrocarbon receptor, related factors, and xenobiotic metabolizing enzymes in murine embryos. *J Reprod Dev* 2005; **51**(5): 593–605.

52. Tetel MJ, Giangrande PH, Leonhardt SA, McDonnell DP, Edwards DP. Hormone-dependent interaction between the amino- and carboxyl-terminal domains of progesterone receptor in vitro and in vivo. *Mol Endocrinol* 1999; **13**(6): 910–24.

53. Gillespie RF, Gudas LJ. Retinoid regulated association of transcriptional co-regulators and the polycomb group protein SUZ12 with the retinoic acid response elements of Hoxa1, RARbeta(2), and Cyp26A1 in F9 embryonal carcinoma cells. *J Mol Biol* 2007; **372**(2): 298–316.

54. Higashimoto K, Kuhn P, Desai D, Cheng X, Xu W. Phosphorylation-mediated inactivation of coactivator-associated arginine methyltransferase 1. *Proc Natl Acad Sci USA* 2007; **104**(30): 12 318–23.

55. Majumder S, Liu Y, Ford OH, 3rd, Mohler JL, Whang YE. Involvement of arginine methyltransferase CARM1 in androgen receptor function and prostate cancer cell viability. *Prostate* 2006; **66**(12): 1292–301.

56. Kraus WL, Kadonaga JT. p300 and estrogen receptor cooperatively activate transcription via differential enhancement of initiation and reinitiation. *Genes Dev* 1998; **12**(3): 331–42.

57. Ikonen T, Palvimo JJ, Janne OA. Interaction between the amino- and carboxyl-terminal regions of the rat androgen receptor modulates transcriptional activity and is influenced by nuclear receptor coactivators. *J Biol Chem* 1997; **272**(47): 29 821–8.

58. Paul BD, Buchholz DR, Fu L, Shi YB. SRC-p300 coactivator complex is required for thyroid hormone-induced amphibian metamorphosis. *J Biol Chem* 2007; **282**(10): 7472–81.

59. Kino T, Ichijo T, Chrousos GP. FLASH interacts with p160 coactivator subtypes and differentially suppresses transcriptional activity of steroid hormone receptors. *J Steroid Biochem Mol Biol* 2004; **92**(5): 357–63.

60. Klinge CM, Jernigan SC, Mattingly KA, Risinger KE, Zhang J. Estrogen response element-dependent regulation of transcriptional activation of estrogen receptors alpha and beta by coactivators and corepressors. *J Mol Endocrinol* 2004; **33**(2): 387–410.

61. Paul BD, Shi YB. Distinct expression profiles of transcriptional coactivators for thyroid hormone receptors during Xenopus laevis metamorphosis. *Cell Res* 2003; **13**(6): 459–64.

62. Hong H, Darimont BD, Ma H. *et al.* An additional region of coactivator GRIP1 required for interaction with the hormone-binding domains of a subset of nuclear receptors. *J Biol Chem* 1999; **274**(6): 3496–502.

63. Nilsson S, Makela S, Treuter E. *et al.* Mechanisms of estrogen action. *Physiol Rev* 2001; **81**(4): 1535–65.

64. Fondell JD. Gene activation by thyroid hormone receptor in vitro and purification of the TRAP coactivator complex. *Methods Mol Biol* 2002; **202**: 195–214.

65. Blanco JC, Minucci S, Lu J. *et al.* The histone acetylase PCAF is a nuclear receptor coactivator. *Genes Develop* 1998; **12**(11): 1638–51.

66. Shibata H, Spencer TE, Onate SA. *et al.* Role of co-activators and co-repressors in the mechanism of steroid/thyroid receptor action. *Recent Prog Horm Res* 1997; **52**: 141–64; discussion 164–5.

67. Peterson TJ, Karmakar S, Pace MC, Gao T, Smith CL. The silencing mediator of retinoic acid and thyroid hormone receptor (SMRT) corepressor is required for full estrogen receptor alpha transcriptional activity. *Mol Cell Biol* 2007; **27**(17): 5933–48.

68. Smith CL, O'Malley BW. Coregulator function: a key to understanding tissue specificity of selective receptor modulators. *Endocr Rev* 2004; **25**(1): 45–71.

69. Inoshita H, Masuyama H, Hiramatsu Y. The different effects of endocrine-disrupting chemicals on estrogen receptor-mediated transcription through interaction with coactivator TRAP220 in uterine tissue. *J Mol Endocrinol* 2003; **31**(3): 551–61.

70. Font de Mora J, Brown M. AIB1 is a conduit for kinase-mediated growth factor signaling to the estrogen receptor. *Mol Cell Biol* 2000; **20**(14): 5041–7.

71. Grossmann C, Freudinger R, Mildenberger S, Husse B, Gekle M. EF domains are sufficient for nongenomic mineralocorticoid receptor actions. *J Biol Chem* 2008; **283**(11): 7109–16.

72. Cato ACB, Nestl A, Mink S. Rapid actions of steroid receptors in cellular signaling pathways. *Sci STKE* 2002; **2002**(138): re9.

73. Losel R, Wehling M. Nongenomic actions of steroid hormones. *Nat Rev Mol Cell Biol* 2003; **4**(1): 46–55.

74. Boonyaratanakornkit V, Scott MP, Ribon V. *et al.* Progesterone receptor contains a proline-rich motif that directly interacts with SH3 domains and activates c-Src family tyrosine kinases. *Mol Cell* 2001; **8**(2): 269–80.

75. Wyckoff MH, Chambliss KL, Mineo C. *et al.* Plasma membrane estrogen receptors are coupled to endothelial nitric-oxide synthase through G alpha. *J Biol Chem* 2001; **276**(29): 27 071–6.

76. Song RXD, McPherson RA, Adam L. *et al.* Linkage of rapid estrogen action to MAPK Activation by ER - Shc Association and Shc Pathway Activation. *Mol Endocrinol* 2002; **16**(1): 116–27.

77. Haynes MP, Sinha D, Russell KS. *et al.* Membrane estrogen receptor engagement activates endothelial nitric oxide synthase via the PI3-Kinase-Akt pathway in human endothelial cells. *Circ Res* 2000; **87**(8): 677–82.

78. Kousteni S, Bellido T, Plotkin LI. *et al.* Nongenotropic, sex-nonspecific signaling through the estrogen or androgen receptors: dissociation from transcriptional activity. *Cell* 2001; **104**(5): 719–30.

79. Barletta F, Wong C-W, McNally C. *et al.* Characterization of the interactions of estrogen receptor and MNAR in the activation of cSrc. *Mol Endocrinol* 2004; **18**(5): 1096–108.

80. Moraes LA, Swales KE, Wray JA. *et al.* Nongenomic signaling of the retinoid X receptor through binding and inhibiting Gq in human platelets. *Blood* 2007; **109**(9): 3741–4.

81. Improta-Brears T, Whorton AR, Codazzi F. *et al.* Estrogen-induced activation of mitogen-activated protein kinase requires mobilization of intracellular calcium. *Proc Natl Acad Sci USA* 1999; **96**(8): 4686–91.

82. Pietras RJ, Szego CM. Endometrial cell calcium and oestrogen action. *Nature* 1975; **253**(5490): 357–9.

83. Perret S, Dockery P, Harvey BJ. 17 beta-oestradiol stimulates capacitative Ca2+ entry in human endometrial cells. *Mol Cell Endocrinol* 2001; **176**(1–2): 77–84.

84. Morley P, Whitfield JF, Vanderhyden BC, Tsang BK, Schwartz JL. A new, nongenomic estrogen action: the rapid release of intracellular calcium. *Endocrinology* 1992; **131**(3): 1305–12.

85. Tesarik J, Mendoza C. Nongenomic effects of 17 beta-estradiol on maturing human oocytes: relationship to oocyte developmental potential. *J Clin Endocrinol Metab* 1995; **80**(4): 1438–43.

86. Ropero AB, Alonso-Magdalena P, Ripoll C, Fuentes E, Nadal A. Rapid endocrine disruption: Environmental estrogen actions triggered outside the nucleus. *J Steroid Biochem Mol Biol* 2006; **102**(1–5): 163–9.

87. Watson CS, Bulayeva NN, Wozniak AL, Alyea RA. Xenoestrogens are potent activators of nongenomic estrogenic responses. *Steroids* 2007; **72**(2): 124–34.

88. Masuhiro Y, Mezaki Y, Sakari M. *et al.* Splicing potentiation by growth factor signals via estrogen receptor phosphorylation. *Proc Natl Acad Sci USA* 2005; **102**(23): 8126–31.

89. Kato S, Endoh H, Masuhiro Y. *et al.* Activation of the estrogen receptor through phosphorylation by mitogen-activated protein kinase. *Science* 1995; **270**(5241): 1491–4.

90. Joel PB, Traish AM, Lannigan DA. Estradiol and phorbol ester cause phosphorylation of serine 118 in the human estrogen receptor. *Mol Endocrinol* 1995; **9**(8): 1041–52.

91. Campbell RA, Bhat-Nakshatri P, Patel NM. *et al.* Phosphatidylinositol 3-kinase/AKT-mediated activation of estrogen receptor alpha: a new model for anti-estrogen resistance. *J Biol Chem* 2001; **276**(13): 9817–24.

92. Bulayeva NN, Watson CS. Xenoestrogen-induced ERK-1 and ERK-2 activation via multiple membrane-initiated signaling pathways. *Environ Health Perspect* 2004; **112**(15): 1481–7.

93. Stoica GE, Franke TF, Moroni M. *et al.* Effect of estradiol on estrogen receptor-alpha gene expression and activity can be modulated by the ErbB2/PI 3-K/Akt pathway. *Oncogene* 2003; **22**(39): 7998–8011.

94. Razandi M, Pedram A, Greene GL, Levin ER. Cell membrane and nuclear estrogen receptors (ERs) originate from a single transcript: studies of ERalpha and ERbeta expressed in Chinese hamster ovary cells. *Mol Endocrinol* 1999; **13**(2): 307–19.

95. Song RX, Barnes CJ, Zhang Z. *et al.* The role of Shc and insulin-like growth factor 1 receptor in mediating the translocation of estrogen receptor alpha to the plasma membrane. *Proc Natl Acad Sci USA* 2004; **101**(7): 2076–81.

96. Yang SH, Liu R, Perez EJ. *et al.* Mitochondrial localization of estrogen receptor beta. *Proc Natl Acad Sci USA* 2004; **101**(12): 4130–5.

97. Maggiolini M, Vivacqua A, Fasanella G. *et al.* The G protein-coupled receptor GPR30 mediates c-fos up-regulation by 17{beta}-estradiol and phytoestrogens in breast cancer cells. *J Biol Chem* 2004; **279**(26): 27008–16.

98. Albanito L, Sisci D, Aquila S. *et al.* Epidermal growth factor induces G protein-coupled receptor 30 expression in estrogen receptor-negative breast cancer cells. *Endocrinology* 2008; **149**(8): 3799–808.

99. Brailoiu E, Dun SL, Brailoiu GC. *et al.* Distribution and characterization of estrogen receptor G protein-coupled receptor 30 in the rat central nervous system. *J Endocrinol* 2007; **193**(2): 311–21.

100. Lagrange AH, Ronnekleiv OK, Kelly MJ. Modulation of G protein-coupled receptors by an estrogen receptor that activates protein kinase A. *Mol Pharmacol* 1997; **51**(4): 605–12.

101. Le Mellay V, Grosse B, Lieberherr M. Phospholipase C beta and membrane action of calcitriol and estradiol. *J Biol Chem* 1997; **272**(18): 11 902–7.

102. Lu Q, Pallas DC, Surks HK. *et al.* Striatin assembles a membrane signaling complex necessary for rapid, nongenomic activation of endothelial NO synthase by estrogen receptor alpha. *Proc Natl Acad Sci USA* 2004; **101**(49): 17 126–31.

103. Wyckoff MH, Chambliss KL, Mineo C. *et al.* Plasma membrane estrogen receptors are coupled to endothelial nitric-oxide synthase through Galpha(i). *J Biol Chem* 2001; **276**(29): 27 071–6.

104. Razandi M, Pedram A, Merchenthaler I, Greene GL, Levin ER. Plasma membrane estrogen receptors exist and function as dimers. *Mol Endocrinol* 2004; **18**(12): 2854–65.

105. Christ M, Gunther A, Heck M. *et al.* Aldosterone, not estradiol, is the physiological agonist for rapid increases in cAMP in vascular smooth muscle cells. *Circulation* 1999; **99**(11): 1485–91.

106. Ravnskjaer K, Kester H, Liu Y. *et al.* Cooperative interactions between CBP and TORC2 confer selectivity to CREB target gene expression. *Embo J* 2007; **26**(12): 2880–9.

107. Canesi L, Lorusso LC, Ciacci C. *et al.* Environmental estrogens can affect the function of mussel hemocytes through rapid modulation of kinase pathways. *Gen Comp Endocrinol* 2004; **138**(1): 58–69.

108. Yoneda T, Hiroi T, Osada M, Asada A, Funae Y. Non-genomic modulation of dopamine release by bisphenol-A in PC12 cells. *J Neurochem* 2003; **87**(6): 1499–508.

109. Filardo EJ, Thomas P. GPR30: a seven-transmembrane-spanning estrogen receptor that triggers EGF release. *Trends Endocrinol Metab* 2005; **16**(8): 362–7.

110. Thomas P, Pang Y, Filardo EJ, Dong J. Identity of an estrogen membrane receptor coupled to a G protein in human breast cancer cells. *Endocrinology* 2005; **146**(2): 624–32.

111. Thomas P, Dong J. Binding and activation of the seven-transmembrane estrogen receptor GPR30 by environmental estrogens: a potential novel mechanism of endocrine disruption. *J Steroid Biochem Mol Biol* 2006; **102**(1–5): 175–9.

112. Funakoshi T, Yanai A, Shinoda K, Kawano MM, Mizukami Y. G protein-coupled receptor 30 is an estrogen receptor in the plasma membrane. *Biochem Biophys Res Commun* 2006; **346**(3): 904–10.

113. Pedram A, Razandi M, Levin ER. Nature of functional estrogen receptors at the plasma membrane. *Mol Endocrinol* 2006; **20**(9): 1996–2009.

114. Manavathi B, Kumar R. Steering estrogen signals from the plasma membrane to the nucleus: two sides of the coin. *J Cell Physiol* 2006; **207**(3): 594–604.

115. Shen K, Novak RF. DDT stimulates c-erbB2, c-met, and STATS tyrosine phosphorylation, Grb2-Sos association, MAPK phosphorylation, and proliferation of human breast epithelial cells. *Biochem Biophys Res Commun* 1997; **231**(1): 17–21.

116. Kahlert S, Nuedling S, van Eickels M. *et al.* Estrogen receptor alpha rapidly activates the IGF-1 receptor pathway. *J Biol Chem* 2000; **275**(24): 18 447–53.

117. Klaassen C, Amdiur M, Doull J. *Casarett and Doull's Toxicology: The Basic Scienc of Poisons.* New York: McGraw-Hill, 2001.

118. Norman A, Litwack G. *Hormones.* New York: Academic Press, 1987.

119. Damstra TBS, Bergman A, Kavlock R, Der Draak V. (eds). *WHO Global Asssessment of the State-of-the-Science of Endocrine Disruptors.* World Health Organization, 2002.

120. Bader D, Riskin A, Vafsi O. *et al.* Alpha-fetoprotein in the early neonatal period – a large study and review of the literature. *Clin Chim Acta* 2004; **349**(1–2): 15–23.

121. Parker KL, Schimmer BP. Transcriptional regulation of the genes encoding the cytochrome P-450 steroid hydroxylases. *Vitam Horm* 1995; **51**: 339–70.

122. Cai W, Benitez R, Counsell RE. *et al.* Bovine adrenal cortex transformations of mitotane [1-(2- chlorophenyl)-1-(4-chlorophenyl)-2,2-dichloroethane; o,p'-DDD] and its p,p'- and m,p'-isomers. *Biochem Pharmacol* 1995; **49**(10): 1483–9.

123. Martz F, Straw JA. Metabolism and covalent binding of 1-(o-chlorophenyl)-1-(p-chlorophenyl)-2,2-dichloroethane (o,p,'-DDD). Correlation between adrenocorticolytic activity and metabolic activation by adrenocortical mitochondria. *Drug Metab Dispos* 1980; **8**(3): 127–30.

124. Alavanja MC, Samanic C, Dosemeci M. *et al.* Use of agricultural pesticides and prostate cancer risk in the Agricultural Health Study cohort. *Am J Epidemiol* 2003; **157**(9): 800–14.

125. Mahajan R, Bonner MR, Hoppin JA, Alavanja MC. Phorate exposure and incidence of cancer in the agricultural health study. *Environ Health Perspect* 2006; **114**(8): 1205–9.

126. Usmani KA, Rose RL, Hodgson E. Inhibition and activation of the human liver microsomal and human cytochrome P450 3A4 metabolism of testosterone by deployment-related chemicals. *Drug Metab Dispos* 2003; **31**(4): 384–91.

127. Usmani KA, Cho TM, Rose RL, Hodgson E. Inhibition of the human liver microsomal and human cytochrome P450 1A2 and 3A4 metabolism of estradiol by deployment-related and other chemicals. *Drug Metab Dispos* 2006; **34**(9): 1606–14.

128. Sterling KM, Jr., Cutroneo KR. Constitutive and inducible expression of cytochromes P4501A (CYP1A1 and CYP1A2) in normal prostate and prostate cancer cells. *J Cell Biochem* 2004; **91**(2): 423–9.

129. Finnstrom N, Bjelfman C, Soderstrom TG. *et al.* Detection of cytochrome P450 mRNA transcripts in prostate samples by RT-PCR. *Eur J Clin Invest* 2001; **31**(10): 880–6.

130. Lawson T, Kolar C. Human prostate epithelial cells metabolize chemicals of dietary origin to mutagens. *Cancer Lett* 2002; **175**(2): 141–6.

131. Prins G. Endocrine disruptors and prostate cancer risk. *Endocrin Relat Cancer* 2008; 15: 649–56.

132. Prins GS, Korach KS. The role of estrogens and estrogen receptors in normal prostate growth and disease. *Steroids* 2008; **73**(3): 233–44.

133. Schurmeyer T, Nieschlag E. Effect of ketoconazole and other imidazole fungicides on testosterone biosynthesis. *Acta Endocrinol (Copenh)* 1984; **105**(2): 275–80.

134. Waller DP, Martin A, Vickery BH, Zaneveld LJ. The effect of ketoconazole on fertility of male rats. *Contraception* 1990; **41**(4): 411–17.

135. Heckman WR, Kane BR, Pakyz RE, Cosentino MJ. The effect of ketoconazole on endocrine and reproductive parameters in male mice and rats. *J Androl* 1992; **13**(3): 191–8.

136. Bhasin S, Sikka S, Fielder T. *et al.* Hormonal effects of ketoconazole in vivo in the male rat: mechanism of action. *Endocrinology* 1986; **118**(3): 1229–32.

137. Kellis JT Jr, Vickery LE. Inhibition of human estrogen synthetase (aromatase) by flavones. *Science* 1984; **225**(4666): 1032–4.

138. Akingbemi BT, Sottas CM, Koulova AI, Klinefelter GR, Hardy MP. Inhibition of testicular steroidogenesis by the xenoestrogen bisphenol A is associated with reduced pituitary luteinizing hormone secretion and decreased steroidogenic enzyme gene expression in rat Leydig cells. *Endocrinology* 2004; **145**(2): 592–603.

139. Chen S, Oh S-R, Phung S. *et al.* Anti-aromatase activity of phytochemicals in white button mushrooms (*Agaricus bisporus*). *Cancer Res* 2006; **66**(24): 12 026–34.

140. Wilson JD. Role of dihydrotestosterone in androgen action. *Prostate Suppl* 1996; **6**: 88–92.

141. Lo S, King I, Allèra A, Klingmüller D. Effects of various pesticides on human 5[alpha]-reductase activity in prostate and LNCaP cells. *Toxicol in Vitro* 2007; **21**(3): 502–8.

142. Kester MH, Bulduk S, Tibboel D. *et al.* Potent inhibition of estrogen sulfotransferase by hydroxylated PCB metabolites: a novel pathway explaining the estrogenic activity of PCBs. *Endocrinology* 2000; **141**(5): 1897–900.

143. Harris RM, Wood DM, Bottomley L. *et al.* Phytoestrogens are potent inhibitors of estrogen sulfation: implications for breast cancer risk and treatment. *J Clin Endocrinol Metab* 2004; **89**(4): 1779–87.

144. Qian YM, Song WC. Regulation of estrogen sulfotransferase expression in Leydig cells by cyclic adenosine 3',5'-monophosphate and androgen. *Endocrinology* 1999; **140**(3): 1048–53.

145. Waddington CH. *Endeavor* 1942; **1**: 18–20.

146. Fraga MF, Ballestar E, Paz MF. *et al.* Epigenetic differences arise during the lifetime of monozygotic twins. *Proc Natl Acad Sci USA* 2005; **102**(30): 10 604–9.

147. Holliday R, Pugh JE. DNA modification mechanisms and gene activity during development. *Science* 1975; **187**(4173): 226–32.

148. Riggs AD. X inactivation, differentiation, and DNA methylation. *Cytogenet Cell Genet* 1975; **14**(1): 9–25.

149. Fatemi M, Pao MM, Jeong S. *et al.* Footprinting of mammalian promoters: use of a CpG DNA methyltransferase revealing nucleosome positions at a single molecule level. *Nucleic Acids Res* 2005; **33**(20): e176.

150. Allis C, Jenuwein, T, Reinberg, D. In Caparros M, ed. *Epigenetics*. Cold Springs Harbor: Cold Springs Harbor Laboratory Press, 2007.

151. Jackson-Grusby L, Beard C, Possemato R. *et al.* Loss of genomic methylation causes p53-dependent apoptosis and epigenetic deregulation. *Nat Genet* 2001; **27**(1): 31–9.

152. Li E, Bestor TH, Jaenisch R. Targeted mutation of the DNA methyltransferase gene results in embryonic lethality. *Cell* 1992; **69**(6): 915–26.

153. Lei H, Oh SP, Okano M. *et al.* De novo DNA cytosine methyltransferase activities in mouse embryonic stem cells. *Development* 1996; **122**(10): 3195–205.

154. Okano M, Bell DW, Haber DA, Li E. DNA methyltransferases Dnmt3a and Dnmt3b are essential for de novo methylation and mammalian development. *Cell* 1999; **99**(3): 247–57.

155. Okano M, Xie S, Li E. Dnmt2 is not required for de novo and maintenance methylation of viral DNA in embryonic stem cells. *Nucleic Acids Res* 1998; **26**(11): 2536–40.

156. Hermann A, Schmitt S, Jeltsch A. The human Dnmt2 has residual DNA-(cytosine-C5) methyltransferase activity. *J Biol Chem* 2003; **278**(34): 31 717–21.

157. Santos F, Hendrich B, Reik W, Dean W. Dynamic reprogramming of DNA methylation in the early mouse embryo. *Dev Biol* 2002; **241**(1): 172–82.

158. Jenuwein T. The epigenetic magic of histone lysine methylation. *Febs J* 2006; **273**(14): 3121–35.

159. Quivy V, Calomme C, Dekoninck A. *et al.* Gene activation and gene silencing: a subtle equilibrium. *Cloning Stem Cells* 2004; **6**(2): 140–9.

160. Jenuwein T, Allis CD. Translating the histone code. *Science* 2001; **293**(5532): 1074–80.

161. Martin C, Zhang Y. Mechanisms of epigenetic inheritance. *Curr Opin Cell Biol* 2007; **19**(3): 266–72.

162. Pluemsampant S, Safronova OS, Nakahama K, Morita I. Protein kinase CK2 is a key activator of histone deacetylase in hypoxia-associated tumors. *Int J Cancer* 2008; **122**(2): 333–41.

163. Garcia-Bassets I, Kwon YS, Telese F. *et al.* Histone methylation-dependent mechanisms impose ligand dependency for gene activation by nuclear receptors. *Cell* 2007; **128**(3): 505–18.

164. Blazquez M, Koornneef M, Putterill J. Flowering on time: genes that regulate the floral transition. Workshop on the molecular basis of flowering time control. *EMBO Rep* 2001; **2**(12): 1078–82.

165. Kucharski R, Maleszka J, Foret S, Maleszka R. Nutritional control of reproductive status in honeybees via DNA methylation. *Science* 2008; **319**(5871): 1827–30.

166. Schaefer CB, Ooi SKT, Bestor TH, Bourc'his D. Epigenetic decisions in mammalian germ cells. *Science* 2007; **316**(5823): 398–9.

167. Sanz LA, Chamberlain S, Sabourin JC. *et al.* A mono-allelic bivalent chromatin domain controls tissue-specific imprinting at *Grb10*. *Embo J* 2008 **27**: 2523–32.

168. Alworth LC, Howdeshell KL, Ruhlen RL. *et al.* Uterine responsiveness to estradiol and DNA methylation are altered by fetal exposure to diethylstilbestrol and methoxychlor in CD-1 mice: effects of low versus high doses. *Toxicol Appl Pharmacol* 2002; **183**(1): 10–22.

169. Dolinoy DC, Huang D, Jirtle RL. Maternal nutrient supplementation counteracts bisphenol A-induced DNA hypomethylation in early development. *Proc Natl Acad Sci USA* 2007; **104**(32): 13 056–61.

170. Anway MD, Rekow SS, Skinner MK. Transgenerational epigenetic programming of the embryonic testis transcriptome. *Genomics* 2008; **91**(1): 30–40.

171. Waalkes MP, Liu J, Chen H. *et al.* Estrogen signaling in livers of male mice with hepatocellular carcinoma induced by exposure to arsenic in utero. *J Natl Cancer Inst* 2004; **96**(6): 466–74.

172. Li S, Washburn KA, Moore R. *et al.* Developmental exposure to diethylstilbestrol elicits demethylation of estrogen-responsive lactoferrin gene in mouse uterus. *Cancer Res* 1997; **57**(19): 4356–9.

173. Welshons WV, Thayer KA, Judy BM. *et al.* Large effects from small exposures. i. mechanisms for endocrine-disrupting chemicals with estrogenic activity. *Environ Health Perspect* 2003; **111**(8): 994.

174. Varayoud J, Ramos JG, Bosquiazzo VL, Munoz-de-Toro M, Luque EH. Developmental exposure to bisphenol a impairs the uterine response to ovarian steroids in the adult. *Endocrinology* 2008; **149**(11): 5848–60.

175. Li S, Ma L, Chiang T. *et al.* Promoter CpG methylation of Hox-a10 and Hox-a11 in mouse uterus not altered upon neonatal diethylstilbestrol exposure. *Mol Carcin* 2001; **32**(4): 213–19.

176. Ho SM, Tang WY, Belmonte de Frausto J, Prins GS. Developmental exposure to estradiol and bisphenol A increases susceptibility to prostate carcinogenesis and epigenetically regulates phosphodiesterase type 4 variant 4. *Cancer Res* 2006; **66**(11): 5624–32.

177. Newbold RR, Bullock BC, McLachlan JA. Uterine adenocarcinoma in mice following developmental treatment with estrogens: a model for hormonal carcinogenesis. *Cancer Res* 1990; **50**(23): 7677–81.

178. Newbold RR, Jefferson WN, Grissom SF. *et al.* Developmental exposure to diethylstilbestrol alters uterine gene expression that may be associated with uterine neoplasia later in life. *Mol Carcin* 2007; **46**(9): 783–96.

179. Tang WY, Newbold R, Mardilovich K. *et al.* Persistent hypomethylation in the promoter of nucleosomal binding protein 1 (Nsbp1) correlates with overexpression of Nsbp1 in mouse uteri

neonatally exposed to diethylstilbestrol or genistein. *Endocrinology* 2008; **149**(12): 5922–31.

180. Crews D. Epigenetics and its implications for behavioral neuroendocrinology. *Front Neuroendocrinol* 2008; **29**(3): 344–57.

181. Champagne FA. Epigenetic mechanisms and the transgenerational effects of maternal care. *Front Neuroendocrinol* 2008; **29**(3): 386–97.

182. Steinberg RM, Walker DM, Juenger TE, Woller MJ, Gore AC. Effects of perinatal polychlorinated biphenyls on adult female rat reproduction: development, reproductive physiology, and second generational effects. *Biol Reprod* 2008; **78**(6): 1091–101.

183. Anway MD, Leathers C, Skinner MK. Endocrine disruptor vinclozolin induced epigenetic transgenerational adult-onset disease. *Endocrinology* 2006; **147**(12): 5515–23.

184. Anway MD, Cupp AS, Uzumcu M, Skinner MK. Epigenetic transgenerational actions of endocrine disruptors and male fertility. *Science* 2005; **308**(5727): 1466–9.

185. Nilsson EE, Anway MD, Stanfield J, Skinner MK. Transgenerational epigenetic effects of the endocrine disruptor vinclozolin on pregnancies and female adult onset disease. *Reproduction* 2008; **135**(5): 713–21.

# Developmental exposures and implications for early and latent disease

Retha R. Newbold and Jerrold J. Heindel

## Introduction

A complex series of events is involved in the development of the mammalian fetus and neonate; in order to go from a single cell to a fully developed organism containing over one trillion cells composed of over 300 different cell types at birth, a number of well-orchestrated events are required. Processes including cell division, proliferation, differentiation, and migration are all involved and are closely regulated by hormones that communicate information between specializing cells, tissues, and organs. Over the past 50-plus years, embryonic and fetal development was thought to occur by the "unfolding of a rigid genetic program" where environmental factors played no significant role (for review see *Soto et al.* [1]). However, this strict interpretation of developmental events has been challenged because numerous experimental and epidemiologic studies point out the developmental plasticity of the fetus and neonate. In fact, it is becoming increasingly apparent that environmental factors such as nutrition, and external stressors and toxicants can dramatically alter developmental programming signals. This represents a major paradigm shift in developmental biology/toxicology and focuses attention on the role of environmental factors in fetal growth and development. It is now clear that the placenta is not a completely impenetrable barrier protecting and insulating the fetus from the outside world and that, in many cases, the fetus and neonate are more sensitive than the adult to the same environmental insults.

In 1992, Professor Howard Bern coined the term "the fragile fetus" to denote the extreme vulnerability of a developing organism to perturbation by environmental chemicals, in particular those with hormone-like activity [2]. He pointed out that rapid cell proliferation and cell differentiation coupled with complex patterns of cell signaling contributed to its unique sensitivity. Further, fetuses and neonates have a high metabolic rate as compared with adults, and liver metabolism is not completely developed; fetuses also have an under-developed immune system, lack many detoxifying enzymes, and the blood–brain barrier is not fully functional, making them prone to chemical insult. Exposure to environmental chemicals during development can result in fetal death in the most severe cases, or structural malformations and/or functional alterations in the embryo or fetus. Unlike adult exposures that can result in reversible – activational – alterations, developmental exposure to environmental chemicals or other factors during critical windows of differentiation can cause irreversible – organizational – consequences. Some of these consequences, like birth defects, can be seen immediately: prenatal exposure to thalidomide, a drug used to treat maternal anxiety and depression, resulted in limb deformities in the exposed offspring; this chemical is probably the best-known example of a prenatal teratogen. Other consequences of developmental exposure may not be seen until much later in life [3]: prenatal exposure to the potent synthetic estrogen diethylstilbestrol (DES) which was prescribed to prevent miscarriage, is a well-known example where a multitude of adverse consequences were not seen until later in life [4]. In fact, the full extent of the consequences of this chemical exposure is still unfolding as the DES population ages.

The realization that developmental exposure to drugs and chemicals like DES can cause permanent functional changes that are not overtly toxic like ionizing radiation or teratogenic like thalidomide, yet result in increased susceptibility to disease/dysfunction later in life, has led to a new field of toxicology called "the developmental origins of disease."

*Environmental Impacts on Reproductive Health and Fertility*, ed. T. J. Woodruff, S. J. Janssen, L. J. Guillette, and L. C. Giudice. Published by Cambridge University Press. © Cambridge University Press 2010.

# The developmental origins of disease/dysfunction

This concept was first used in the field of nutrition, where epidemiologic studies found that "low birth weight" babies resulting from poor nutrition of their mothers had latent appearance of disease in adult life which included increased susceptibility to non-communicable diseases, coronary heart disease, obesity/overweight, type 2 diabetes, osteoporosis, and metabolic dysfunction [5]. Subsequently, chronic stress during development was also associated with similar latent responses; for example, experimental studies using macaque monkeys demonstrated that early life stress resulted in obesity and increased incidences of metabolic diseases later in life [6]. Maternal smoking, another fetal stressor, was also linked to the development of obesity and disease later in life [7]. These studies represent some examples in the literature that have led to a substantial research effort focusing on perinatal influences and subsequent chronic disease [8].

Supporting evidence for this concept independently developed in the field of environmental chemical exposure, specifically developmental toxicology, where it was recognized that between 2 and 5% of all live births have major developmental abnormalities. Up to 40% of these defects have been estimated to result from maternal exposures to harmful environmental agents that impact the intrauterine environment [9,10]. Although a spectrum of adverse effects can occur ranging from fetal death or frank structural malformations, to functional defects which may not be readily apparent, the latter may be the most common and those that result in increased susceptibility to disease/dysfunction later in life. These defects are the most difficult to detect because the length of time may be years between exposure and detection of the abnormality. However, numerous examples in experimental animals and wildlife populations document that perinatal exposure to endocrine-disrupting chemicals (EDCs) can alter the developing organism and cause long-term effects including infertility/subfertility, retained testes, altered puberty, premature menopause, and increased cancer rates (for reviews, see Colborn *et al.* and Crain *et al.* [11,12]). Taken together, nutritional studies describing an association of restricted fetal growth with the subsequent development of obesity and metabolic diseases, and experimental toxicology studies showing a correlation of prenatal exposure to EDCs with multiple long-term adverse effects, provide an attractive framework to understand delayed effects of toxicant exposures.

For example, the "developmental origins of disease and dysfunction" paradigm now incorporates features that are common to both nutritional and environmental exposure studies; these features are further outlined:

- Time-specific (vulnerable window) and tissue-specific effects can occur with both nutritional and environmental chemical exposures.
- The initiating in utero environmental insult (nutritional or environmental chemical) can act alone or in concert with other environmental stressors. That is, there could be an in utero exposure that would lead by itself to pathophysiology later in life or there could be in utero exposure combined with a neonatal exposure (same or different environmental stressor(s)) or adult exposure that would trigger or exacerbate the pathophysiology.
- The pathophysiology can manifest as: the occurrence of a disease that otherwise would not have happened; an increase in risk for a disease that would normally be of lower prevalence; either an earlier onset of a disease that would normally have occurred or an exacerbation of the disease.
- The pathophysiology can have a variable latent period from onset in the neonatal period, to early childhood, to puberty, to early adulthood to late adulthood depending on the environmental stressor, time of exposure, and tissue/organ affected.
- Either altered nutrition and/or exposure to environmental chemicals can lead to aberrant developmental programming that permanently alters gland, organ, or system potential. These states of altered potential or compromised function (regardless of the stressor – nutritional or chemical exposure) are likely to result from epigenetic changes e.g. altered gene expression due to effects on imprinting, and the underlying methylation-related protein-DNA relationships associated with chromatin remodeling. The end result is an individual that is sensitized such that it will be more susceptible to certain diseases later in life.
- The effect of either developmental nutrition or environmental chemical exposures can be transgenerational, affecting future generations.

93

- While the focus of nutritional changes during development has been on low birthweight, effects of in utero exposure to toxic environmental chemicals or nutritional changes can occur in the absence of reduced birthweight. The lack of a specific easily measurable biomarker like birthweight makes it more difficult to assess developmental effects. Thus, for both exposures, new more sensitive biomarkers of exposure are needed.

- Extrapolation of risk from both nutritional studies and environmental exposures can be difficult because effects need not follow a monotonic dose–response relationship. Nutritional effects which result in low birthweight are different from those that result in high birthweight. Similarly, low-dose effects of environmental chemicals may not be the same as the effects that occur at higher doses. Also, the environmental chemical and/or nutritional effects may have an entirely different effect on the embryo, fetus, or perinatal organism, compared with the adult.

- Exposure of one individual to an environmental stressor (environmental chemical or nutritional or combinations) may have little effect, whereas another individual will develop overt disease or dysfunctions due to differences in genetic background including genetic polymorphisms.

- The toxicant (or nutritional)-induced pathogenic responses are most likely the result of altered gene expression or altered protein regulation associated with altered cell production and differentiation that are involved in the interactions between cell types and the establishment of cell lineages. These changes can lead to abnormal morphological and/or functional characteristics of the tissues, organs, and systems. These alterations could be due, at least in part, to altered epigenetics and the underlining methylation-related protein-DNA relationships associated with chromatin remodeling. Effects can occur in a time-specific (i.e. vulnerable window) and/or tissue-specific manner and the changes might not be reversible. The end result is an animal that is sensitized such that it will be more susceptible to specific diseases later in life.

These key concepts are important aspects of the "developmental origins of disease and dysfunction" paradigm. To further examine and to provide additional support for the concept, a well-known example of perinatal chemical exposure which causes latent adverse health effects is described.

# Prenatal exposure to diethylstilbestrol as an example of the developmental origin of disease/dysfunction

Diethylstilbestrol (DES), a synthetic non-steroidal pharmaceutical with estrogenic activity, was heavily prescribed from the late 1940s through the 1970s to women with high-risk pregnancies with the mistaken belief that it would prevent miscarriage and other complications of pregnancy. In 1971, a hallmark report associated prenatal DES treatment with a rare form of reproductive tract cancer, "vaginal clear cell adenocarcinoma," which was detected in a small number (< 0.1%) of adolescent daughters of women who had taken the drug while pregnant [13]. Subsequently, DES was linked to more frequent benign reproductive tract problems in more than 95% of the DES-exposed daughters; reproductive tract malformation and dysfunction, poor pregnancy outcome, and immune system disorders were also some of the reported effects. Likewise, prenatally DES-exposed men experienced a range of reproductive tract abnormalities including hypospadias, microphallus, retained testes, and increased genital-urinary inflammation [4,14,15]. Although increased incidence in prostatic and testicular cancers was proposed, so far the DES-exposed population has not experienced a documented rise in these diseases as compared with unexposed men but rigorous studies await a definitive conclusion.

Thus, DES became a well-documented example of the developmental origin of disease/dysfunction. In fact, it had the dubious distinction of being the first example of a transplacental carcinogen in humans; it was shown to cross the placenta and to induce a direct carcinogenic effect on the developing fetus. Unlike thalidomide which caused immediate observable limb defects, many of the abnormalities caused by DES could not be detected until later in life. Diethylstilbestrol resulted in a major medical catastrophe that continues to unfold today. Although it is no longer prescribed to prevent miscarriage, a major concern remains that, as DES-exposed individuals age and reach the time when the incidence of reproductive organ tumors normally increase, they will show a much higher incidence of lesions than unexposed individuals. An example can be seen in the reports of DES-exposed women who are showing a higher incidence of breast cancer as they age as compared with unexposed individuals [16]. Another concern is that additional organ

**Table 7.1.** Comparative effects of prenatal diethylstilbestrol (DES) exposure in mice and humans: an example of the developmental origins of reproductive disease and dysfunction.

| Abnormality | Male offspring | Female offspring |
|---|---|---|
| Reproductive tract dysfunction | Subfertility/infertility<br>Decreased sperm counts | Subfertility/infertility<br>Poor reproductive outcome<br>Early puberty<br>Menstrual (estrous) cycle irregularities<br>Premature menopause/early reproductive senescence |
| Structural malformations | Microphallus and hypospadias<br>Retained hypoplastic testes<br>Retained müllerian remnants (anatomical feminization) | Oviduct, uterus, cervix, and vagina<br>Paraovarian cysts of mesonephric origin<br>Retained mesonephric remnants |
| Cellular abnormalities | Testicular tumors<br>Tumors in retained müllerian remnants<br>Epididymal cysts<br>Prostatic lesions and inflammation<br>Multigenerational effects (? Humans) | Oviductal proliferative lesions<br>Vaginal adenomyosis and adenocarcinoma<br>Uterine fibroids<br>Uterine cancer (? in humans)<br>Breast cancer (? mice)<br>Multigenerational effects |

systems (urinary, immune, cardiovascular, brain/nervous, gastrointestinal, bone, adipocytes) may be affected. Further, the possibility of multigenerational effects is suggested by experimental animal studies [17] and a case report of an ovarian carcinoma in a DES-exposed granddaughter [18] which suggests that another generation may be at risk for developing health problems associated with DES treatment of their grandmothers. The DES episode is a salient reminder of the potential toxicity and carcinogenicity that may be caused by hormonally active chemicals if exposure occurs during critical windows of susceptibility.

Questions about the mechanisms involved in DES-induced abnormalities prompted the development of numerous experimental animal models to study the adverse effects of estrogens and other EDCs on genital tract differentiation. Since the murine model has been particularly successful in duplicating and predicting many adverse effects observed in humans with similar DES-exposure (for review see Newbold [3]), detailed findings in the animal model follow.

## Diethylstilbestrol murine model to study human disease: critical windows of susceptibility

### Prenatal exposure

Timed pregnant outbred CD-1 mice were treated with DES on days 9–16 of gestation, the major period of organogenesis in the mouse. After birth, the offspring were followed for up to 24 months of age. The doses

of DES range from 0.01–100 µg/kg maternal body weight. The highest dose of DES is equal to or less than that given therapeutically to pregnant women, and the lower DES doses are comparable with exposure to weak estrogenic compounds found in the environment. Diethylstilbestrol exposure during this critical prenatal period of sex differentiation resulted in significant alterations in both female and male offspring [3]. A summary and comparison of the abnormalities observed in prenatally DES-exposed humans and mice are shown in Table 7.1.

In the prenatally DES-exposed females, the frequency of vaginal adenocarcinoma was rare in mice as it was in humans (< 0.1%). However, other regions of the murine reproductive tract were also a target for DES; the cervix was often enlarged and there was a low prevalence of benign (leiomyomas) and malignant (stromal cell sarcomas, leiomyosarcomas) tumors in this area. In the uterus, cystic endometrial hyperplasia was a common finding and, as in the cervix, there was a low incidence of benign (leiomyomas) and malignant (stromal cell sarcomas, leiomyosarcomas) uterine tumors. The ovaries of prenatal DES-treated mice were often cystic and had an enhanced tumor incidence compared with age-matched controls. In addition to cellular changes in reproductive tissues, these DES females had a high incidence of reproductive tract malformations in the oviduct, uterus, and cervix; these malformations were subsequently found in DES humans. Further, they had functional defects including early puberty, subfertility/infertility, and premature reproductive senescence (early menopause) [19].

In the prenatally DES-exposed male mice, 1% of the animals had benign interstitial cell tumors of the testes while 2% had interstitial cell tumors. Interstitial cell tumors have been produced experimentally in certain strains of mice after prolonged treatment with various estrogenic compounds [20] but not after short-term prenatal exposure. Further, the significance of our finding in the prenatal DES model was that there were so many malignant interstitial cell tumors in proportion to the number of benign tumors. In addition, interstitial cell tumors were not common in this strain of mouse.

Since testicular seminoma was reported in prenatally DES-exposed men [4,15], we specifically screened for this lesion in prenatally DES-exposed mice. Seminomas have been experimentally induced in dogs but such germ cell tumors in rodents are very rare. Cryptorchidism is considered to be a predisposing factor for seminoma in dogs and men, but in spite of the high incidence of retained testis in our mouse model (91%), we were not able to demonstrate this particular testicular lesion except in one case of all our historical DES-treated mice. However, a more common lesion resembling adenocarcinoma of the rete testis was observed in 5% mice after in utero DES exposure. To date, no reports of rete adenocarcinoma in humans have been attributed to prenatal DES exposure, but three cases of seminoma reported in DES-exposed men could have been misdiagnosed since seminoma has to be ruled out before a diagnosis of rete adenocarcinoma can be made. This requires further study.

The association of prenatal DES exposure and the development of testicular tumors in men has become a subject of much controversy over the last few years; some reports, specifically addressing factors for cancer of the testis, list prenatal DES exposure as a risk factor, whereas other studies show no relationship to hormonal treatment during pregnancy. However, the data in our experimental mouse model support the idea that DES-treated males are at a greater risk for testicular tumors than unexposed males.

In addition to the testes, tumors were observed in retained embryonic structures (müllerian remnants) in 8% of the DES-exposed mice; tumors in embryonic-derived wolffian tissue were rare other than in the rete testis. Inflammation and squamous metaplasia of the prostate were seen in our DES-exposed mice and have been reported in similarly exposed humans.

Taken together, these data in female and male mice suggest that in utero exposure to DES caused a multitude of reproductive tract abnormalities including a low, but significant, increase in reproductive tract tumors; structural (malformations) and functional (subfertility/infertility) effects were also commonly observed depending on the dose.

## Neonatal exposure

Since experimental studies from a number of laboratories suggested developmental exposure to DES during only neonatal life resulted in a high incidence of vaginal abnormalities [21,22], the effects of DES in females were compared following prenatal and neonatal treatment. Using the same animal model, newborn CD-1 mice were treated with DES (2 µg/pup per day) on days 1–5. Neonatal exposure resulted in a high incidence (90–95%) of uterine cancer at 18 months [23]. Other species including rats [24] and hamsters [25] also have a high incidence of uterine tumors following neonatal treatment with DES. Thus, the neonatal mouse model replicates tumors seen in other experimental animal models and is possibly predictive of the carcinogenic potential of estrogenic chemicals in the uterus of women as they age because many of the developmental processes that occur neonatally in mice actually occur prenatally in women. This points out an important maxim in developmental studies: the stage of tissue differentiation is more important in predicting adverse effects of environmental insults than the chronological age of the organism. This is further verified by our study comparing sensitive windows of DES exposure in experimental animals and humans; for two endpoints, retained testes and vaginal neoplasia, the best fit for incidence of lesions in the two species occurred when stage of tissue differentiation at the time of treatment was compared rather than specific age [26].

Thus, developmental exposure (prenatal or neonatal) to DES resulted in increased incidences of reproductive tract abnormalities including tumors (benign and malignant). In general, prenatal treatment caused a high incidence of malformation and a low, but significant, increase in reproductive tract tumors; whereas neonatal treatment caused a low incidence of malformation, but a high incidence of reproductive tract neoplasia. Predictably, this supports the developmental maximum described where it is apparent that the timing of exposure and the stage of tissue differentiation determine the subsequent resulting abnormalities. Further, since many developmental events that occur in the mouse during prenatal and neonatal life happen entirely prenatally in humans, the prenatal plus neonatal mouse model can be useful in predicting what happens prenatally in humans. In humans, the timing of exposure during gestation was also shown to be an important factor for cancer risk in DES-exposed daughters; research showed that exposure early in pregnancy was associated with a greater risk for vaginal adenocarcinoma than exposure later in pregnancy [4,15].

# Early effects: childhood disease/ dysfunction following developmental exposure

## Reproductive tract malformations

Cryptorchid (retained) testes were common problems observed in both experimental animal models and boys following prenatal exposure to DES [14]. Likewise, hypospadias and microphallus were reported. These findings have been used as a guide to look for similar changes following exposure to other environmental chemicals and numerous examples now suggest these birth defects are not limited to DES. In fact, a whole body of literature has developed describing studies of EDC effects on the developing male genital tract and these effects are referred to as "the testicular dysgenesis syndrome" to denote the effects on multiple tissues and reproductive endpoints. Early life exposures and these particular abnormalities are covered in detail in Chapter 11.

Recently, another study showed for the first time a statistical link between prenatal exposure to phthalates and ano-genital distance (AGD) in boys [27]. Ano-genital distance is considered a sensitive marker of anti androgen activity in the development of the rodent genital tract. This marker is sexually dimorphic and androgen dependent in both humans and rodents. Swan and colleagues observed that boys born to mothers with phthalate metabolites present in their urine were at higher risk of impaired testicular descent and shorter AGD. A similar effect has been observed in experimental animals and a "phthalate syndrome" which includes testicular, epididymal, and gubernacular cord agenesis has been described [28]. Although the mechanisms of phthalate disruption of male sex differentiation are different from those caused by the estrogen DES, many resulting abnormalities are similar because DES dampens the effects of androgens which masculinize the male genital tract during development and differentiation. This idea points out the multiple routes and mechanisms that can be involved in abnormal differentiation of reproductive tract tissues.

# Altered puberty (early or delayed)

Puberty is marked by the development of secondary sex characteristics, accelerated growth, behavioral changes, and finally attainment of the ability to reproduce. There is general agreement that the age of puberty is getting earlier for both boys and girls, and this has been attributed to exposure to environmental chemicals especially EDCs during prenatal and/or early childhood life [29]. Many of these chemicals can mimic the effects of DES. Although DES is a potent estrogen, low doses have been successfully used to study the effects of other environmental estrogens. In addition to DES [14], studies using experimental animals and wildlife point to numerous examples of chemicals such as pesticides [30], PCBs [30], polybrominated biphenols [31], and bisphenol-A [32] which are associated with early puberty; many of these same chemicals have been associated with signs of early puberty in girls. Interestingly, some chemicals have been reported to have opposite effects; examples include lead [33] and endosulfan [34], which have been associated with delayed puberty. Multiple mechanisms, many involving alterations in the hypothalamic–pituitary–gonadal axis, can be responsible for altered timing of pubertal events. For a more in-depth discussion of environmental chemical effects on puberty, see Chapter 9. The timing of puberty is important for numerous societal issues but also a risk factor for diseases later in life especially those that are influenced by hormones. For example, the total duration of estrogen exposure during a woman's life has been linked with her chance of developing breast cancer; thus early puberty combined with late menopause causes the highest risk.

## Obesity

Another example of developmental exposure being associated with childhood health and disease can be seen with the link of EDCs and obesity. Obesity and overweight have increased in prevalence dramatically over the past two to three decades. It is now reaching epidemic proportions in the USA. Common causes have usually been attributed to high calorie/fat diets and lack of exercise combined with a genetic predisposition for the disease. However, the alarming rise in obesity can not be solely explained by these factors; an environmental component must be involved. A recent hypothesis by Baillie-Hamilton [35] suggests that exposure to environmental chemicals during critical stages of adipogenesis (neonatal life) is contributing to the obesity epidemic. Experimental animal studies support her theory; developmental exposure to numerous chemicals including DES and other estrogens [36], tributyl tin [37], and bisphenol-A [32] have shown increases in weight and adipocity. The term "obesogens" has been coined for environmental chemicals that stimulate fat accumulation [37]. Childhood obesity is a significant human health problem because most obese children grow up to be obese adults; and further, it is such a difficult disease to treat.

Obesity and overweight are known to have adverse health effects, and to impact the risk and prognosis for a number of serious medical conditions such as type 2 diabetes, hyperinsulinemia, insulin resistance, coronary heart disease, high blood pressure, stroke, gout, liver disease, asthma and pulmonary problems, gall bladder disease, kidney disease, reproductive problems, osteoarthritis, and some forms of cancer [38,39]. Unfortunately, these illnesses are starting to be more frequently reported in obese and overweight children whereas in the past, these were diseases of older adults. Health professionals warn that the current generation of children may be the first in history to experience a shorter life expectancy than their parents due to the impact of obesity-related diseases.

# Latent effects: adult disease/ dysfunction following developmental exposure

## Menstrual cycle irregularities

Alterations in the menstrual cycle such as shortened or prolonged length, abnormal bleeding between cycles, lack of ovulation, absence of menstruation, etc. can result in subfertility and/or infertility. It may also be involved in multiple other health problems since the controlling endocrine system is responsible for communicating cellular signals throughout the body. Exposures to numerous chemicals such as lead, dioxins, and PCBs have been linked to menstrual cycle irregularities in women; however, most of the data involve exposure as adults, not developmental exposures. Investigators are just now starting to evaluate the effects of fetal and early neonatal exposure to chemicals, especially some EDCs, to determine if menstrual cycle irregularity is a reproductive endpoint that may be affected. However, we know from experimental animals where estrous cycle irregularities have been documented and from prenatally DES-exposed women that

the menstrual cycle is a likely targeted process that will be adversely affected.

## Endometriosis

Endometriosis is a disease of menstruating species and is characterized by ectopic sites of endometrial growth following retrograde menstruation. While estrogen is a risk factor for endometriosis, progesterone may play a role in protecting women from the development and progression of the disease. In addition, endometriosis is an invasive process that requires degradation of the extracellular matrix, a process that has been reported to be associated with expression and action of members of the matrix metalloproteinase family [40]. As discussed by these investigators [40], since some degree of retrograde menstruation occurs in nearly all normally cycling women, genetic and/or environmental factors must play a role in the etiology of the disease. This laboratory has developed an animal model of endometriosis and has shown that female mice exposed to 2,3,7,8-tetrachlorodibenzo-$p$-dioxin (TCDD) in utero and again during the development of reproductive potential show a progressive loss of progesterone receptor (PR-A and PR-B) expression. Further, they report the ability of TCDD exposure to reduce PR expression in stromal cells and increase matrix metalloproteinases by both stromal and epithelial cells, which could explain the development of endometriosis. This work is not only an example of developmental exposure leading to disease later in life but also highlights the fact that developmental exposure "sets the stage" for subsequent exposures to be more effective (a two-hit model of the developmental basis of disease).

## Fibroids (leiomyomata)

Uterine leiomyomas, commonly called fibroids, are tumors of smooth muscle origin which cause pain, bleeding, infertility, and pregnancy complications; they are the leading indication for hysterectomy. Fibroids are the most common type of tumor in women over 30 years of age and estimated incidence rates are that as many as 77% of women of reproductive age are afflicted with the disease. In mice, early life exposure to DES has been reported to cause fibroid development in adult animals [19]. Data from our DES mouse model have shown that these tumors occur in approximately 9% of the DES-treated mice as compared to < 1% incidence in unexposed animals. Interestingly, we have also shown an association of fibroids with prenatal DES treatment in humans [41]. Our data with both DES-exposed mice and humans indicate a role for prenatal estrogen exposure in the etiology of uterine fibroids. This is a relatively new area of research that awaits information from effects of other EDCs in both human and other experimental animal models.

There is, however, another animal model relevant to developmental estrogen exposure and fibroid development. Studies using the Eker rat which contains a defective tumor suppressor gene have shown increased susceptibility to uterine fibroids following early life exposure to DES [42]. The defective gene resulted in reprogramming of the myometrium leading to an increase in expression of estrogen-responsive genes. Later in life, these neonatal DES-exposed rats have increased tumor suppressor gene penetrance that correlates with increased tumor size and multiplicity. This is discussed in detail in Chapter 6. This effect of DES in the Eker rat is an example of gene–environment interactions during development.

Together these data suggest that uterine fibroids observed in women of reproductive age may originate during development and early life, and that altered uterine programming due to exposure to environmental estrogens may play a role in their etiology.

## Prostatic and breast cancer

The increase in cancer rates especially the two hormonally related diseases prostatic and breast cancer has been a central premise in the endocrine disruptor hypothesis for years [11,43]. Since estrogens are known risk factors for the development of breast cancer, it is likely that exposures to EDCs with estrogenic activity can adversely affect the developing mammary gland. Evidence to support a link between EDC exposure and subsequent mammary cancer comes from numerous animal studies including developmental exposure to bisphenol-A [1], dioxin [44], and DES [45]. Epidemiologic studies also support a link since women exposed to DES during prenatal development have a statistically significant increase in breast cancer rates [16]. This increase was detected only as the women aged (40 years plus) and reached a time at which breast cancer is usually diagnosed; thus, fetal exposure can have long-term latent effects in the adult.

Similar associations have been proposed for prostate cancer. Prostate development and differentiation is known to be under the control of androgens and is sensitive to perturbation by estrogenic chemicals. Again, developmental exposure to DES provides an excellent example in experimental animal models [46]. However, studies with other environmental chemicals such as BPA and dioxin also show that the developing prostate can be disrupted if exposure occurs during prenatal life [47]. Further, a recent study shows that developmental exposure to BPA can alter the programming of the prostate so that it is more sensitive to environmental insult later in life and result in increased prostate disease and tumors [48]. This increase in susceptibility is attributed to epigenetic mechanisms and is further discussed in Chapter 14.

Together these data are consistent with the hypothesis that developmental exposure to chemicals with hormone-like activity may increase the risks of breast and prostate cancer.

## Multigenerational effects

Perhaps the most compelling data for an association of developmental exposure and multigenerational effects comes from experimental studies of methoxychlor (an estrogenic pesticide) and vinclozolin (an antiandrogenic fungicide given by intra-peritoneal injection at high doses) in male mice exposed on gestational days 8–15 [49]. In utero exposure to these chemicals caused infertility in a small percent of the exposed animals after 90 days of age and reduced sperm counts in 90% of the animals along with immune abnormalities, kidney disease, prostate lesions, and cancer; however, most importantly, these effects were transmitted through the male germ line for at least four generations. The transgenerational effects were only seen when exposure correlated with critical developmental processes such as germ cell methylation in the differentiating testes. In addition, the effect was not seen with flutamide, another androgen receptor antagonist indicating some chemical specificity for the effect [50].

Other experimental studies have previously reported effects that persisted through two generations including dioxin in the mammary gland, and DES in male and female reproductive tract tissues and gonads [17]. Interestingly, there has been a case report of ovarian neoplasia in a young girl whose grandmother was exposed to DES during development [18] and several other transgenerational epidemiology studies with DES [51–53]. These transgenerational exposures if proven to extend to other environmental toxicants could have a major impact on public health. This area of scientific investigation definitely needs further study.

# Mechanisms involved in the adverse effects of developmental exposure

It is easy to understand how an environmental chemical like DES with estrogenic activity, for example, can stimulate estrogen-sensitive gene expression at the wrong time if the cells are exposed to the agent when estrogen levels are usually low and estrogen-sensitive genes are not active. However, it is not clear why some of these activated genes remain active long after the estrogenic stimulus is removed. This is the situation that occurs during the developmental basis of disease paradigm. Environmental agents are present only for a specific time during development (in utero or neonatally) but their effects are felt throughout life. The mechanisms that are responsible for this phenomenon are termed "programming or epigenetic regulation of gene activity". Epigenetics literally means "on top of genetics" and deals with chemical modifications of DNA and chromatin that affect genome function (transcription, replication, recombination, etc.). The epigenetic code comprises several interconnected, interdependent codes that orchestrate genome activity together with RNA interference [54]. At the DNA level, DNA can be methylated at CpG islands (areas of concentrated CpG repeats) due to DNA methyltransferases. Methyl-binding protein-binding proteins then bind to these sites and attract other proteins, with the result that there is a change in chromatin structure, leading to a silencing of the methylated gene. On the other hand, hypomethylation of genes can generate increased and inappropriate gene expression [55]. At the chromatin level, nucleosomal proteins, histones, can be covalently modified via acetylation, phosphorylation, methylation, ubiquination, or adenosine diphosphate ribosylation or combinations. These modifications encompass what is termed the histone code and they control gene expression by controlling DNA availability [56, 57]. Hyperacetylation of chromatin proteins leads to open DNA and transcriptional activation. DNA methylation of histones can lead to either compaction and gene silencing or activation depending on the site of methylation. These epigenetic marking systems work synergistically and cooperatively to remodel chromatin, thereby determining whether a gene is active or silenced. DNA methylation, histone deacetylation, and histone methylation all lead to gene silencing.

These epigenetic marks are laid down during development and are responsible for the genetic programming that leads to the development of different types of cells and tissues. During development, the loss and subsequent re-establishment of the epigenetic marks in the fetus and embryo comprise a critically sensitive period during which the system is subject to perturbation. Thus, development is a sensitive time for alterations due to environmental exposures. Indeed it is proposed that developmental exposures to environmental chemicals may have long-term effects on the expression of various genes by interacting with epigenetic mechanisms and altering chromatin conformation and transcription factor accessibility. While exposure to environmental agents may not result in any physical signs of toxicity, at the genome level, these exposures can alter the genetic programming of cells (alter the gene expression pattern controlled by the epigenetic code) leading to tissues with functional changes that are then sensitive to disease or dysfunction later in life. The exact mechanism whereby environmental agents can alter the epigenome is still under investigation but some possibilities include alteration of DNA methyltransferases and alteration of gene expression during the time of epigenetic programming. There are now a significant number of environmental agents that can alter epigenetic programming when exposure occurs during development [55, 58].

# Summary

The data included in this review support the idea that brief exposure early in development to environmental chemicals, in particular those with hormone-like activity, are contributing to childhood disease and dysfunction such as birth defects and malformations, altered timing of puberty, and non-reproductive problems like obesity. Further, exposure to these chemicals during critical stages of development may also have long-term latent effects that are not observed until much later in life such as menstrual irregularities, subfertility/infertility, uterine fibroids, early reproductive senescence, and some types of cancer including breast and prostate cancer. Of utmost importance, new studies suggest multigenerational effects may also be seen which would indicate our grandchildren would be affected by chemical exposure of their grandparents. Together these data show the extreme sensitivity of the developing organism and point out the need for identification and avoidance of EDCs, and additional studies on the mechanisms involved in their adverse effects so that future generations may look forward to a healthy future.

## Acknowledgments

This research was supported, in part, by the Intramural Research Program of the NIH, National Institute of Environmental Health Sciences.

## References

1. Soto AM, Maffini MV, Sonnenschein C. Neoplasia as development gone awry: the role of endocrine disruptors. *Int J Androl* 2008; **31**(2): 288–93.

2. Bern HA. The fragile fetus. In Colborn T, Clement C, ed. *Alterations in Sexual and Functional Development: The Wildlife/Human Connection*. Princeton, NJ: Princeton Science Publishing, 1992 9–15.

3. Newbold R. Lessons learned from perinatal exposure to diethylstilbestrol (DES). *Toxicol Appl Pharmacol* 2004; **199**: 142–50.

4. National Institute of Health (NIH). DES Research Update, NIH Publication No. 00–4722. Bethesda, MD, 1999.

5. Barker DJ, Eriksson JG, Forsen T, Osmond C. Fetal origins of adult disease: strength of effects and biological basis. *Int J Epidemiol* 2002; **31**(6): 1235–9.

6. Kaufman D, Banerji MA, Shorman I. *et al.* Early-life stress and the development of obesity and insulin resistance in juvenile bonnet macaques. *Diabetes* 2007; **56**(5): 1382–6.

7. Levin ED. Fetal nicotinic overload, blunted sympathetic responsivity, and obesity. *Birth Defects Res A Clin Mol Teratol* 2005; **73**(7): 481–4.

8. Gluckman PD, Hanson MA, Pinal C. The developmental origins of adult disease. *Matern Child Nutr* 2005; **1**(3): 130–41.

9. Heindel JJ. Role of exposure to environmental chemicals in the developmental basis of reproductive disease and dysfunction. *Semin Reprod Med* 2006; **24**(3): 168–77.

10. Heindel JJ. Role of exposure to environmental chemicals in the developmental basis of disease and dysfunction. *Reprod Toxicol* 2007; **23**(3): 257–9.

11. Colborn T, Dumanoski D, Myers JP. *Our Stolen Future*. Penguin Books USA, Inc., 1996.

12. Crain DA, Janssen SJ, Edwards TM. *et al.* Female reproductive disorders: the roles of endocrine-disrupting compounds and developmental timing. *Fertil Steril* 2008; **90**(4): 911–40.

13. Herbst AL, Ulfelder H, Poskanzer DC. Adenocarcinoma of the vagina: association of maternal stilbestrol therapy with tumor appearance in young women. *N Eng J Med* 1971; **284**: 878–9.

14. Herbst AL, Bern HA. *Developmental Effects of Diethylstilbestrol (DES) in Pregnancy*. New York: Hieme-Stratton, Inc., 1981.

15. Giusti RM, Iwamoto K, Hatch EE. Diethylstilbestrol revisited: a review of the long-term health effects. *Ann Intern Med* 1995; **122**(10): 778–88.

16. Hatch EE, Palmer JR, Titus-Ernstoff L. *et al.* Cancer risk in women exposed to diethylstilbestrol in utero. *J Am Med Assoc.* 1998; **280**(7): 630–4.

17. Newbold RR, Padilla-Banks E, Jefferson WN. Adverse effects of the model environmental estrogen diethylstilbestrol are transmitted to subsequent generations. *Endocrinology* 2006; **147** (Suppl 6): S11–17.

18. Blatt J, Van Le L, Weiner T, Sailer S. Ovarian carcinoma in an adolescent with transgenerational exposure to diethylstilbestrol. *J Pediatr Hematol Oncol* 2003; **25**(8): 635–6.

19. Newbold RR. Cellular and molecular effects of developmental exposure to diethylstilbestrol: implications for other environmnetal estrogens. *Environ Health Perspect* 1995; **103**(7): 83–7.

20. Huseby RA. Estrogen-induced Leydig cell tumor in the mouse: a model system for the study of carcinogenesis and hormone dependency. *J Toxicol Environ Health Suppl* 1976; **1**: 177–92.

21. Bern HA, Mills KT, Ostrander PL. *et al.* Cervicovaginal abnormalities in BALB/c mice treated neonatally with sex hormones. *Teratology* 1984; **30**(2): 267–74.

22. Iguchi T, Takase M, Takasugi N. Development of vaginal adenosis-like lesions and uterine epithelial stratification in mice exposed perinatally to diethylstilbestrol. *Proc Soc Exp Biol Med* 1986; **181**(1): 59–65.

23. Newbold RR, Bullock BC, McLachlan JA. Uterine adenocarcinoma in mice following developmental treatment with estrogens: a model for hormonal carcinogenesis. *Cancer Res* 1990; **50**(23): 7677–81.

24. Rothschild TC, Calhoon RE, Boylan ES. Effects of diethylstilbestrol exposure in utero on the genital tracts of female ACI rats. *Exp Mol Pathol* 1988; **48**(1): 59–76.

25. Leavitt WW, Evans RW, Hendry WJ 3rd. Etiology of DES-induced uterine tumors in the Syrian hamster. *Adv Exp Med Biol* 1981; **138**: 63–86.

26. Hogan MD, Newbold RR, McLachlan JA. Extrapolation of teratogenic responses observed in laboratory animals to humans. *Branbury Report 26: Development Toxicology: Mechanisms and Risk*. New York: Cold Spring Harbor Laboratory, 1987.

27. Swan SH, Main KM, Liu F. *et al.* Decrease in anogenital distance among male infants with prenatal phthalate exposure. *Environ Health Perspect* 2005; **113**(8): 1056–61.

28. Gray Jr LE, Foster Pmd. Significance of experimental studies for assessing adverse effects of endocrine-disrupting chemicals. *Pure Appl Chemistry* 2003; **75**: 2125–41.

29. Buck Louis GM, Gray LE, Jr, Marcus M. *et al.* Environmental factors and puberty timing: expert panel research needs. *Pediatrics* 2008; **121** (Suppl. 3): S192–207.

30. Gladen BC, Ragan NB, Rogan WJ. Pubertal growth and development and prenatal and lactational exposure

to polychlorinated biphenyls and dichlorodiphenyl dichloroethene. *J Pediatr* 2000; **136**(4): 490–6.

31. Blanck HM, Marcus M, Tolbert PE. *et al.* Age at menarche and tanner stage in girls exposed in utero and postnatally to polybrominated biphenyl. *Epidemiology* 2000; **11**(6): 641–7.

32. Rubin BS, Murray MK, Damassa DA, King JC, Soto AM. Perinatal exposure to low doses of bisphenol A affects body weight, patterns of estrous cyclicity, and plasma LH levels. *Environ Health Perspect* 2001; **109**(7): 675–80.

33. Selevan SG, Rice DC, Hogan KA. *et al.* Blood lead concentration and delayed puberty in girls. *N Engl J Med* 2003; **348**(16): 1527–36.

34. Saiyed H, Dewan A, Bhatnagar V. *et al.* Effect of endosulfan on male reproductive development. *Environ Health Perspect* 2003; **111**(16): 1958–62.

35. Baillie-Hamilton PF. Chemical toxins: a hypothesis to explain the global obesity epidemic. *J Altern Complement Med* 2002; **8**(2): 185–92.

36. Newbold RR, Padilla-Banks E, Jefferson WN, Heindel JJ. Effects of endocrine disruptors on obesity. *Int J Androl* 2008; **31**(2):201–8.

37. Grun F, Watanabe H, Zamanian Z. *et al.* Endocrine-disrupting organotin compounds are potent inducers of adipogenesis in vertebrates. *Mol Endocrinol* 2006; **20**(9): 2141–55.

38. Collins S. Overview of clinical perspectives and mechanisms of obesity. *Birth Defects Res A Clin Mol Teratol* 2005; **73**(7): 470–1.

39. Mokdad AH, Ford ES, Bowman BA. *et al.* Prevalence of obesity, diabetes, and obesity-related health risk factors, 2001. *J Am Med Assoc* 2003; **289**(1): 76–9.

40. Nayyar T, Bruner-Tran KL, Piestrzeniewicz-Ulanska D, Osteen KG. Developmental exposure of mice to TCDD elicits a similar uterine phenotype in adult animals as observed in women with endometriosis. *Reprod Toxicol* 2007; **23**(3): 326–36.

41. Baird DD, Newbold RR. Prenatal diethylstilbestrol (DES) exposure is associated with uterine leiomyoma development. *Reprod Toxicol* 2005; **20**(1): 81–4.

42. Cook JD, Davis BJ, Cai SI. *et al.* Interaction between genetic susceptibility and early-life environmental exposure determines tumor-suppressor-gene penetrance. *Proc Natl Acad Sci USA* 2005; **102**: 8644–9.

43. Colborn T, vom Saal FS, Soto AM. Developmental effects of endocrine-disrupting chemicals in wildlife and humans. *Environ Health Perspect* 1993; **101**(5): 378–84.

44. Fenton SE, Hamm JT, Birnbaum LS, Youngblood GL. Persistent abnormalities in the rat mammary gland following gestational and lactational exposure to 2,3,7,8-tetrachlorodibenzo-p-dioxin (TCDD). *Toxicol Sci* 2002; **67**(1): 63–74.

45. Boylan ES, Calhoon RE. Transplacental action of diethylstilbestrol on mammary carcinogenesis in female rats given one or two doses of 7,12-dimethylbenz(a) anthracene. *Cancer Res* 1983; **43**(10): 4879–84.

46. Newbold RR, McLachlan JA. Neoplastic and non-neoplastic lesions in male reproductive organs following perinatal exposure to hormones and related substances. In Mori T, Nagasawa H, eds. *Toxicity of Hormones in Perinatal Life*. Boca Raton, FL: CRC Press, Inc., 1988, 89–109.

47. vom Saal FS, Timms BG, Montano MM. *et al.* Prostate enlargement in mice due to fetal exposure to low doses of estradiol or diethylstilbestrol and opposite effects at high doses. *Proc Natl Acad Sci USA* 1997; **94**: 2056–61.

48. Prins GS, Tang WY, Belmonte J, Ho SM. Developmental exposure to bisphenol A increases prostate cancer susceptibility in adult rats: epigenetic mode of action is implicated. *Fertil Steril* 2008; **89** (Suppl. 2): e41.

49. Anway MD, Cupp AS, Uzumcu M, Skinner MK. Epigenetic transgenerational actions of endocrine disruptors and male fertility. *Science* 2005; **308**(5727): 1466–9.

50. Anway MD, Rekow SS, Skinner MK. Comparative anti-androgenic actions of vinclozolin and flutamide on transgenerational adult onset disease and spermatogenesis. *Reprod Toxicol* 2008; **26**(2): 100–6.

51. Klip H, Verloop J, van Gool JD. *et al.* Hypospadias in sons of women exposed to diethylstilbestrol in utero: a cohort study. *Lancet* 2002; **359**(9312): 1102–7.

52. Brouwers MM, Feitz WF, Roelofs LA. *et al.* Hypospadias: a transgenerational effect of diethylstilbestrol? *Hum Reprod* 2006; **21**(3): 666–9.

53. Titus-Ernstoff L, Troisi R, Hatch EE. *et al.* Offspring of women exposed in utero to diethylstilbestrol (DES): a preliminary report of benign and malignant pathology in the third generation. *Epidemiology* 2008; **19**(2): 251–7.

54. Gallou-Kabani C, Vige A, Junien C. Lifelong circadian and epigenetic drifts in metabolic syndrome. *Epigenetics* 2007; **2**(3): 137–46.

55. Ho SM, Tang WY. Techniques used in studies of epigenome dysregulation due to aberrant DNA methylation: an emphasis on fetal-based adult diseases. *Reprod Toxicol* 2007; **23**(3): 267–82.

56. Jones PA, Baylin SB. The fundamental role of epigenetic events in cancer. *Nat Rev Genet* 2002; **3**(6): 415–28.

57. van Driel R, Fransz PF, Verschure PJ. The eukaryotic genome: a system regulated at different hierarchical levels. *J Cell Sci* 2003; **116**(20): 4067–75.

58. Ho SM, Tang WY, Belmonte de Frausto J, Prins GS. Developmental exposure to estradiol and bisphenol A increases susceptibility to prostate carcinogenesis and epigenetically regulates phosphodiesterase type 4 variant 4. *Cancer Res* 2006; **66**(11): 5624–32.

# Chapter 8

# Wildlife as sentinels of environmental impacts on reproductive health and fertility

Heather J. Hamlin and Louis J. Guillette Jr.

Animals have long served as sentinels of environmental hazards. As early as 1962, Rachel Carson wrote "our fate is connected with the animals" foreshadowing the dual fates of wildlife and humans exposed to synthetic pesticides [1]. The twentieth century marked a turning point in the ability of humans to chemically modify the landscape, and there is a growing body of epidemiologic data linking exposure to environmental contaminants with an array of reproductive maladies in humans including infertility, reduced sperm quality, early puberty onset, reproductive tract abnormalities, and cancer [2, 3].

Animal sentinels have been described as any nonhuman organism that can react to an environmental contaminant before the contaminant can impact humans [4]. Despite predictions offered by wildlife, many contaminants take significant tolls on human populations either because warning signs were ignored, or regulatory intervention did not effectuate a timely response. Although sentinel species data is not expected to be the sole determinative factor in assessing human health concerns, these data can be particularly useful as an additional weight of evidence in risk assessment, as well as to highlight suspect environmental contaminants. Indeed, humans and wildlife share common environments and food chains, and the physiologic and molecular responses to toxic chemicals are often highly conserved among vertebrate species.

While laboratory studies in controlled environments assist in providing causal links and dose–response relationships, laboratory animals are often genetically similar and responses under these conditions do not reflect the genetic and environmental diversity more reflective of human exposure conditions. In addition, wildlife studies provide information on the interactive effects of chemical mixtures and reflect "real-world" data.

In this chapter we will provide examples of how environmental chemicals have impacted wildlife populations and the implications these studies have for human reproductive disorders.

## Lessons from wildlife: past, present and future

### The Great Lakes wildlife sentinels

Since the 1950s, 16 top predator species including birds, mammals, fish, and reptiles in the Laurentian Great Lakes have exhibited reproductive impairments. Health assessments showed these animals to have a suite of developmental and reproductive effects including thyroid dysfunction, decreased fertility, birth deformities, feminization of males, defeminization of females, and behavioral abnormalities [5]. These effects were attributed to high concentrations of organochlorine pesticides and industrial chemicals found in these animals' tissues. These observations led to the gathering of a multidisciplinary group of scientists in 1991, which came to the conclusion that contaminants measured in humans were well within the range at which developmental and reproductive effects were seen in wildlife populations. Since many of the effects observed in the affected animals were directed by the endocrine system, the group termed the phenomenon *endocrine disruption*, and recommended that chemical testing should begin to include hormonal activity in vivo [5].

Because wildlife are often highly mobile and widely dispersed, health assessments are often limited to stages of the life cycle that are less mobile. Unlike mammalian embryos, the eggs of birds, reptiles, and other oviparous vertebrates are independent metabolic systems whereby persistent lipophilic contaminants such

*Environmental Impacts on Reproductive Health and Fertility*, ed. T. J. Woodruff, S. J. Janssen, L. J. Guillette, and L. C. Giudice. Published by Cambridge University Press. © Cambridge University Press 2010.

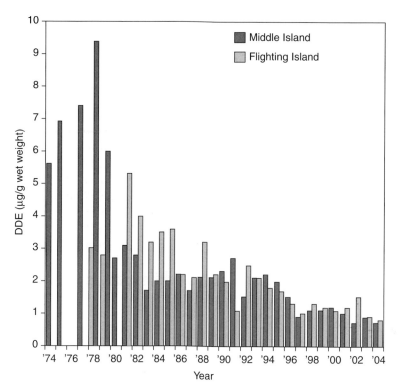

**Fig. 8.1.** Changes in dichlordiophenyl-dichloroethylene (DDE) concentration in herring gull eggs from 1974–2004 in the US Great Lakes. (Redrawn from data collected by Canadian Wildlife Service – http://www.epa.gov/med/grosseile_site/indicators/gulleggs.html.)

as PCBs, DDE and polychlorinated dibenzo-furans (PCDFs) can be bioconcentrated in the egg yolk, often at levels far exceeding circulating maternal concentrations [6]. Although concentrations of many persistent organochlorines declined rapidly after the use of these compounds was restricted, levels in many species' eggs have not changed significantly in the last two decades (Fig. 8.1). The bald eagle was one of the first North American species widely affected by environmental DDT, paralleling effects seen in raptor species in the UK [7]. Within one year of the widespread application of DDT, wildlife biologists noted considerable reproductive anomalies including failure to return to nesting sites, failure to lay eggs, egg shell thinning, and an inability of many of the eggs to hatch. Even today, bald eagle populations in the Great Lakes region which contain elevated concentrations of DDE and PCBs have lower productivity (total number of fledged young) and success (percent of nests producing at least one fledgling) than less contaminated eagle populations [8].

Other disorders in fish-eating birds of the Great Lakes include embryo mortality, thyroid malfunction, and immunosuppression. In the 1980s, Great Lakes herring gulls had significantly enlarged thyroid glands, and although a direct link could not be made, incidences of goiter decreased at the same time that organochlorine contamination decreased.

Although wildlife biologists were documenting crashes of top predator fish populations in the Great Lakes as early as the 1940s [9], it was not until 1995 that the EPA discovered that dioxin concentrations in Lakes Ontario and Michigan were at levels that eggs and hatchlings of certain fish species could not survive [10]. As a result of regulatory action, concentrations of DDT, dieldrin, PCBs and mirex in the Great Lakes declined significantly in the late 1970s. Chemical concentrations in fish tissues and bird eggs, however, have been decreasing at a much slower rate [11] (Fig. 8.1).

The behavioral and reproductive failures initially noted in Great Lakes wildlife have predicted many of the organochlorine-induced disorders that have now been seen in humans. An accidental contamination of PCBs and PCDFs in cooking oil occurred in Japan in 1968 and Taiwan in 1979. These episodes caused nearly 4000 people to develop symptoms of intoxication, and this population now serves as a human toxicology reference of organochlorine exposure. Boys exposed in utero showed abnormal sperm morphology, reduced sperm motility, and a decreased capacity of sperm to penetrate oocytes. Exposed men also experienced similar changes in sperm function [12, 13]. In females, organochlorine exposure has been associated with endometriosis, a decreased conception rate, spontaneous abortion, and low birthweight [3, 14].

Similar to the Great Lakes herring gulls, humans exposed to organochlorines also experience alterations in thyroid function. Women exposed to PCBs during pregnancy have been shown to experience reduced free thyroxine concentrations [15, 16]. Because thyroid hormones are essential for normal brain function, disruptions in this hormone axis have been proposed as a potential mechanism for neurodevelopmental effects of several organic pollutants [17]. Humans exposed to organochlorine pesticides have been shown to experience reduced intelligence quotients (IQ) and studies have shown that children whose mothers consumed 2–3 meals/month of PCB-contaminated fish from the Great Lakes were more than a year behind their peers in word and reading comprehension [18].

## Lake Apopka, Florida and alligators

The fourth largest lake in Florida, Lake Apopka was once one of central Florida's main attractions, attracting boaters, swimmers, and fishermen alike. Fishing enthusiasts from across the USA came to the lake to fish for large-mouth bass and numerous fishing camps lined the lake's shore. The 1940s marked the beginning of the lake's decline, as muck farming, the repeated draining of thousands of acres of farmland into the lake, filled its waters with nutrients and agricultural chemicals. These nutrients caused algal blooms that prevented sunlight from reaching plant life, which indirectly reduced fish populations. After an ill-fated attempt to restore fish populations in the 1950s, muck farming supplanted recreation, and the nutrient loading continued [19].

About a mile from the lake's southern shore, the Tower Chemical Company produced dicofol, which contained synthesis by-products such as the pesticide DDT and its degradation product DDE. In 1980, a chemical spill caused large quantities of dicofol and sulfuric acid to run into the lake from an adjoining stream. The site of the Tower Chemical disaster is now listed as one of the US EPA Superfund sites, which are contaminated sites in the USA that are identified as being harmful to human health and the environment. This chemical spill, in concert with agricultural runoff and a sewage treatment facility associated with the city of Winter Garden, has made Lake Apopka one of the most contaminated lakes in Florida [19].

In the 1990s, studies of the lake's alligator populations began to reveal juvenile male alligators with abnormal gonads, abnormally small phallus size, and depressed plasma testosterone concentrations which were comparable to those of females from an uncontaminated reference lake. Juvenile females had abnormal ovarian morphology, large numbers of polyovular (multioocytic) follicles, and plasma 17β-estradiol concentrations nearly two times greater than females from a reference site [20]. Additionally, gonadal steroidogenesis was unresponsive to stimulation with luteinizing hormone, suggesting that the gonads of the juveniles had been permanently modified in ovo, and that normal steroidogenesis was no longer possible.

When alligator eggs were brought back to the laboratory for incubation and viability studies, embryos and neonates exhibited much higher mortality rates than those from reference lakes [21]. Although several hypotheses were raised to explain the notable differences seen at Apopka, such as a poor nesting environment or age structure of the breeding population, none of these parameters contributed significantly to the poor egg viability observed. These observations, combined with studies showing elevated concentrations of many organochlorines, including DDE, in Apopka alligator eggs [6], suggested that contaminants could be the major contributing factor for low egg viability [22].

The evidence provided by Lake Apopka alligators strongly suggests that environmental contaminants are responsible for the adverse reproductive effects. But alligators and humans are decidedly different animals. Could alligators and humans share the same physiologic fate when exposed to similar environmental contaminants? After all, alligators and humans, like most vertebrates, share similar molecular, biochemical, and cellular processes, and the steroidogenic pathways leading to an appropriately functioning reproductive system share many common pathways. Could humans exposed to pesticides and other chemicals that can alter endocrine function also experience alterations in circulating hormone concentrations, reduced phallus size, and other feminizing conditions? It appears so. More than a decade after the discoveries in alligators, human researchers discovered that the sons of women who were occupationally exposed to greenhouse pesticides during pregnancy showed significant reductions in serum testosterone concentrations, testicular volume, and penile length [23]. In addition, these children had lower concentrations of inhibin B, a hormone secreted by the Sertoli cells which inhibits FSH production, and a corresponding increase in circulating FSH versus that of boys whose mothers were not occupationally exposed to pesticides. Similar to the alligator studies, these results suggest that the gonadal cells were adversely affected during embryonic development, permanently altering normal steroidogenesis. Further, a study examining neonatal sons of mothers that came to a "well baby clinic" observed that boys of mothers with elevated, but environmentally relevant, phthalate levels had reduced ano-genital distances and smaller penis volumes [24]. These studies support the biology that demonstrates that much of the underlying molecular and cellular endocrinology related to genital development and growth is similar among vertebrate species, including humans [25].

## Tributyltin and marine mollusks

Research examining the effectiveness of tributyltin (TBT) as a wood preservative began in the late 1950s and followed with its extensive use as an antifouling and biocide agent in marine paints and aquatic wood [26, 27] and as a pesticide on high-value food crops [28]. As early as 1970, wildlife studies were emerging describing shell thinning and reproductive impairments in mollusks exposed to TBT [29, 30].

A significant body of literature now exists linking TBT exposure with an irreversible reproductive abnormality in marine mollusks termed imposex – the imposition of sex characteristics from one sex to the other. Female mollusks exposed to low concentrations of environmental TBT can develop a penis, vas deferens, and seminiferous tubules. Many marine gastropods located in organotin-polluted areas are unable to reproduce due to a blockage of the oviduct by vas deferens, and in some species oogenesis has been supplanted with spermatogenesis [31]. Approximately 150 species of gastropods affected with imposex have been identified throughout the world [32]. These reproductive maladies have led to population declines and in some cases mass extinction [33, 34].

Although the use of TBT, as well as other organotins, has been banned or severely restricted for some uses (e.g. anti fouling paint) in several countries, including the USA, these regulations have not prevented TBT from moving rapidly up the food chain, affecting both fish and marine mammals [35, 36, 37]. Many fish species contaminated with TBT are routinely consumed by humans, including tuna, salmon, mackerel, and cod, contributing to nearly 38% of the total organotin exposure by humans [35].

In certain species of fish such as medaka, studies have shown that TBT exposure leads to concentration-dependent mortality and impaired embryonic development including tail deformities, hemorrhage, and abnormal eye development [38]. Salmon exposed to TBT showed alterations to multiple genes critical to hormone signaling, gamete formation, and liver clearance including estrogen receptors, androgen receptor β, vitellogenin, CYP1A1, and CYP3A [39].

Tributyltin's negative affects on reproduction are not limited to aquatic animals and studies with rats exposed to TBT have shown decreased testes weights, prostate atrophy, and reduced sperm counts. More importantly, the effects of TBT in the $F_2$ generation can be greater than that in the $F_1$ generation [40], which has been attributed to the ability of TBT to be transferred via the placenta to the fetus.

Tributyltin exposure in humans has been implicated in a number of physiologic impairments. Although the rising world wide incidence of obesity is due in large part to high-calorie modern diets coupled with reduced activity, it is certain that genetic variation affects the degree of individual weight gain [41, 42]. In animal models, prenatal exposure to TBT leads to being 15% heavier later in life [41].

Although humans are routinely exposed to TBT through both aquatic and terrestrial sources, interest in TBT as a potential human toxicant was the result of a culmination of wildlife sentinels, signaling a milieu of reproductive and developmental abnormalities. A study examining butyltin compounds in central Michigan residents found 70% of participants to possess detectable plasma concentrations of TBT, with reported plasma concentrations as high as 85 ng/ml [43]. Because TBT is persistent in the environment and accumulates through the food chain, reservoir sources may contribute substantially to human exposure for some time to come.

## Nitrate: a global contaminant

Groundwater provides the drinking water for more than half of US residents, and is the sole source of drinking water for many rural communities [44]. The chemicals in groundwater often reflect regional sources, although many chemicals can travel great distances affecting locales far removed from the original source. The groundwater in areas of heavy agricultural activity often has a distinct water quality signature composed of nitrate, potassium, calcium, magnesium, and chloride [45]. Nitrate in particular can persist in groundwater for decades and can reach very high concentrations from the yearly accumulation of non-point sources such as the seasonal application of fertilizers, manure, and lime. Although fertilizers often contain nitrate directly, the nitrogen from manure and other sources can be converted to nitrate in the soil where it then leaches into the water table (see Fig. 8.2). Urban areas are also susceptible to nitrate contamination through the application of fertilizers to lawns and golf courses, as well as airborne nitrogen from coal- and oil-burning electric utilities and automobiles. World wide, humans fix 160 million tons of nitrogen per year, of which 83 million tons is used as agricultural fertilizer (see Fig. 8.3). This nitrogen loading has dramatically increased the nitrogen burden on rivers, lakes, shallow seas, and human water supplies. Studies have shown that parts of the western, midwestern and northeastern USA are at high risk of nitrate groundwater contamination [46].

The US drinking water standard is currently 10 mg/L $NO_3$-N. This limit was originally established solely based on prevention of methemoglobinemia in infants (blue baby syndrome) [47]. New studies are emerging, however, which show physiological responses to nitrate other than methemoglobinemia [48]. A study of male mosquitofish living in nitrate-contaminated springs in Florida showed that increasing nitrate (up to 5 mg/L $NO_3$-N) was negatively correlated with total sperm count and positively correlated with testicular weight and gonopodium length (a modified anal fin used to transfer sperm to the female) [49]. The increased testicular weight was attributed to a long-term compensatory response of the testis to nitrate, which resulted in testicular hypertrophy. Female mosquitofish showed a significant negative association between nitrate and embryo weight and rate of reproductive activity [50]. The nitrate concentrations associated with the altered reproductive effects seen in these studies were half that of the current US drinking water standard.

Nitrate has been shown to elicit its effects through several documented mechanisms (see review by Guillette and Edwards [51]). Some of these mechanisms are suggested to interfere with steroid clearance in the liver. Thus, if nitrates are reducing steroid clearance, they are likely modifying the clearance of many

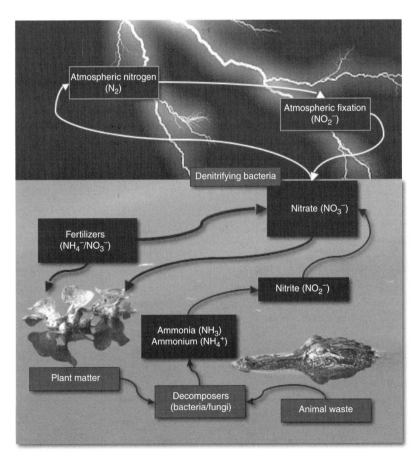

**Fig. 8.2.** Nitrogen cycle. Fertilizers and human fixation of nitrogen (e.g. fossil fuel use, large animal production facilities) are a major contributor to increasing nitrate levels in surface waters that serve as major sources of drinking water and aquatic environments for wildlife.

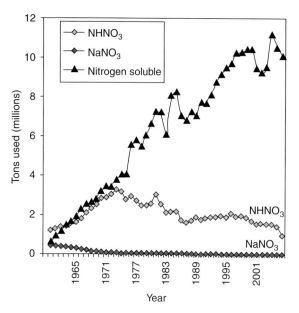

**Fig. 8.3.** Changes in use of selective forms of nitrogen-based fertilizer in the USA from 1965–2006. Data from USDA (http://www.ers.usda.gov/data/fertilizeruse/).

drugs and other chemicals that are metabolized by this enzyme system.

A retrospective analysis of Florida's alligators reveals that nitrate could also have played a role in the observed reproductive dysfunctions [51]. Results of regression analysis indicate that lake water nitrogen was inversely correlated with plasma testosterone in both male and female alligators. Conversely, plasma 17β-estradiol concentrations showed a positive relationship with lake water nitrogen in males, although this relationship was not as strong in females.

Nitrate reacts with other chemicals (amines and amides) to form carcinogenic compounds (N-nitroso compounds), of which over 80 have been found to be carcinogens and associated with at least 15 cancers including stomach, lung, esophageal, bone, skin, thyroid, liver, kidney, and brain.

Each year humans consume approximately 25 million tons of protein nitrogen, a figure expected to reach 40–45 million tons by 2025. There is increasing evidence that agricultural non-point source pollution is the leading source of water quality impact to freshwater systems, including drinking water sources. Given the emerging reproductive effects shown in wildlife, and the increasing epidemiologic evidence for human reproductive disorders, increased efforts should be made to limit the nitrate burden on our land and water

systems, and ensure that the effects of nitrate contamination do not worsen.

# Amphibians and agricultural pesticides

In recent decades, amphibian populations have suffered alarming population declines and there is a growing body of evidence that environmental pesticides are contributing to this decline [52], which has been experienced by more than 40% of the world's 5743 amphibian species [53]. Pesticide application often occurs in spring and early summer, a time that coincides with the breeding season of many amphibian species. Field studies examining amphibians exposed to pesticides have had mixed findings. While some field studies have found limited effects [54], other studies have found considerable developmental and reproductive disorders associated with pesticide exposure.

The San Joaquin Valley of California is heavily exposed to pesticides, receiving about 60% of the total pesticide usage in the state. A study of Pacific treefrogs (*Hyla regilla*) residing in this area concluded that agricultural pesticides reduced cholinesterase activity in treefrog tadpoles [55]. Cholinesterase is an enzyme that catalyzes the hydrolysis of an important neurotransmitter, acetylcholine, which is necessary to allow a cholinergic neuron to return to its resting state. Because of its essential functions in brain and other tissues, chemicals that interfere with cholinesterase action have the potential to be potent neurotoxins. A high occurrence of hind limb deformities were recorded in frog and toad species residing in agricultural areas exposed to pesticide runoff in Quebec, Canada [56]. A study of habitats in Florida characterized by differing degrees of agricultural activity showed resident toads (*Bufo marinus*) to have dose-dependent gonadal and morphological feminization [57] (Fig. 8.4). Male toads living in the agricultural areas possessed varying degrees of intersex gonads, feminized coloration, demasculinized forearm widths, and reduced testosterone concentrations. Since plasma steroid concentrations and secondary sexual traits are likely to correlate with reproductive success, the toads exposed to agricultural areas, and presumably associated pesticides, are also likely to have altered reproductive success.

The adverse reproductive responses to agricultural pesticides likely extends far beyond that of amphibian and other wildlife populations. Much of the food that is grown in these agricultural areas eventually ends up on the tables of humans, and people working

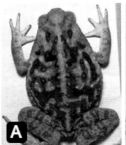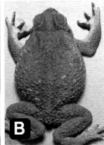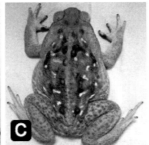

**Fig. 8.4.** Abnormalities in secondary sexual traits of male *Bufo marinus* from agricultural sites. Normal female (A), normal male (B), and intersex toad from an agricultural site (C). (Photographs courtesy of Krista McCoy.)

in agricultural fields are exposed further still. A study assessing the geographic variation in semen quality among US citizens found residents of Missouri to have significantly reduced sperm concentrations [58] versus residents of other US regions. This prompted further assessments to determine a possible root cause. Stored urine samples from the Missouri males were used to provide estimates of the men's exposure to pesticides used in the region. The study found that men with higher concentrations of certain pesticides, including alachlor, diazinon, and atrazine were more likely to have poor semen quality [59]. Later studies in other countries have supported these findings [60].

While correlations such as these cannot definitively determine the cause of the poor semen quality, laboratory studies support an association with pesticides and reduced semen quality as well as other reproductive dysfunctions. The pesticide chlorpyrifos causes reduced testes weight, sperm count, and serum testosterone concentration in male rats [61]. The pesticide methoxychlor (MXC) is an insecticide that was developed to replace DDT. Methoxychlor has been shown to stimulate estrogen-like responses in the liver and increase the regulation of genes responsible for liver clearance in fish. In the testes, MXC down-regulates steroidogenic acute regulatory protein (StAR) expression, which is considered the rate-limiting step in steroidogenesis [62]. Methoxychlor has been shown to inhibit follicular development in female rats as well as directly stimulate anti-müllerian hormone in the ovary [63]. Other organochlorine-induced reproductive dysfunctions in females include reduced ovulation rate, increased gestation length, estrogenic stimulation of the vagina, and reduced ovarian cyclicity (see review by Tiemann [64]).

The adverse effects of some pesticides, like the fungicide vinclozolin, can be transmitted through the male germ line. Studies with female rats exposed to vinclozolin during pregnancy showed prostate inflammation in the sons which was evident only after the sons reached puberty. Since the effects seen in the male

pups occurred long after vinclozolin should have been cleared from their bodies, this indicates that vinclozolin could have epigenetic effects that could transcend multiple generations. In humans, prostate inflammation affects approximately 9% of men and for 90% of those men, the cause of the inflammation is unknown.

A study of peripubertal girls from Mexico revealed that girls living in areas that used modern agricultural practices, including the use of pesticides, exhibited larger breasts than those of girls living in areas free of modern agricultural activity. In addition, girls from the modern agricultural areas did not display a well-defined relationship between breast size and mammary gland development, whereas girls from traditional ranching areas showed a positive relationship [65].

## Polar bears, penguins, and pesticides

Ratios of DDT to DDE in Adélie penguins have decreased significantly since the 1960s. This indicates that the pesticide burden seen in the penguins is likely due to old, rather than new, contaminant sources. However, DDT in Adélie penguins from the Western Antarctic region has not decreased for more than 30 years, indicating the possibility of a current reservoir source of DDT [66]. Measurable amounts of DDT have been reported in glacier meltwater [67] and both Arctic and Antarctic water bodies that receive glacial runoff exhibit elevated pesticide levels. Measurements of the glaciers themselves reveals a considerable DDT burden, implicating glacier runoff as a likely reservoir source of DDT. These studies reveal a new and compelling consequence of global warming.

During a 1996 polar bear research expedition, researchers discovered two yearling cubs traveling with their mother [68]. The cubs had a normal vaginal opening, which was accompanied by a 20 mm penis containing a baculum (a penis bone found in many mammalian species). DNA results revealed no evidence of a Y chromosome, and because the researchers could not observe their internal gonads and could therefore not determine if the cubs were true hermaphrodites, they

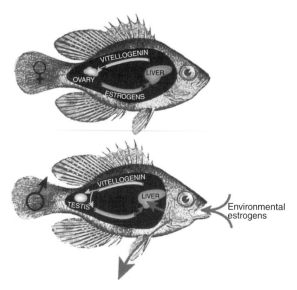

**Fig. 8.5.** Vitellogenesis has been used as a biomarker of estrogen exposure in male and female fish. Females will normally make vitellogenin (VTG), a yolk precursor protein, in the liver following stimulation by ovarian estrogens. In contrast, males do not synthesize VTG unless they are exposed to an exogenous estrogenic chemical.

were classified as pseudohermaphrodites, individuals with genital, but not gonadal, ambiguity. In 1990, and again in 1997, female polar bears were discovered with abnormal genital morphology in the form of excessive clitoral hypertrophy with a glans-like distal end. Researchers theorized that the most likely explanation for the genital malformations and pseudohermaphroditism was ingestion of androgenic compounds by the mother during pregnancy. Laboratory experiments have confirmed that exposure of the fetus to organochlorine pesticides can alter organ differentiation [69] and organs with receptors for gonadal hormones, such as the external genitalia, are especially at risk [70].

# Wildlife biomarkers of contaminant exposure

The notion that wildlife could have suffered adverse reproductive health effects from exposure to endocrine disruptors has led to a surge in the development of in vitro assays to screen for endocrine disruptors. However, in vivo systems have more direct application to wildlife, and arguably human populations, since they reflect the multiplicity of mechanistic pathways, and a wide range of physiological responses. In this regard, they are more predictive of real-life exposure. Wildlife biomarkers commonly used include vitellogenesis, amniote egg assays, and several others (see review by Tyler *et al.* [71]).

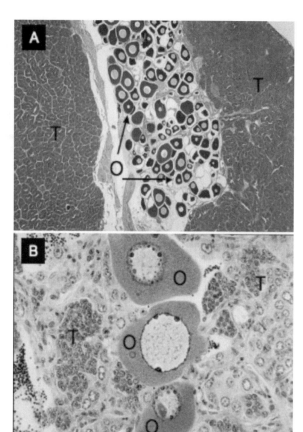

**Fig. 8.6.** Exposure of male fish (roach: *Rutilus rutilus*) to estrogenic and anti androgenic sewage effluents leads to the development of ovotestes in a large number of individuals. Ovotestes can be composed of large regions of oocytes (A) or regions with just a few oocytes lying among the seminepherous tubules (B). T, testicular tissues; O, oocytes (Photographs courtesy of Sue Jobling.)

Vitellogenesis is the process by which vitellogenin (VTG) is produced by the liver and is sequestered in the yolk of amniote eggs (Fig. 8.5). It is a major precursor of egg yolk proteins and acts as a nutrient to support embryonic development. Vitellogenins are considered to have similar characteristics among both vertebrates and invertebrates. Since the production of VTG is estrogen dependent, it is usually restricted to females. Under normal circumstances little, if any, VTG is detected in the plasma of males. However, males are capable of VTG production, and exposure to estrogens, both natural and synthetic, can trigger its expression. Vitellogenin production in males is now one of the most widely used biomarkers to establish estrogenic exposure in fish and shellfish (see review by Matozzo *et al.* [72]).

Other markers such as gonadal intersex, altered sex ratios, and sensitivity of sex differentiation have also

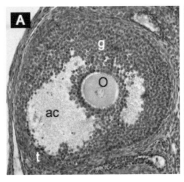 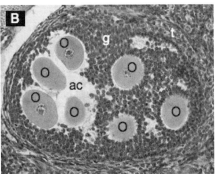

**Fig. 8.7.** Mammalian (mouse) ovarian follicles displaying a normal morphology (A) or abnormal multioocytic morphology (B) induced by neonatal DES exposure. O, oocyte; ac, antral cavity; g, granulosa; t, theca.

been used to assess the effects of hormone mimics. There is increasing evidence for endocrine disruption in fish populations, including gonadal intersex, altered sex ratios, reduced gonad size, abnormal gonadal cells, and male vitellogenin induction, living downstream of sewage treatment effluent across the world (see review by Jobling and Tyler [73]). Most of the effluents tested in the USA, and almost all effluents in the UK, have been shown to be estrogenic and anti androgenic, and capable of inducing a host of adverse reproductive effects. The lack of estrogenicity in a few sewage treatment effluents in the USA has been attributed to heavy dilution or extensive sewage treatment processes at those sites.

The presence of intersex, gonadal characteristics of both ovary and testes in the same individual, has also served as a common marker of contaminant exposure (Fig. 8.6). Although intersex has been documented in numerous fish and shellfish species, the roach, a cyprinid fish found throughout the UK and Europe, is one of the most extensively studied. At several sites downstream from sewage discharges in the UK, virtually all of the male roach populations were reported to have some degree of intersex [74], as well as oocytes within a predominantly male testes, and altered plasma sex steroid concentrations. Small groups of wild roach in UK rivers have been found that are not able to produce gametes at all due to the severity of the disruption [75].

An emerging model system which is gaining popularity as a biomarker of environmental exposure is the development of multioocytic (polyovular) follicles (MOFs) [76]. Normally one oocyte is found in each follicle, however, abnormal follicles may contain multiple oocytes (Fig. 8.7) and this condition can be induced by exposure to estrogenic contaminants. Wildlife studies reveal that MOFs have been shown to occur at a very high frequency in female alligators exposed to environmental contaminants [3, 20].Given the conserved

nature of folliculogenesis, similar responses could be observed in human populations as well.

In mammals, the effects of environmental contaminants have largely focused on disruptions of the gonad. In females, some of the most common indices of xenoestrogen exposure include reductions in ovary and follicle size, epithelial height of uterine cells, lordosis behavior, serum gonadotropin patterns, and ovulation frequency. In males the most common endpoints involve testicular endpoints including number and morphology of Sertoli cells, sperm number and motility, and the ability of the sperm to penetrate oocytes. Gonadal aromatase activity has often been used as a marker for both males and females. Behavioral changes and ano-genital distance have also been used to assess exposure to estrogens and anti-androgens, respectively.

## Are we listening?

Over 9000 birds were reportedly "dropping from the sky" in a seaside community in Australia, and the diagnosis was lead poisoning from a uniquely toxic form of lead [77]. The source was traced back to lead transport activities at a local port, which had begun less than two years earlier. Researchers then found lead carbonate in local drinking water supplies and in the residents themselves. The effects of lead toxicity are well known, and include neurological, cardiovascular, and reproductive damage. Had it not been for the birds acting as the "canaries in the coal mine" the presence of the lead would likely not have been discovered, leading to a potentially tragic outcome.

The clues provided by wildlife have heralded many of the reproductive dysfunctions later seen in humans. Often these parallels were drawn decades after the reproductive anomalies were evident in wildlife. Typical laboratory protocols for assessing chemical safety generally involve high-dose exposures, an approach which has been argued will efficiently identify as many adverse responses as possible.

Wildlife and laboratory studies involving endocrine-disrupting chemicals, however, have shown us that many adverse effects have a tendency to be cryptic at birth, for example, and low-dose, environmentally relevant exposures can have long-lasting, latent (not appearing until years or life stages later) and/or generational effects. It is clear that many of the effects shown in wildlife populations mirror those in human populations. New data are emerging in wildlife that could indicate the need for closer investigation into the reticent effects human populations could be facing. The question is: "Will we listen – and respond – to what the wildlife sentinels are telling us?"

## Summary

Wildlife studies provide a critical link for the vast array of epidemiologic evidence of contaminant-induced reproductive dysfunction. Wildlife populations exposed to environmental contaminants are showing signs of behavioral, developmental, and reproductive dysfunction. Wildlife sentinels continue to predict that decades of environmental abuse could be contributing to the dramatic increase in human reproductive disorders including infertility, reduced semen quality, early puberty onset, and gonadal abnormalities.

The information we gain from wildlife assessments is often a gross underestimate of the occurrence or severity of health effects of a given population, because the individuals observed are the survivors. Therefore, the information offered by wildlife sentinels highlights a chronic and compelling need for scientists, healthcare professionals, legislators, and the public at large to mobilize to identify links between contaminant-induced reproductive dysfunction in wildlife and its implications for human reproductive disorders.

## References

1. Carson, R. *Silent Spring*. Boston, MA: Houghton Mifflin Co., 1962.
2. Toppari J, Larsen, J, Christiansen, P. Male reproductive health and environmental xenoestrogens. *Environ Health Perspect* 1996; **104** (Suppl 4): 741–803.
3. Crain DA, Janssen SJ, Edwards TM. *et al*. Female reproductive disorders: the roles of endocrine disrupting compounds and developmental timing. *Fertil Steril* 2008; **90**: 911–40.
4. Stahl RG Jr. Can mammalian and non-mammalian "sentinel species" data be used to evaluate the human health implications of environmental contaminants. *Hum Ecol Risk Assess* 1997; **3**: 329–35.
5. Colborn T, Clement C, eds. *Chemically-Induced Alterations in Sexual and Functional Development: The Wildlife/Human Connection*. Princeton, NJ: Princeton Scientific, 1992.
6. Heinz GH, Percival HF, Jennings ML. Contaminants in American alligator eggs from lakes Apopka, Griffin and Okeechobee, Florida. *Environ Monit Assess* **1991; 16**: 277–85.
7. Ratcliffe DA. Decrease in eggshell weight in certain birds of prey. *Nature* 1967; **215**: 208–10.
8. Bowerman WW, Best DA, Giesy JP. *et al*. Associations between regional differences in polychlorinated biphenyls and dichlorodiphenyldichloroethylene in blood of nestling bald eagles and reproductive productivity. *Env Toxicol Chem* 2003; **22**: 371–6.
9. Colborn TE, Davidson A, Green SN. *et al. Great Lakes, Great Legacy?* Washington, DC: The Conservation Foundation, 1991.
10. Rolland RM, Gilbertson M, Peterson RE, eds. Chemically Induced Alterations in Functional Development and Reproduction of Fishes. Proceedings from a session at the 1995 Wingspread Conference. Society of Environmental Toxicology and Chemistry (SETAC), Pensacola, FL, 1995.
11. Colborn T, Thayer K. Aquatic ecosystems: harbingers of endocrine disruption. *Ecol Applic* 2000; **10**: 949–57.
12. Guo YL, Hsu PC, Hsu CC, Lambert GH. Semen quality after prenatal exposure to polychlorinated biphenyls and dibenzofurans. *Lancet* 2000; **356**: 1240–1.
13. Hsu PC, Huang, W Yao WJ. *et al*. Sperm changes in men exposed to polychlorinated biphenyls and dibenzofurans. *J Am Med Assoc* 2003; **289**: 2943–4.
14. Toft G, Hagmar L, Giwercman A, Bonde JP. Epidemiological evidence on reproductive effects of persistent organochlorines in humans. *Reprod Toxicol* 2004; **19**: 5–26.
15. Chevrier J, Eskenazi B, Holland N, Bradman N, Barr DB. Effects of exposure to polychlorinated biphenyls and organochlorine pesticides on thyroid function during pregnancy. *Am J Epidemiol* 2008; **168**: 298–310.
16. Herbstman JB , Sjodin A, Apelberg BJ. *et al*. Birth delivery mode modifies the associations between prenatal polychlorinated biphenyl (PCB) and polybrominated diphenyl thyroid hormone levels. *Environ Health Perspect* 2008; **116**: 1376–82.
17. Porterfield SP. Thyroidal dysfunction and environmental chemicals – potential impact on brain development. *Environ Health Perspect* 2000; **108**: 433–8.
18. Jacobson JL, Jacobson SW. Intellectual impairment in children exposed to polychlorinated biphenyls in utero. *N Engl J Med* 1996; **335**: 783–9.
19. Schelske C, Brezonik P. Can Lake Apopka be restored? In *Restoration of Aquatic Ecosystems: Science, Technology and Public Policy*. Washington, DC: National Academy of Sciences, 393–8.

20. Guillette LJ Jr, Gross TS, Masson GR. *et al.* Developmental abnormalities of the gonad and abnormal sex hormone concentrations in juvenile alligators from contaminated and control lakes in Florida. *Environ Health Perspect* 1994; **102**: 680–8.

21. Woodward AR, Jennings ML, Percival HF, Moore CT. Low clutch viability of American alligators on Lake Apopka, Fl. *Science* 1993; **56**: 52–63.

22. Rauschenberger RH, Wiebe JJ, Sepulveda MS, Scarborough JE, Gross TS. Parental exposure to pesticides and poor clutch viability in American alligators. *Environ Sci Tech* 2007; **41**: 5559–63.

23. Andersen HR, Schmidt IM, Grandjean P. *et al.* Impaired reproductive development in sons of women occupationally exposed to pesticides during pregnancy. *Environ Health Perspect* 2008; **116**: 566–72.

24. Swan SH, Main KM, Liu F. *et al.* Decrease in anogenital distance among male infants with prenatal phthalate exposure. *Environ Health Perspect* 2005; **113**: 1056–61.

25. Seifert AW, Harfe B, Cohn, MJ. Origin of the penile urethra and the proximodistal fate of the urethral epithelium. *Dev Biol* 2006; **295**: 459.

26. Hof T, Luijten JGA. Organotin compounds as wood preservatives. *Timb Technol* 1959; **67**: 83–4.

27. Walters CS. Problems and practices in wood preservation, 1958–9. *For Prod J* 1960; **10**: 73–81.

28. Appel KE. Organotin compounds: toxicokinetic aspects. *Drug Metab Rev* 2004; **36**: 763–86.

29. Babler SJM. The occurrence of a penis-like outgrowth behind the right tentacle in spent female of *Nucella lapillus* (L.) *Proc Malacol Soc Lond* 1970; **39**: 231–3.

30. Stroganov NS, Danil'chenko OP, Amochaeva EI. Changes in developmental metabolism of the mollusk lymnaea stagnalis under the effect of tributyltin chloride in low concentrations. *Biologicheskie Nauki* 1977; **20**: 75–8.

31. Matthiessen P, Gibbs PE, 1998. Critical appraisal of the evidence for tributyltin-mediated endocrine disruption in mollusks. *Environ Toxicol Chem* 1998; **17**: 37–43.

32. Matthiessen P, Reynoldson T, Billinghurst Z. *et al.* Field assessment for endocrine disruption in invertebrates. In deFur P, Crane M, Ingersoll C, Tattersfield L, eds. *Endocrine Disruption in Invertebrates: Endocrinology, Testing and Assessment.* Pensacola, FL: SETAC Press, 1999:199–270.

33. Bryan GW, Gibbs PE, Hummerstone LG, Burt GR. The decline of the gastropod Nucella lapillus around the south-west of England: evidence for the effect of tributyltin from anti-fouling paints. *J Mar Biol Assoc UK* 1986; **66**: 611–40.

34. ten Hallers-Tjabbes CC, Kemp JF, Boon JP. Imposex in whelks *Buccinum undatum* from the open North Sea: relation to shipping traffic intensities. *Mar Pollut Bull* 1994; **28**: 311–13.

35. Guérin T, Sirot V, Volatier JL, Leblanc JC. Organotin levels in seafood and its implications for health risk in high-seafood consumers. *Sci Tot Environ* 2007; **388**: 66–77.

36. Harino H, Ohji M, Wattayakorn G, et al.. Accumulation of organotin compounds in tissues and organs of stranded whales along the coasts of Thailand. *Arch Environ Contam Toxicol* 2007; **53**: 119–25.

37. Harino H, Ohji M, Wattayakorn G. *et al.* Accumulation of organotin compounds in tissues and organs of dolphins from the coasts of Thailand. *Arch Environ Contam Toxicol* 2008; **54**: 145–53.

38. Hano T, Oshima Y, Kim SG. *et al.* Tributyltin causes abnormal development in embryos of medaka, *Oryzias latipes. Chemosphere* 2007; **69**: 927–33.

39. Mortensen AS, Arukwe A. Modulation of xenobiotic biotransformation system and hormonal responses in Atlantic salmon (*Salmo salar*) after exposure to tributyltin (TBT). *Comp Biochem Physiol C* 2007; **145**: 431–41.

40. Omura M, Ogata R, Kubo K. *et al.* Two-generation reproductive toxicity study of tributyltin chloride in male rats. *Toxicol Sci* 2001; **64**: 224–32.

41. Grün F, Blumberg B. Environmental obesogens: organotins and endocrine disruption via nuclear receptor signaling. *Endocrinology* 2006; **147**: S50–5.

42. Iguchi T, Watanabe H, Ohta Y, Blumberg B. Developmental effects: oestrogen-induced vaginal changes and organotin-induced adipogenesis. *Int J Androl* 2008; **31**: 1–6.

43. Kannan K, Senthilkumar K, Giesy JP. Occurrence of butyltin compounds in human blood.. *Environ Sci Technol* 1999; **33**: 1776–9.

44. Solley WB, Peirce RR, Perlman HA. *Estimated Use of Water in the United States in 1990.* Reston, VA: U.S. Geological Survey, 1993; Circular 1081.

45. Hamilton PA, Shedlock RJ. *Are Fertilizers and Pesticides in the Ground Water?* Reston, VA: U.S. Geological Survey, 1992; Circular 1080.

46. Nolan BT, Ruddy BC, Hitt KJ, Helsel DR. Risk of nitrate in groundwaters of the United States – a national perspective. *Environ Sci Technol* 1977; **31**: 2229–36.

47. Fewtrell L. Drinking-water nitrate, methemoglobinemia, and global burden of disease: a discussion. *Environ Health Perspect* 2004; **112**: 1371–4.

48. Hamlin HJ, Moore BC, Edwards TM. *et al.* Nitrate induced elevations in circulating sex steroid concentrations in female Siberian sturgeon (*Acipenser baeri*) in commercial aquaculture. *Aquaculture* 2008; **281**: 118–25.

49. Edwards TM, Guillette LJ Jr. Reproductive characteristics of male mosquitofish (*Gambusia holbrooki*) from nitrate-contaminated springs in Florida. *Aquat Toxicol* 2007; **85**: 40–7.

113

50. Edwards TM, Miller HD, Guillette LJ Jr. Water quality influences reproduction in female mosquitofish (*Gambusia holbrooki*) from eight Florida springs. *Environ Health Perspect* 2006; **114**: 69–75.

51. Guillette LJ Jr, Edwards TM. Is nitrate an ecologically relevant endocrine disruptor in vertebrates? *Integr Comp Biol* 2005; **45**: 19–27.

52. Hayes TB, Case P, Chui S. *et al.* Pesticide mixtures, endocrine disruption, and amphibian declines: are we underestimating the impact? *Environ Health Perspect* 2006; **114**: 40–50.

53. Stuart SN, Chanson JS, Cox NA. *et al.* Status and trends of amphibian declines and extinctions worldwide. *Science* 2004; **306**: 1783–6.

54. Murphy MB, Hecker M, Coady KK. *et al.* Atrazine concentrations, gonadal gross morphology and histology in ranid frogs collected in Michigan agricultural areas. *Aquat Toxicol* 2006; **76**: 230–45.

55. Sparling DW, Fellers GM, McConnell LL. Pesticides and amphibian population declines in California, USA. *Environ Toxicol Chem* 2001; **20**: 1591–5.

56. Ouellet M, Bonin J, Rodrigue J, DesGranges J, Lair S. Hindlimb deformities (ectromelia, ectrodactyly) in free-living anurans from agricultural habitats. *J Wild Dis* 1997; **33**: 95–104.

57. McCoy KA, Bortnick LJ, Campbell CM. *et al.* Agriculture alters gonadal form and function in the toad *Bufo marinus*. *Environ Health Perspect* 2008; **116**: 1526–32.

58. Swan SH, Brazil C, Drobnis EZ. *et al.* Geographic differences in semen quality of fertile U.S. males. *Environ Health Perspect* 2003; **111**: 414–20.

59. Swan SH. Semen quality in fertile US men in relation to geographical area and pesticide exposure. *Int J Androl* 2006; **29**: 62–8.

60. Recio-Vega R, Ocampo-Gomez G, Borja-Aburto VH, Moran-Martinez J, Cebrian-Garcia ME. Organophosporous pesticide exposure decreases sperm quality: association between sperm parameters and urinary pesticide levels. *J Appl Toxicol* **28**: 674–80.

61. Joshi SC, Mathur R, Gulati N. Testicular toxicity of chlorpyrifos (an organophosphate pesticide) in albino rat. *Toxicol Ind Health* 2007; **23**: 439–44.

62. Blum JL, Nyagode BA, James MO, Denslow ND. Effects of the pesticide methoxychlor on gene expression in the liver and testes of the male largemouth bass (*Micropterus salmoides*). *Aquat Toxicol* 2008; **86**: 459–69.

63. Uzumcu M, Kuhn PE, Marano JE, Armenti, AE, Passantino L. Early postnatal methoxychlor exposure inhibits folliculogenesis and stimulates anti-Müllerian hormone production in the rat ovary. *J Endocrinol* 2006; **191**: 549–58.

64. Tiemann U. In vivo and in vitro effects of the organochlorine pesticides DDT, TCPM, methoxychlor, and lindane on the female reproductive tract of mammals: a review. *Reprod Toxicol* 2008; **25**: 316–26.

65. Guillette EA, Conard C, Lares F. *et al.* Altered breast development in young girls from an agricultural environment. *Environ Health Perspect* 2006; **114**: 471–5.

66. Geisz HN, Dickhut RM, Cochran MA, Fraser WR, Ducklow HW. Melting glaciers: a probable source of DDT to the Antarctic marine ecosystem. *Environ Health Perspect* 2008; Doi 10.1021/es702919n.

67. Chiuchiolo AL, Dickhut RM, Cochran MA, Ducklow HW. Persistent organic pollutants at the base of the Antarctic marine food web. *Environ Sci Technol* 2004; **38**: 3551–7.

68. Wiig O, Derocher A E, Cronin MM, Skaare JU. Female pseudohermaphrodite polar bears at Svalbard. *J Wildl Dis* 1998; **34**: 792–6.

69. Colborn T, Vom Saal FS, Soto AM. Developmental effects of endocrine-disrupting chemicals in wildlife amid humans. *Environ Health Perspect* 1993; **101**: 378–84.

70. Wang MH, Baskin LS. Endocrine disruptors, genital development and hypospadias. *J Androl* 2008; **29**: 499–505.

71. Tyler CR, Jobling S, Sumpter JP. Endocrine disruption in wildlife: a critical review of the evidence. *Crit Rev Toxico* 1998; **28**: 319–61.

72. Matozzo V, Gagne F, Marin MG, Ricciardi F, Blaise C. Vitellogenin as a biomarker of exposure to estrogenic compounds in aquatic invertebrates: a review. *Environ Int* 2008; **34**: 531–45.

73. Jobling S, Tyler CR. Endocrine disruption in wild freshwater fish. *Pure Appl Chem.* **75**: 2219–34.

74. Jobling S, Nolan M, Tyler CR, Brighty G, Sumpter JP. Widespread sexual disruption in wild fish. *Environ Sci Tech* 1998; **32**: 2498–506.

75. Jobling S, Coey S, Whitmore JG. *et al.* Wild intersex roach (*Rutilus rutilus*) have reduced fertility. *Biol Reprod* 2002; **67**: 515–24.

76. Guillette LJ Jr, Moore BC. Environmental contaminants, fertility, and multioocytic follicles: a lesson from wildlife. *Semin Reprod Med* 2006; **24**: 134–41.

77. Gulson B, Korsch M, Matisons M *et al.* Re-entrained lead carbonate as the main source of lead in blood of children from a seaside community: an example of local birds as "canaries" in the mine. *Environ Health Perspect* Published online October 23, 2008 (doi: 10.1289/ehp. 11577).

# Environmental contaminants and effects on timing and progression of human pubertal development

Annette Mouritsen, Julie Damm, Lise Aksglaede, Kaspar Sørensen, and Anders Juul

## Normal puberty

Puberty is defined as the transition from childhood to adolescence and is associated with the development of secondary sexual characteristics, accelerated growth, behavioral changes, and finally the attainment of adult reproductive capacity.

Pubertal development is initiated by activation of the hypothalamic–pituitary–gonadal (HPG) axis. Activation of the HPG axis is caused by changes in levels of neurotransmitters such as an increase in glutamate stimulation and a decrease in GABA inhibition of these groups of neurons. It is still not known whether or not it is the increase of the stimulation or the decrease of the inhibition that is the main event leading to the activation of the HPG axis. The level of the neuropeptide kisspeptin is also increased and directly activates the gonadotropin-releasing hormone (GnRH) neurons. Kisspeptin has an important role in the initiation of GnRH secretion in puberty.

At 3 months of postnatal life, the pituitary–gonadal axis is activated for the first time. Thus, infant boys and girls have high follicle-stimulating hormone (FSH) and luteinizing hormone (LH) levels which stimulate gonadal hormone production [1]. At 6 months of age the HPG axis is silenced again, and remains in a quiescent stage until puberty when the HPG axis is reactivated. The reason for this first activation of the HPG axis (also termed mini-puberty) remains unknown. During childhood the HPG axis appears to have a high sensitivity for negative feedback of estrogen, meaning that very low levels of estrogen (or other factors/hormones) are capable of suppressing the gonadotropins until puberty, where this restraint of the hypothalamic–pituitary axis is removed (for review see Aksglaede et al. [2]).

The hypothalamic GnRH pulse generator is stimulated by central and peripheral factors (like leptin), and stimulates the pituitary release of the gonadotropins, FSH and LH.

In girls, secretion of gonadotropins stimulates ovarian estradiol (E2) production, which in turn initiates breast development (thelarche) and, subsequently, uterine/endometrial maturation. Simultaneous with the pituitary–gonadal activation, the adrenal glands increase the secretion of androgens (adrenarche), which results in pubic hair growth (pubarche) approximately 6 months after breast budding. Development of pubic hair is an effect of androgen stimulation; initially from the adrenal gland and subsequently also from the ovaries. The raised level of adrenal androgens is seen already at approximately 6 years of age and continues to increase until menarche, after which a levelling off is observed. The adrenarche is responsible for the initiation of pubic hair development and growth of the axillary hair. Development of pubic hair therefore does not reflect activation of the HPG axis, although pubic hair may never be fully completed in subjects who lack in ovarian function.

The first menstruation (menarche) occurs as a late pubertal event, approximately 2 years after the onset of puberty. The three notable characteristics that have been used to indicate puberty in human females (which are different from pubertal markers in non-human animals) are thelarche, pubarche, and menarche. Evaluation of pubertal onset and progression in girls include the use of Tanner stages [3] for breast (stages B1–B5) and pubic hair (stages PH1–PH5) development. The female Tanner stages are specified in Fig. 9.1a and 9.1b. Thus, while menarche is clinically easier to determine, early breast development is a more sensitive and earlier pubertal index.

In boys, the first clinical evidence of pubertal development, caused by release of gonadotropins, is an

*Environmental Impacts on Reproductive Health and Fertility*, ed. T. J. Woodruff, S. J. Janssen, L. J. Guillette, and L. C. Giudice. Published by Cambridge University Press. © Cambridge University Press 2010.

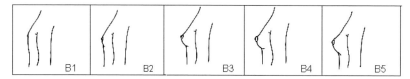

**Fig. 9.1a.** Tanner stages [3]. Breast stage in girls:
B1: Pre-adolescent; elevation of papilla only.
B2: Breast bud stage; elevation of breast and papilla as a small mound, enlargement of areola diameter.
B3: Further enlargement of breast and areola, with no separation of their contours.
B4: Projection of areola and papilla to form a secondary mound above the level of the breast.
B5: Mature stage; projection of papilla only, due to recession of the areola to the general contour of the breast.

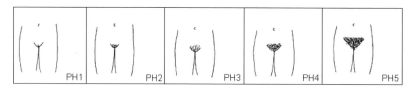

**Fig. 9.1b.** Tanner stages [3]. Pubic hair stage in girls:
PH1: Pre-adolescent; the vellus over the pubes is not further developed than that over the anterior abdominal wall, i.e. no pubic hair.
PH2: Sparse growth of long, slightly pigmented, downy hair, straight or only slightly curled, appearing chiefly along the labia.
PH3: Considerably darker, coarser, and more curled. The hair spreads sparsely over the junction of the pubes.
PH4: Hair is now adult in type, but the area covered by it is still considerably smaller than in most adults. There is no spread to the medial surface of the thighs.
PH5: Adult in quantity and type, distributed as an inverse triangle of the classically feminine pattern. Spread to the medial surface of the thighs.

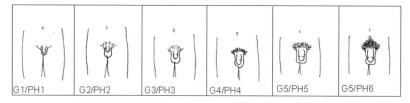

**Fig. 9.1c.** Tanner stages [4]. Genitalia and pubic hair stage in boys:
G1: Pre-adolescent; testes, scrotum, and penis are about the same size and proportion as in early childhood.
G2: The scrotum and testes have enlarged and there is a change in the texture of the scrotal skin. There is also some reddening of the scrotal skin.
G3: Growth of the penis has occurred, at first mainly in length but with some increase in breadth.
G4: Penis further enlarged in length and breadth with development of glans. Testes and scrotum further enlarged. There is also further darkening of the scrotal skin.
G5: Genitalia adult in size and shape. No further enlargement takes place after Stage 5 is reached. Pubic hair stage:
PH1 Pre-adolescent. The velus over the pubes is no further developed than that over the abdominal wall, i.e. no pubic hair.
PH2: Sparse growth of long, slightly pigmented, downy hair, straight or only slightly curled, appearing chiefly at the base of the penis.
PH3: Considerably darker, coarser, and more curled. The hair spreads sparsely over the junction of the pubes.
PH4: Hair is now adult in type, but the area covered by it is still considerably smaller than in most adults. There is no spread to the medial surface of the thighs.
PH5: Adult in quantity and type, and is described in the inverse triangle. There can be spread to the medial surface of the thighs.
PH6: Pubic hair spreads further beyond the triangular pattern.

increase in testicular volume above 3 ml, consistent with genital stage 2 according to Tanner's criteria. This change can only be observed by thorough evaluation at physical examination including the assessment of testicular volume by orchidometry or ultrasound (alternatively testicular length can be measured using a ruler), and the use of Tanner stages [4] for genital (stages G1–G5) and pubic hair (stages PH1–PH6) development. The male Tanner stages are specified in Fig. 9.1c.

As for girls, developmental increase in adrenal androgen secretion (adrenarche) occurs independently of the pituitary–gonadal activation. In contrast to menarche in girls, no specific event can reliably be recalled to time male pubertal development when taking a medical history in boys. Age at first ejaculation is a very unprecise estimate, but can be estimated by analysis of morning urine for the presence of spermatozoa (spermaturia).

Late pubertal phenomena in boys include the pubertal growth spurt (especially determination of age at peak height velocity; PHV) and age at voice break. Voice break and PHV occur at a mean age of 14 years, thus several years after puberty is initiated.

In both sexes, E2 stimulates longitudinal bone growth directly at the level of the growth plate and indirectly via stimulation of increased growth hormone and insulin-like growth factor secretion (for review see Parent *et al.* [5]).

In humans, a striking variability in the timing of puberty is observed among children despite relatively similar life conditions. This variability is dependent on environmental as well as genetic factors.

## Environmental aspects of puberty

Certainly fat mass plays an important role for timing of puberty. Many human studies have shown a positive relation between prepubertal body fat, primarily measured by body mass index (BMI) or skinfold thickness, and onset of puberty as determined by the onset of the growth spurt or in girls by breast development or menarche, or in boys the age at voice break [6–10]. Taken together, these studies suggest that pubertal onset in both sexes may depend on fat mass, although to a higher degree in girls. Other factors, in addition to body fatness, may theoretically be involved in the changes towards earlier sexual maturation, which we are currently witnessing. Less physical activity, insulin-resistance, and changed dietary habits could be involved. Furthermore, exposure to endocrine-disrupting chemicals (EDCs) from the environment could be a candidate factor.

## Genetic aspects of puberty

Several studies have evaluated age at menarche in mono- and dizygotic twins and unanimously found a very high degree of heritability. Kirk *et al.* [11] found a heritability estimate (h2) of 0.50 based on 1373 monozygotic and 1310 dizygotic twin sister pairs. Altogether these studies imply a strong genetic influence on the timing and progression of puberty. Isolated cases of point mutations in selected genes have illustrated such genes are important for puberty. As an example, mutations in *GPR54*, a G protein-coupled receptor gene, cause autosomal recessive idiopathic hypogonadotropic hypogonadism in humans and mice [12]. Conversely, an activating mutation in *GPR54* was recently demonstrated in a girl with precocious puberty [13]. Despite the fact that the kisspeptin–GPR54 system is essential

for normal GnRH physiology and for puberty, common genetic polymorphisms in the GPR54-kisspeptin system do not seem to explain the large variation in pubertal timing [14]. Several genetic studies using association or linkage approaches have suggested several candidate genes associated with variations in age at menarche. These genes include the estrogen receptor gene (ER-α), sex hormone binding globulin (SHBG) gene, androgen receptor gene (AR), and in the estrogen-metabolizing genes – the CYP family genes (CYP450). Such association studies suggested associations between age at menarche and loci related to genes encoding SHBG (*17q13*), CYP 17 (*10q24*) and GPR54 (*19p13*). Nevertheless, a recent genome-wide linkage scan study for quantitative trait loci associated with age at menarche in 2462 women from 402 pedigrees did not support this [15, 16]. Thus, so far no single "puberty gene" has been identified.

## Secular trend in onset and progression of puberty

Most data on timing of sexual maturation depend on studies of girls and age at menarche. These studies suggest a decline in the average age of menarche in the USA over the period from the 1850s to the 1950s [17, 18], which was attributed to improvements in general health, nutrition, and other living conditions over this time frame.

Two large epidemiological studies (PROS and NHANES III) indicate that American girls enter puberty much earlier than what was previously seen. The Pediatric Research in Office Settings (PROS) study was a cross-sectional study on the timing of sexual maturation in girls (assessed pubic hair, breast development, and menarche) on a large (n = 17 077), racially diverse population aged 3–12 years from 1992–93 [19]. The PROS study reported average age at B2 as 9.96 years for Whites and 8.87 years for Blacks, PH2 as 10.51 years for Whites and 8.78 years for Blacks, and menarche as 12.88 years for Whites and 12.16 years for Blacks. These values are lower than any of the studies of preceding years. The average B2 in PROS was approximately 0.6–1.2 years lower and the average PH2 was ~0.5–1.4 years lower than the values from older US studies [15, 20, 21]. In 2002 and 2003, several papers based on pubertal timing in girls from the third National Health and Examination Survey (NHANES III) collected from 1988 to 1994 on children ages 8–19 years were published [10, 22–24]. In this study, age at pubertal

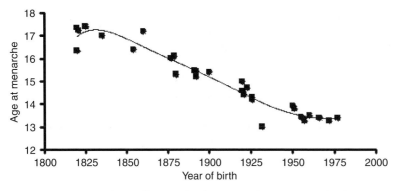

**Fig. 9.2.** Age at menarche in different studies from Denmark according to calendar year. A significant decrease in menarcheal age occurs until the 1960s. Hereafter an apparent halt in the trend towards earlier menarche is seen. (Data are derived from Olesen *et al.* [30])

maturation was slightly higher compared with what was found in PROS, but the majority of authors have interpreted the NHANES III and PROS findings on early puberty as corroborative. In conclusion, the PROS and the NHANES III findings clearly suggest an earlier age of onset of breast and pubic hair development in the US girls in the 1980–90s compared with US data from the 1930–40s, whereas age at first menstrual bleeding occurred only 0.4 years earlier compared with previous studies. Thus, the duration of pubertal development seems to have increased [25–27].

In Europe, a similar decline in age at pubertal maturation has been observed during the last two centuries. As an example, in Denmark the mean menarcheal age has declined from approximately 17 years during the nineteenth century to approximately 13 years today (Fig. 9.2). Examination of menarcheal age in the same region of Denmark in 1965–66 and 1982–83 found a decrease from 13.4 to 13.0 years [28]. A subsequent study from 1996 from the same region demonstrated a halt in the secular trend towards earlier menarche [29]. However, Olesen and coworkers [30] found a renewed decline in mean menarcheal age in a group of Danish textile workers, suggesting that age at menarche could fall even further in Denmark. There are fewer studies that have been able to study the possible secular trend on pubertal onset, as breast palpation is rarely carried out in such studies. A clinical study from the Copenhagen area (carried out in 1991–92) [31] revealed that age at breast development was similar to that reported from Denmark in 1962 [32]. Thus, no apparent secular trend in pubertal onset or progression could be detected from 1962 to 1991–92. Importantly, age at sexual maturation was much later in Denmark compared with what was reported in the American studies (PROS and NHANES III) carried out at the same time.

Genes cannot account for the secular changes in timing of puberty due to the fact that the reported changes in timing of puberty are detected over a few decades. It is therefore more likely that environmental factors play a role in the secular trend.

## Precocious puberty

Traditionally, precocious puberty (PP) is defined as the occurrence of glandular breast tissue or pubic hair before the age of 8–9 years in girls. Menarche is also an important marker used for assessing puberty in girls, although it represents a relatively late pubertal phenomenon (mean age at menarche is 13 years).

Compared with a national study from 1961 [33], a recent nationwide register-based study detected a much higher incidence and prevalence (10–15 times higher) of girls diagnosed with precocious puberty in Denmark in 1994–2001 [34] compared with the data from 1961. The incidence of PP subdivided by gender and age at diagnosis was approximately 0.5 per 10 000 in girls who were younger than 2 years, decreasing to levels below 0.05 per 10 000 in girls aged 2–4 years, thereafter gradually rising to 8 per 10 000 for girls aged 5–9 years. For boys who were younger than 8 years, the incidence was very low (< 1 per 10 000) and increased only slightly to 1–2 per 10 000 in boys aged 8–10 years. The prevalence of PP was approximately 20–23 per 10 000 in girls [34].

Most commonly precocious puberty is of central origin and without known etiology in most girls. By contrast, a significant proportion of boys with central precocious puberty have an underlying pathology. Girls with precocious puberty present with clinical signs of puberty (breast, pubic hair, body odor), growth acceleration, advanced bone age (from X-ray of hand and wrist), and a pubertal LH response (> 6 IU/I) during a

GnRH test. Ultrasonography of ovaries may assist the diagnosis, and in cases of central precocious puberty, a brain MR is performed to rule out CNS pathology. Treatment with a GnRH agonist in such children can, when initiated before 8 years of age in girls, successfully arrest pubertal maturation and increase final height, which may otherwise be compromised.

The demonstrated secular trend towards earlier pubertal onset in US girls has prompted some clinicians to suggest a lowering of the age by which precocious puberty should be defined. Thus, some authors suggest that the limit from which additional diagnostic workup should take place should be lowered to 7 years in White girls, and to 6 years in Black girls. However, controversy exists, as others have claimed that CNS pathologies will be overlooked in 6–8-year-old girls with precocious puberty who would no longer be evaluated properly if revised diagnostic criteria were used.

## Endocrine disrupters and timing of puberty

The possible environmental influences on premature sexual maturation have primarily been studied in populations in which increased incidence of precocious breast development was reported, or by linking exposure data to recorded ages at menarche in exposed populations. These studies are referenced in Table 9.1.

An epidemic of premature thelarche was reported from an Italian school in 1977. Breast enlargement were detected in approximately one third of 3–5-year-old boys and girls, and in 62% of the 6–17-year-old girls from the Via Folli school in the Milan area [35, 36]. Although no estrogen contamination was detected when samples of school meals were tested, an uncontrolled supply of poultry and beef was suspected as the most likely case of this outbreak. Subsequent studies of estrogenic activities in meat products revealed that 150 out of 450 tested food samples had estrogenic activity and detectable DES levels in all samples [37]. Eight children developed gynecomastia in a small village in Bahrain in 1981 [38]. It turned out that all children drank milk from a cow, which had been treated with estrinyl 6 months prior to the first case report. The gynecomastia resolved spontaneously upon slaughter of the cow. Isolated cases of gynecomastia in children have been reported upon accidental exposures to maternal estrogen gels, oral contraceptives, as well as to repeated topical exposure to lavender and tea tree oils [39].

A cross-sectional study of peripubertal girls from Taqui valley of Sonora in Mexico demonstrated that girls from valley towns, areas using modern agricultural practices including the use of pesticides, exhibited more breast tissue compared with girls from Yaqui foothills, where traditional ranching occurs [40]. Likewise, a high incidence of precocious puberty was reported from the Viareggio area in Tuscany with a high density of small industries, navy yards and greenhouses, as compared with surrounding major cities (Livorno, Lucca, Massa, and Pisa) [41]. Both studies represent marked regional variability in the prevalence of precocious puberty within small geographical areas, suggesting differences in exposure to environmental toxins to play a role. However, direct exposure measures were not included in these two studies. In a smaller follow-up study from Tuscany, Massart and coworkers found detectable serum levels of the mycotoxin, zearalenone and its congener, in 6 out of 32 girls with precocious puberty but in none of the 31 controls [42].

The first study to report an association between timing of puberty and developmental exposure to persistent organic pollutants was conducted among a cohort of individuals exposed to brominated flame retardants [43]. An industrial accident resulted in the contamination of cattle feed with polybrominated biphenyls (PBBs) and widespread human exposure through consumption of meat and dairy products. The daughters of women who consumed contaminated farm products were evaluated. Interestingly, girls who were exposed in utero to high concentrations (> 7 ppb) and who were breastfed reported menarche a full year earlier than unexposed girls (< 1 ppb) or girls who were exposed in utero but not breastfed [43].

Increased exposure to persistent PCB congeners has been reported in fishing populations, especially populations whose diet include marine species high in the food chain such as subjects living in the Faroe Islands, where pilot whale is part of the traditional diet. Prenatal exposure to PCBs and its association to spermaturia and reproductive hormones was evaluated in Faroese boys. Despite a wide range of exposure to PCBs, no definite associations with the timing of puberty in boys were reported [44]. Prenatal dioxin exposure was associated with delayed breast development and delayed age at first ejaculation in a small longitudinal cohort (n = 33; 18 girls) [45].

Exposure to lead has been associated with delayed puberty in girls. In a population-based study of 2186 girls (NHANES III), blood lead concentrations of 3 μg/dL

**Table 9.1.** Summary of relationship between exposure and pubertal development

| Compound | Study population | Study area | Methods | Main findings | Reference |
|---|---|---|---|---|---|
| **Perinatal exposure** | | | | | |
| DDE PCBs | 151 girls | Michigan angler cohort of fish-eating mothers with serum DDE levels at time of pregnancy up to 25 µg/L | Retrospective study. Telephone interviews. In utero exposure calculated from maternal serum levels | Reduced age at menarche by 1 year associated with an increase in in utero DDE exposure of 15 µg/L | [49] |
| DDE PCBs | 316 girls 278 boys | North Carolina cohort with DDE concentrations up to 4 µg/g fat | Prospective study. Mail questionnaires. Concentrations in mother's milk and maternal serum | No association with pubertal stages | [48] |
| PBBs | 327 girls | Michigan food chain contamination | Prospective study. Questionnaires. In utero exposure extrapolated from maternal serum levels at the time of the accident | Earlier age at menarche and earlier pubic hair stage in breastfed girls with in utero PBB exposure above 7 ng/g serum | [43] |
| PCBs | 196 boys | Faroese birth cohort | Prospective study. Clinical and physical examination. Concentrations in cord blood | No effect on pubertal stages or testicular volume | [44] |
| PCBs PCDFs | 55 boys | Yucheng | Prospective study. Clinical and physical examination. Maternal serum levels | Reduced penile length | [58] |
| PCDD/F | 18 girls 15 boys | Amsterdam/ Zaandam area | Longitudinal follow up. Concentrations in breast milk | Delayed breast development and age at first ejaculation | [45] |
| **Pubertal exposure** | | | | | |
| DDE | 26 immigrant girls 15 native Belgian girls | Precocious puberty patients (Belgium) | Patients study. Interviews/physical examination. Serum measurements | High levels of plasma DDE in immigrant girls compared to Belgian native controls | [50] |
| PCBs Dioxin measured by CALUX | 80 boys and 120 girls | One rural and two urban villages in Belgium | Cross-sectional study. Physical examination. Pubertal serum levels | Retarded pubertal development associated with higher PCB exposure in boys Retarded breast development associated with higher dioxin levels in girls | [57] |

| Compound | Subjects | Setting | Study | Findings | Reference |
|---|---|---|---|---|---|
| PCB Bisphenol-A Phytoestrogens | 192 girls | New York, inner-city girls | Cross-sectional study. Physical examination. Urinary phytoestrogen and bisphenol-A. Blood lead and PCB (subset) | Phytoestrogens associated with delayed breast development. No effect of bisphenol-A and PCB | [59] |
| Dioxins | 282 girls exposed pre-pubertal | Seveso | Archived serum levels from time of the accident and extrapolated to age at menarche | No effect on age at menarche | [60] |
| Lead | 2186 girls | NHANES III cross-sectional study | Cross-sectional study. Physical examination. Blood lead levels | Delayed pubertal development (breast and pubic hair stage), delayed age at menarche associated with blood lead > 3 µg/dL | [46] |
| Lead | 1235 girls | NHANES III cross-sectional study | Cross-sectional study. Physical examination. Blood lead levels | Delayed attainment of menarche and pubic hair growth | [24] |
| Lead | 489 boys | Cross-sectional study, Chapaevsk, Russia | Cross-sectional study. Physical examination. Blood lead levels | Delayed pubertal onset | [47] |
| Endosulfan | 117 boys 90 controls | Indian village with high levels of endosulfan used as pesticide | Cross-sectional study. Physical examination. Serum levels | Delayed sexual maturation (Tanner stages) | [61] |
| Phthalates | 41 girls with premature breast development 35 controls | Puerto Rico | Case control study. Physical examination Serum analysis | Higher levels of DEHP and MEHP in serum of patients | [53] |
| DBP DEHP | 110 precocious girls 100 controls | Shanghai | Case control study. Ultrasonographies of uterus and ovaries. Serum analysis | Higher levels of DBP and DEHP in patients | [55] |

DDE, dichlorodiphenyldichloroethylene; PCBs, polychlorinated biphenyls; PBBs, polybrominated biphenyls; PCDFs, polychlorinated dibenzo-furans; PCDDs, polychlorinated dibenzo-dioxins; DBP, di-n-butyl phthalate; DEHP, di-(2-ethylhexyl) phthalate; MEHP, mono-(2-ethylhexyl) phthalate.

were associated with significant delays in development of breast and pubic hair and menarche compared to concentrations of 1 µg/dL [46]. Similar results were reported by Wu *et al.* [24]. Furthermore, blood lead concentrations were associated with pubertal delay in a cross-sectional study of 489 Russian boys [47].

Some studies have evaluated pubertal development in children who were exposed to DDT and its metabolite DDE. Gladen and coworkers [48] conducted a prospective cohort study of boys and girls residing in North Carolina in relation to DDE concentrations previously measured in the mothers' serum as well as in cord serum. There was no association between maternal DDE concentrations with age at menarche in their daughters, but an association of higher in utero or lactational exposure to DDT/DDE and earlier breast and pubic hair development was suggested (although not statistically significant). In 2004 Vasiliu and colleagues reported on significantly earlier menarche among girls with an increased in utero exposure to DDT/DDE in a Michigan angler cohort [49].

Krstevska-Konstantinova *et al.* [50] measured DDE concentration among girls with precocious puberty who were born in Belgium compared with those who were foreign born, and found that the foreign-born girls had significantly higher levels of DDE than native-born girls with precocious puberty. However, a proper control group was not included in that study (i.e. DDE levels in foreign-born girls without precocious puberty). Recently, Ouyang and colleagues [51] reported on a significant dose–response relation between serum DDT/DDE concentrations and earlier menarche in Chinese textile workers. However, some controversy exists as others failed to demonstrate any association between DDT exposure and age at sexual maturation [52].

Colon *et al.* [53] studied premature thelarche in girls exposed to phthalate esters. Significantly higher phthalate serum levels were found among the 44 girls with premature thelarche compared with 35 prepubertal control girls. The authors concluded that the findings were suggestive of a possible association between phthalate exposure and premature breast development in girls. Interpretation of these findings may be limited by concerns about the analytical method of measuring the phthalate parent compound instead of its metabolites [54]. A recent study from China found increased serum levels of DBP and DEHP in 110 girls with precocious puberty compared with 100 prepubertal controls [55]. Thus, more studies are needed to conclude on the possible association between phthalate exposure and risk of precocious puberty.

# Possible mechanisms of action

Experimental data from animal models of human puberty have shown that numerous ubiquitous environmental chemicals such as DES, DDT, and PCBs, as well as contemporary-use chemicals such as bisphenol-A and phthalates have detrimental effects on female reproduction (for review see Crain *et al.* [56]). The mechanisms for EDC-induced puberty can theoretically be (1) a central maturation of the hypothalamus/pituitary or (2) a peripheral action directly at the levels of the ovary or breast. Numerous laboratory animal studies indicate that prenatal exposure to natural and synthetic estrogens can accelerate puberty. In rodents, vaginal opening is the earliest visible sign of puberty occurring in response to elevated estrogens. Early vaginal opening (VO) or reduced number of days between VO and estrus is seen in rodents prenatally exposed to estradiol, the synthetic estrogen DES, phytoestrogens, many plasticizers, or bisphenol-A.

Prepubertal exposure to estrogens may induce early breast development, and conversely exposure to compounds that block estrogen action may delay breast development. Dioxin has an antiestrogenic effect on breast development, and exposure of girls to PCBs with dioxin-like activity results in retarded breast development [57].

Despite numerous experimental studies showing the influence of endocrine disrupters on pubertal maturation, limited data exist in humans. However, a number of human studies clearly support findings in animals. Delineating the role of particular endocrine disrupters in promoting early puberty is complicated by the fact that humans are exposed to a cocktail of different EDCs, each of which could have a different effect on puberty and its timing.

# References

1. Chellakooty M, Schmidt IM, Haavisto AM. *et al.* Inhibin A, inhibin B, follicle-stimulating hormone, luteinizing hormone, estradiol, and sex hormone-binding globulin levels in 473 healthy infant girls. *J Clin Endocrinol Metab* 2003; **88**: 3515–20.
2. Aksglaede L, Juul A, Leffers H, Skakkebaek NE, Andersson AM. The sensitivity of the child to sex steroids: possible impact of exogenous estrogens. *Hum Reprod Update* 2006; **12**: 341–9.
3. Marshall WA, Tanner JM. Variations in pattern of pubertal changes in girls. *Arch Dis Child* 1969; **44**: 291–303.
4. Marshall WA, Tanner JM. Variations in the pattern of pubertal changes in boys. *Arch Dis Child* 1970; **45**: 13–23.

5. Parent AS, Teilmann G, Juul A. *et al.* The timing of normal puberty and the age limits of sexual precocity: variations around the world, secular trends, and changes after migration. *Endocr Rev* 2003; **24**: 668–93.

6. Adair L S, Gordon-Larsen P. Maturational timing and overweight prevalence in US adolescent girls. *Am J Public Health* 2001; **91**: 642–4.

7. He Q, Karlberg J. BMI in childhood and its association with height gain, timing of puberty, and final height. *Pediatr Res* 2001; **49**: 244–51.

8. Freedman DS, Khan LK, Serdula MK. *et al.* Relation of age at menarche to race, time period, and anthropometric dimensions: the Bogalusa Heart Study. *Pediatrics* 2002; **110**: e43.

9. Juul A, Magnusdottir S, Scheike T, Prytz S, Skakkebaek NE. Age at voice break in Danish boys: effects of pre-pubertal body mass index and secular trend. *Int J Androl* 2007; **30**: 537–42.

10. Anderson SE, Dallal GE, Must A. Relative weight and race influence average age at menarche: results from two nationally representative surveys of US girls studied 25 years apart. *Pediatrics* 2003; **111**: 844–50.

11. Kirk KM, Blomberg SP, Duffy DL. *et al.* Natural selection and quantitative genetics of life-history traits in Western women: a twin study. *Evolution* 2001; **55**: 423–35.

12. Seminara SB, Messager S, Chatzidaki EE. *et al.* The GPR54 gene as a regulator of puberty. *New Engl J Med* 2003; **349**: 1614–27.

13. Teles MG, Bianco SD, Brito VN. *et al.* A GPR54-activating mutation in a patient with central precocious puberty. *New Engl J Med* 2008; **358**: 709–15.

14. Luan X, Zhou Y, Wang W. *et al.* Association study of the polymorphisms in the KISS1 gene with central precocious puberty in Chinese girls. *Eur J Endocrinol* 2007; **157**: 113–18.

15. Reynolds EL, Wines JV. Individual differences in physical changes associated with adolescence in girls. *Am J Dis Child* 1948; **75**: 329–50.

16. Guo Y, Shen H, Xiao P. *et al.* Genomewide linkage scan for quantitative trait loci underlying variation in age at menarche. *J Clin Endocrinol Metab* 2006; **91**: 1009–14.

17. Zacharias L, Wurtman RJ. Age at menarche. Genetic and environmental influences. *New Engl J Med* 1969; **280**: 868–75.

18. Wyshak G, Frisch RE. Evidence for a secular trend in age of menarche. *New Engl J Med* 1982; **306**: 1033–5.

19. Herman-Giddens ME, Slora EJ, Wasserman RC. *et al.* Secondary sexual characteristics and menses in young girls seen in office practice: a study from the Pediatric Research in Office Settings network. *Pediatrics* 1997; **99**: 505–12.

20. Nicolson AB, Hanley C. Indices of physiological maturity: derivation and interrelationships. *Child Dev* 1953; **24**: 3–38.

21. Lee PA. Normal ages of pubertal events among American males and females. *J Adolesc Health Care* 1980; **1**: 26–9.

22. Sun SS, Schubert CM, Chumlea WC. *et al.* National estimates of the timing of sexual maturation and racial differences among US children. *Pediatrics* 2002; **110**: 911–19.

23. Chumlea WC, Schubert CM, Roche AF. *et al.* Age at menarche and racial comparisons in US girls. *Pediatrics* 2003; **111**: 110–13.

24. Wu T, Buck GM, Mendola P. Blood lead levels and sexual maturation in U.S. girls: the Third National Health and Nutrition Examination Survey, 1988–1994. *Environ Health Perspect* 2003; **111**: 737–41.

25. Euling SY, Herman-Giddens ME, Lee PA. *et al.* Examination of US puberty-timing data from 1940 to 1994 for secular trends: panel findings. *Pediatrics* 2008; **121** (Suppl. 3): S172–91.

26. Euling SY, Selevan SG, Pescovitz OH, Skakkebaek NE. Role of environmental factors in the timing of puberty. *Pediatrics* 2008; **121** (Suppl. 3): S167–71.

27. Buck Louis GM, Gray LE, Jr., Marcus M. *et al.* Environmental factors and puberty timing: expert panel research needs. *Pediatrics* 2008; **121** (Suppl. 3): S192–207.

28. Helm, P., Helm S. Decrease in menarcheal age from 1966 to 1983 in Denmark. *Acta Obstet Gynecol Scand* 1984; **63**: 633–5.

29. Helm P. Grolund L. A halt in the secular trend towards earlier menarche in Denmark. *Acta Obstet Gynecol Scand* 1998; **77**: 198–200.

30. Olesen AW, Jeune B, Boldsen JL. A continuous decline in menarcheal age in Denmark. *Ann Hum Biol* 2000; **27**: 377–86.

31. Juul A, Teilmann G, Scheike T. *et al.* Pubertal development in Danish children: comparison of recent European and US data. *Int J Androl* 2006; **29**: 247–55.

32. Andersen E. Skeletal maturation of Danish school children in relation to height, sexual development, and social conditions. *Acta Paediat Scand* 1968; Suppl.

33. Thamdrup E. *Precocious sexual development. A clinical study of 100 children*. Doctoral thesis, 1961.

34. Teilmann G, Pedersen CB, Jensen TK, Skakkebaek NE, Juul A. Prevalence and incidence of precocious pubertal development in Denmark: an epidemiologic study based on national registries. *Pediatrics* 2002; **116**: 1323–8.

35. Scaglioni S, Di Pietro C, Bigatello A, Chiumello G. Breast enlargement at an Italian school. *Lancet* 1978; **1**: 551–2.

36. Fara GM, Del Corvo G, Bernuzzi S. *et al.* Epidemic of breast enlargement in an Italian school. *Lancet* 1979; **2**: 295–7.

37. Loizzo A, Gatti GL, Macri A. *et al.* Italian baby food containing diethylstilbestrol: three years later. *Lancet* 1984; **1**: 1014–15.

38. Kimball AM, Hamadeh R, Mahmood RA. *et al.* Gynaecomastia among children in Bahrain. *Lancet* 1981; **1**: 671–2.

39. Henley DV, Lipson N, Korach KS, Bloch CA. Prepubertal gynecomastia linked to lavender and tea tree oils. *New Engl J Med* 2007; **356**: 479–85.

40. Guillette EA, Conard C, Lares F. *et al.* Altered breast development in young girls from an agricultural environment. *Environ Health Perspect*, **114**, 471–5.

41. Massart F, Seppia P, Pardi D. *et al.* High incidence of central precocious puberty in a bounded geographic area of northwest Tuscany: an estrogen disrupter epidemic? *Gynecol Endocrinol* 2005; **20**: 92–8.

42. Massart F, Meucci V, Saggese G, Soldani G. High growth rate of girls with precocious puberty exposed to estrogenic mycotoxins. *J Pediatr* 2008; **152**: 690–5.

43. Blanck HM, Marcus M, Tolbert PE. *et al.* Age at menarche and tanner stage in girls exposed in utero and postnatally to polybrominated biphenyl. *Epidemiology* 2000; **11**: 641–7.

44. Mol NM, Sorensen N, Weihe P. *et al.* Spermaturia and serum hormone concentrations at the age of puberty in boys prenatally exposed to polychlorinated biphenyls. *Eur J Endocrinol* 2002; **146**: 357–63.

45. Leijs MM, Koppe JG, Olie K. *et al.* Delayed initiation of breast development in girls with higher prenatal dioxin exposure; a longitudinal cohort study. *Chemosphere* 2008; **73**: 999–1004.

46. Selevan SG, Rice DC, Hogan KA. *et al.* Blood lead concentration and delayed puberty in girls. *New Engl J Med* 2003; **348**: 1527–36.

47. Hauser R, Sergeyev O, Korrick S. *et al.* Association of blood lead levels with onset of puberty in Russian boys. *Environ Health Perspect* 2008; **116**: 976–80.

48. Gladen BC, Ragan NB, Rogan WJ. Pubertal growth and development and prenatal and lactational exposure to polychlorinated biphenyls and dichlorodiphenyl dichloroethene. *J Pediatr*, 2000; **136**: 490–6.

49. Vasiliu O, Muttineni J, Karmaus W. In utero exposure to organochlorines and age at menarche. *Hum Reprod* 2004; **19**: 1506–12.

50. Krstevska-Konstantinova M, Charlier C, Craen M. *et al.* Sexual precocity after immigration from developing countries to Belgium: evidence of previous exposure to organochlorine pesticides. *Hum Reprod* 2001; **16**: 1020–6.

51. Ouyang F, Perry MJ, Venners SA. *et al.* Serum DDT, age at menarche, and abnormal menstrual cycle length. *Occup Environ Med* 2005; **62**: 878–84.

52. Denham M., Schell LM, Deane G. *et al.* Relationship of lead, mercury, mirex, dichlorodiphenyldichloroethylene, hexachlorobenzene, and polychlorinated biphenyls to timing of menarche among Akwesasne Mohawk girls. *Pediatrics* 2005; **115**: e127–34.

53. Colon I, Caro D, Bourdony CJ, Rosario O. Identification of phthalate esters in the serum of young Puerto Rican girls with premature breast development. *Environ Health Perspect* 2000; **108**: 895–900.

54. McKee RH. Phthalate exposure and early thelarche. *Environ Health Perspect* 2004; **112**: A541–3.

55. Qiao L, Zheng L, Cai D. [Study on the di-n-butyl phthalate and di-2-ethylhexyl phthalate level of girl serum related with precocious puberty in Shanghai]. *Wei Sheng Yan Jiu* 2007; **36**: 93–5.

56. Crain DA, Janssen SJ, Edwards TM. *et al.* Female reproductive disorders: the roles of endocrine-disrupting compounds and developmental timing. *Fertil Steril* 2008; **90**: 911–40.

57. Den Hond E, Roels HA, Hoppenbrouwers K. *et al.* Sexual maturation in relation to polychlorinated aromatic hydrocarbons: Sharpe and Skakkebaek's hypothesis revisited. *Environ Health Perspect* 2002; **110**: 771–6.

58. Guo YL, Lambert GH, Hsu CC, Hsu MM. Yucheng: health effects of prenatal exposure to polychlorinated biphenyls and dibenzofurans. *Int Arch Occup Environ Health* 2004; **77**: 153–8.

59. Wolff MS, Britton JA, Boguski L. *et al.* Environmental exposures and puberty in inner-city girls. *Environ Res* 2008; **107**: 393–400.

60. Warner M, Samuels S, Mocarelli P. *et al.* Serum dioxin concentrations and age at menarche. *Environ Health Perspect* 2004; **112**: 1289–92.

61. Saiyed H, Dewan A, Bhatnagar V. *et al.* Effect of endosulfan on male reproductive development. *Environ Health Perspect* 2003; **111**: 1958–62.

# Environmental contaminants and impacts on healthy and successful pregnancies

Rémy Slama and Sylvaine Cordier

## Introduction

### Public health relevance of healthy and successful pregnancies

While there have been important declines in perinatal and maternal death rates over the last decades in some countries, rates remain manifold higher in non-industrialized compared with industrialized countries [1]. Moreover, other adverse pregnancy outcomes carry an important public health burden. This is in particular the case for preterm delivery, which is associated with increased neonatal morbidity and mortality; it also carries long-term consequences, as preterm and very preterm births are associated with increased frequencies of neurodevelopmental and behavioral adverse events such as cerebral palsy, cognitive and school difficulties, or altered pulmonary function in childhood and adolescence [2]. According to the *developmental origins of health and disease* (DOHaD) hypothesis, environmental exposures during development may increase the risk of chronic disease in childhood and adulthood, such as metabolic syndrome or cardiovascular disease [3]. Altered fetal growth is probably one marker of these environmental or nutritional aggressions, and birthweight has been shown to be associated with adult illness [3]. Because of the methodological challenges and the length of follow-up necessary to efficiently assess environmental exposures during pregnancy and their long-term consequences in humans, current knowledge presumably only represents a small part of the long-term burden of disease entailed by pregnancy exposures and the associated adverse pregnancy outcomes.

### Scope of this chapter

We will focus on adverse events occurring between fertilization (excluding fecundity troubles) and birth

(Fig. 10.1). We will refer to unintentional fetal losses as early fetal losses (or spontaneous abortions) if these occur within 20 weeks after the date of the last menstrual period and as stillbirths after 20 gestational weeks. Preterm birth is defined as a birth before 37 gestational weeks. Fetal growth is usually assessed from birthweight, combined with information on gestational duration in order to distinguish it from preterm delivery; it is either treated as a continuous outcome (in which case changes in mean gestational age-adjusted birthweight in association with exposure are considered), or dichotomized by comparing birthweight to gestational age- and sex-specific birthweight distribution in a reference population, which allows identifying small-for-gestational age (SGA) births. Congenital malformations and secondary sex ratio (the proportion of male offspring among all births, a value usually close to 0.51) are other considered outcomes. Relevant exposures of either parent-to-be can occur over a larger time period, from the preconceptional period until birth. Effects of prenatal exposures on health in childhood or adulthood (e.g. cancer occurrence) will not be considered here.

In assessing the evidence for environmental effects on healthy and successful pregnancies, our primary focus will be on epidemiologic studies. Considering the support from animal experiments is an important criterion to judge the plausibility of epidemiologic results, but a systematic review of the toxicological evidence is beyond the scope of this chapter.

Adapting a hierarchy already proposed [4], the level of evidence regarding the effect of each given environmental factor on each outcome will be classified as *sufficient* (several good quality studies by different groups, or an expert panel already considered the level of proof as sufficient), *limited* (evidence is suggestive of

*Environmental Impacts on Reproductive Health and Fertility*, ed. T. J. Woodruff, S. J. Janssen, L. J. Guillette, and L. C. Giudice. Published by Cambridge University Press. © Cambridge University Press 2010.

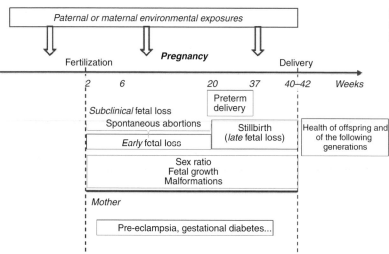

**Fig. 10.1.** Overview of the pregnancy outcomes considered (health of offspring after birth not covered here).

an association, e.g. based on one good quality study), or *inadequate* (available studies are of insufficient quality, consistency or statistical power to permit a conclusion regarding the presence or absence of an association). If the reported effect sizes were imprecise, as can be judged from their confidence intervals, "negative" studies (i.e. not showing statistically significant associations) have not been viewed as contradicting reports in favor of an association [5].

## Some challenges in the study of environmental effects on pregnancy

The application of environmental epidemiology to human reproduction can be seen as the attempt to study the effect of silent exposures on events that often remain hidden. Indeed, most of what occurs to the embryo or the fetus is hidden during pregnancy, and will usually only become visible at delivery. Specific techniques (such as ultrasonography) can allow unveiling of part of the ongoing events. A consequence of these techniques is that medical interventions are performed on some of the pregnancies with a poor diagnosis, which will distort the "normal" course of the pregnancy. For example, some pregnancies are ended by a cesarian section, which are difficult to handle in studies with gestational duration as an outcome. In addition, the start of the period at risk (the pregnancy) can usually only be detected retrospectively, several weeks after it occurred; the recruitment of couples right before or right after the start of the pregnancy remains an exception, and most studies rely on women recruited during the second half of pregnancy, or after delivery.

The challenges related to exposure assessment include handling efficiently exposures to co-pollutants (*mixture* issue, identification of a relevant proxy measure), defining exposure during the right exposure window, handling possible temporal changes in exposure during pregnancy, and trying to disentangle effects of paternal and maternal exposures. For many environmental contaminants, exposure levels (and possibly internal doses for the many contaminants with a short biological half-life) fluctuate over time, and assessing exposure only once during the pregnancy generally yields a poor picture of the biologically relevant exposure. This is all the more complex since the time window of susceptibility is generally not known, and can in theory be a short period during pregnancy, or even before conception, which implies having to be able to recruit couples when the pregnancy is only a project. Biomarkers of exposure have allowed important progress, but they cannot completely address the above-mentioned issues related to contaminants with strong temporal variability, unless the time-window of sensitivity is short and identified or repeated biological samples are collected. Their use in a population of pregnant women requires specific consideration linked to the fact that pregnancy can accelerate or decelerate the metabolism of some xenobiotics. Contrary to laboratory animals, human populations are rarely exposed to one single pollutant at a time. Epidemiologic research often relies on the "old" toxicologic approach of considering environmental pollutants one at a time (ignoring co-exposures), or treating co-exposures as nuisance terms (e.g. as adjustment factors whose effect needs to be removed). This fits well with the approach currently used to regulate pollutants, but might not be as efficient as treating mixtures as a whole to identify causes of adverse health outcomes [6].

# A historical example: effects of maternal smoking on the course of pregnancy

Maternal smoking increases the risk of subclinical fetal loss, ectopic pregnancy, fetal loss [7], stillbirth, sudden infant death syndrome [8], and preterm and very preterm birth not mediated by gestational hypertension [9]; it induces a decrease of about 10–20 g in term birthweight for each cigarette smoked daily; it probably induces an increase in the risk of congenital malformations such as oral clefts or digestive system anomalies [10] and a reduction in the risk of preeclampsia [11]. Maternal smoking level has little day-to-day variations, can be efficiently assessed by a simple retrospective questionnaire to the mother (this may be less true today, at a time when many women are aware of its dangers) and has large effects. The situation is by far more challenging in terms of exposure assessment for most of the environmental contaminants that we will now consider.

# Air pollutants

Air pollution is a mixture of thousands of compounds, which vary in nature and concentration with season and location. Epidemiologic studies only assess a few of these compounds (usually those for which a regulatory level exists, which may not correspond to those really affecting health), which may be correlated with the other constituents of the air pollution mixture differently in each season and location. This may limit between-study consistency in associations with health outcomes.

In this section, we will focus on pollutants whose sources are mainly in the outdoor air. The primary focus will be on "criteria" air pollutants such as particulate matter (PM), carbon monoxide (CO), ozone, nitrogen dioxide ($NO_2$), etc., but studies using a "source-oriented" approach (e.g. those about the health of subjects in relation to the vicinity of traffic or specific industrial sources) will also be mentioned. Some air pollutants with specifically indoor sources are discussed in the sections on ETS and solvents, and the particular case of nuclear waste reprocessing plants is treated in the section on ionizing radiation.

## Fetal loss

A time-series study has reported increased rates of stillbirth (after 28 gestational weeks) in São Paulo (Brazil) in relation to the $NO_2$ levels averaged over the five previous days [12]. In another study in São Paulo relying on a case–control design, exposure to traffic-related air pollution (as assessed by distance-weighted traffic intensity) tended to be associated with an increased risk of stillbirth [13]. A study on association between vicinity to traffic and fetal loss in California has been recently published (Green S *et al.*, Env. Health Perspect, in press). An experiment reported an increased rate of implantation failures in mice in relation to traffic-related air pollution, and a non-significant trend towards an increase in fetal losses [14]. Another experiment in rats showed decreases in the number of pups per litter and in fetal survival in relation to increasing exposure to inhaled benzo-[a]-pyrene, a compound of the PAH (polycyclic aromatic hydrocarbons) family.

## Fetal growth

Many studies reported decrements in mean birthweight adjusted for gestational duration, or increases in the proportion of SGA births in association with air pollution levels during pregnancy [15, 16–18]. The first studies often relied on the air quality monitoring station closest to the home address to estimate air pollution levels, but some studies have also relied on environmental models with finer spatial resolution [19], personal monitoring of fine PM ($PM_{2.5}$, those with an aerodynamical diameter below 2.5 μm) [20], or PAH exposure [21]. In a study in California relying on the network of air quality monitoring stations, an increase by 10 μg/m$^3$ in the mean $PM_{2.5}$ pregnancy average was associated with an adjusted decrease by 38 g (95% confidence interval, 22–55 g) in birthweight [22]. Studies taking account of either spatial or temporal contrasts in exposure (or both) have been conducted, yielding, again, rather consistent findings [23]. Associations have been reported for birthweight, SGA births, but also head circumference and birth length. A study relying on fetal ultrasound measurements suggest that air pollution effects might already be manifest in the first half of pregnancy [24], which does not preclude effects of exposures at the end of pregnancy. These reported effects have some experimental support, in particular from a study in which mice were maintained during gestation in an exposure chamber located at an intersection with heavy traffic in a major Brazilian city [25].

Carbon monoxide, $NO_2$, $PM_{2.5}$ and soot are markers of combustion-related (and in particular traffic-related) air pollutants and are quite consistently associated with altered fetal growth. Therefore, road traffic and other combustion sources appear as the first suspects likely to explain a detrimental effect of air pollution on fetal growth.

## Gestational duration

An increased risk of preterm birth has been reported in association with air pollution levels during pregnancy. In retrospective cohort studies relying on air quality monitoring stations, markers of traffic-related air pollution such as CO [26] and $PM_{2.5}$ have been associated with an increased risk of preterm delivery [27]. A time-series analysis in Pennsylvania also suggested that short-term exposures to $PM_{10}$ (particulate matter with an aerodynamical diameter below 10 μm) and $SO_2$ might increase the risk of preterm birth [28]. An ecologic study took advantage of a natural experiment during the closure of a steel mill, which was accompanied by decreases in $PM_{10}$ levels in the air, as well as PM content in metals. Authors reported decreased rates of preterm births during the closure of the mill in the Utah Valley (USA) followed by an increase after the mill started operating again [29]. No similar temporal trend was observed outside the Utah Valley, further away from the plant. This finding is of importance because the quasi-experimental design of this study makes confounding by spatially varying factors unlikely. Effects of traffic-related air pollutants on preeclampsia risk have been reported (Wu *et al.*, Env. Health Perspect, 2009).

## Congenital malformations

A few studies based on registers of congenital malformations or births in California [30], Texas [31], France [32], the UK [33], and Taiwan [34] have been performed. Ritz *et al.* [30] reported increased risks of cardiac ventricular septal defects in association with CO levels during the second month of pregnancy, which corresponds to a period of rapid fetal heart formation. No monotonous adverse association with CO levels during the first and third months of pregnancy were observed. Ozone second month averages were also associated with aortic artery and valve defects, pulmonary artery and valve anomalies. In a study in Texas, the highest category of average ozone levels during the weeks 3–8 of pregnancy was also associated with odds-ratios of aortic artery and valve defects and odds-ratio of pulmonary artery and valve defects above unity, with large confidence intervals [31]. Results for CO were difficult to compare with the Californian study because average levels were lower in the Texas study and exposure categories differed between studies [31]. Ozone levels during the first or second gestational months were reported to be associated with the risk of cleft lip with or without cleft palate, in a case–control study conducted in Taiwan [34]. The odds-ratio for this malformation reported by the Californian study was consistent with a deleterious effect of ozone levels during the second month of gestation, with broad confidence intervals [30]. A study conducted around solid waste incinerators in the Rhône-Alpes region (France) and relying on a dispersion modeling of the incinerator emissions highlighted an increasing trend of congenital obstructive uropathies with exposure [32]. In Cumbria (north-west England), proximity at birth to an incinerator was associated with increasing risks of heart defects and lethal congenital anomaly, in particular spina bifida [33].

## Sex ratio

So far, one ecologic study in humans in São Paulo reported a decrease in the proportion of male births in association with the $PM_{10}$ levels assessed by the air quality monitoring network [35]. An experiment in which mice were maintained during gestation in an exposure chamber located at an intersection with heavy traffic showed a decrease in the proportion of male pups, compared with mice maintained in filtered chambers [35].

# Environmental tobacco smoke

Tobacco smoke is a mixture of thousands of compounds present in gaseous form or as particulate matter (in the size range between 0.1 and 1 μm). As for many other non-persistent compounds or mixtures, assessment of exposure to environmental tobacco smoke (ETS) is particularly challenging; questionnaires have limitations, and biomarkers such as cotinine (a metabolite of nicotine) are limited by the short half-life of cotinine in the bodies of pregnant women, which is probably around 9 hours [36], compared with about 19 hours in male adults. Overall, the evidence of an effect of ETS is limited for all outcomes but fetal growth and preterm delivery, for which the evidence of an effect can be considered sufficient [37].

## Fetal loss

In a prospective study of newly married couples in which a biomarker of pregnancy was assayed, paternal smoking was associated with an increase in the risk of early pregnancy loss [38]. Such an association may be due to an effect of maternal exposure to ETS or of paternal exposure to tobacco smoke on spermatozoa.

A prospective study reported no increased risk of spontaneous abortion in association with exposure to ETS assessed by questionnaire among non-smokers [39]. One case–control study relying on cotinine assays reported an increased risk of clinical spontaneous abortions in association with cotinine levels among non-smoking women [40]; in spite of a strong study design, several types of rather complex biases might explain such an association [41], so that studies with alternative approaches are warranted.

### Fetal growth

Environmental tobacco smoke exposure, as assessed by a cotinine assay from blood specimens collected during pregnancy, is associated with monotonous decreases in birthweight [37, 42].

### Gestational duration

Several studies relying on biomarkers of exposure reported increased risks of preterm delivery in association with maternal exposure to ETS [37, 42]. No clearly monotonous associations were observed. It must be noted that effects reported for active smoking are relatively small, and differ according to the etiology of preterm birth [9].

### Congenital malformations

Environmental tobacco smoke may be associated with congenital malformations such as non-syndromic oral cleft [43], in line with findings concerning maternal smoking. An increased risk of neural tube defects has also been reported in association with ETS exposure [44]. Studies on the association with the risk of male genital anomalies have shown conflicting results.

### Sex ratio

Smoking of either parent at the time of conception has been reported to entail a decrease in the proportion of male births [45]. Later studies failed to replicate the finding [46].

## Drinking-water pollutants

As for air pollutants, exposure to drinking-water contaminants is widespread and a low increase in risk may contribute to a sizeable proportion of cases of adverse pregnancy outcomes. A number of chemicals are conveyed via drinking water, to which the population is exposed through ingestion, but also through dermal contact or inhalation, when volatile chemicals are released from hot water, during showering for instance. Chemical mixtures likely to be present in public water supplies are those derived from the disinfection step of water treatment (disinfection by-products, or DBPs). In many regions, raw water is also particularly vulnerable to agricultural run offs of fertilizers or pesticides. Presence of these chemicals is not always adequately controlled

during the water treatment process, especially among populations served by private water systems. Microbial contamination will not be considered here.

## Disinfection by-products

While chlorination of public water supplies is a means of controlling infectious diseases, the interaction of chlorine with the organic content of water can generate up to 600 chemical by-products identified to date [47]. The most prevalent classes of compounds are trihalomethanes (THMs) and haloacetic acids. In most countries, surveillance of public water supplies is based on periodic measurement of THMs, considered as markers of the whole mixture. In recent epidemiologic studies, these measurements combined with knowledge of maternal residence during pregnancy and, in some instances, of water uses, are the basis for building exposure indexes. As for atmospheric pollutants, the comparison of the results from various areas is made difficult by the fact that the relative concentrations of DBPs vary between areas, and that the concentration of a very small number of these inter-related pollutants are usually assessed.

### Fetal loss

A prospective study conducted in California suggested an increased risk of spontaneous abortions among women who consumed five or more glasses of cold tap water per day containing $\geq 75\ \mu g/L$ of total THMs; the risk was highest for bromodichloromethane, one of the constituents of the THMs group [48]. These results based on good-quality exposure and outcome assessment were not confirmed by a subsequent study conducted in three USA communities with contrasted exposure using refined exposure characterization [49]. Case–control studies in Canada have reported an increased risk for stillbirths in areas where THMs level was $>80\ \mu g/L$ [50]. No such association was highlighted in a large registry-based study covering three regions in the UK without individual information on drinking, showering, and bathing habits [51].

### Fetal growth

Sixteen studies have been published to date on fetal growth and DBPs [52–54]. Five of these studies used only information on the type of water treatment for exposure characterization, three case–control studies had individual data on water uses [55–57]. Most assessed exposure during the third trimester of pregnancy. Statistically significant associations with low birthweight have been reported in earlier studies while the more recent studies did not confirm this association. Studies on SGA showed more consistent results, the majority reporting increased risks overall. One study showed evidence of an effect measure modification with a genetic variant of the *CYP2E1* gene [56]. Results of the study conducted in three US communities concluded to an elevated risk of SGA babies when maternal exposure to THMs in drinking water exceeded 80 μg/L during the third trimester [58].

### Gestational duration
Studies have quite consistently reported no association between maternal DBP exposure and preterm delivery.

### Congenital malformations
In a meta-analysis of five case–control studies on congenital malformations, Hwang and Jaakkola [59] concluded that their analysis provides evidence for an association with the risk of any birth defect and of neural tube and urinary system defects, whereas evidence regarding cardiac, respiratory defects and oral clefts was heterogeneous and inconclusive. These conclusions were not supported by a registry-based, subsequently published study in England and Wales covering 2.6 million births and using a modeling of THMs data at the place of birth [60].

## Nitrates
Concern regarding impact of exposure to nitrates in drinking water came after the report of cases of methemoglobinemia among infants drinking formula preparation prepared with well water in 1945, an observation that is the basis for the current US standard of 45 mg/L. Nitrate and its metabolite nitrite are precursors in the in vivo formation of N-nitroso compounds, which are potent animal carcinogens.

Overall, the evidence for an impact of high nitrate levels in drinking water on pregnancy outcomes is limited.

### Pregnancy complications
An Australian record-based study reported an association between the risk of prelabor rupture of membranes and increased level of nitrate in water [61].

### Fetal loss
Spontaneous abortions are the main adverse pregnancy outcomes observed among domestic or experimental animals in relation to nitrate exposure. Early case reports in humans supported such an association

but these initial observations were not confirmed by subsequent studies [62].

### Fetal growth, gestational duration
A registry-based study in Prince Edward Island (Canada) reported increased risks of prematurity and intrauterine growth restriction in association with nitrate-nitrogen levels above 3.1 mg/L [63].

### Congenital malformations
Six studies have assessed the association between high nitrate exposure and congenital malformations. Non-significantly increased risks of neural tube defects and cardiac defects have been observed among users of private wells or drinkers of water with higher nitrate levels [64].

## Metals
## Lead

### Fetal loss
In a large study conducted in Mexico City, a doubling in the risk of late fetal death was observed for maternal blood lead levels as low as 5–9 μg/dL [65]. There is also suggestive evidence for high paternal lead exposures (>30 μg/dL blood) to be associated with an increased risk of spontaneous abortions [66].

### Pregnancy complications
There have been several concordant observations that the risk of pregnancy hypertension might be increased among women with blood levels in the order of 10 μg/L. This was confirmed in a study using bone lead as a marker of exposure [67].

### Fetal growth, gestational duration
Findings of recent studies are generally consistent with the hypothesis that maternal lead exposure during pregnancy is inversely related to fetal growth, including infant size at birth, as well as to gestational duration [68]. Similarly, paternal exposures above 25 μg/dL for at least 5 years appear to increase the risks of preterm birth and low birthweight.

### Congenital malformations
There is currently no consistent evidence that parental exposure to lead might lead to an increased risk of congenital malformations.

## Sex ratio

Paternal inorganic lead levels have been reported to entail a dose-related decrease in sex ratio [69].

## Cadmium

Early reports of an impact of maternal cadmium exposure during pregnancy on fetal growth may have been confounded by maternal smoking. More recent studies among non-smoking women found inconsistent associations between maternal exposure to cadmium and markers of fetal growth (birth height or weight) or gestational duration but their conclusions are limited by their small sample size [4].

## Mercury

### Fetal loss

Paternal exposure to inorganic mercury has been associated with an increased risk of spontaneous abortions [70]. Early studies have been conducted among female occupational groups exposed to inorganic mercury but did not reveal an increased risk of spontaneous abortions or congenital malformations associated with mercury exposure at the levels present in these workplaces.

### Gestational duration

An increased risk of very preterm births (< 35 weeks) was reported for mercury levels in maternal hair above 0.55 µg/g [71].

### Health of the newborn

Severe disruption of the developing central nervous system (palsy and retardation) has been observed at birth among children exposed prenatally to poisoning episodes of methylmercury in Minamata, Japan or in Iraq. These effects were observed for maternal hair concentrations of at least 400 µg/g [72]. Insults to the developing central nervous system resulting from prenatal exposure to methylmercury at lower levels are mainly observed during child psychomotor development.

## Arsenic

Exposure to arsenic-contaminated drinking water affects tens of millions of people worldwide and a number of health studies have been conducted, particularly in Bangladesh and West Bengal. Two large cohort studies have shown a small but statistically significant increased risk of fetal death and of congenital malformations among pregnant women who had been exposed from drinking water containing more than 50 µg/L of arsenic [73].

## Pesticides

Pesticides encompass a wide variety of compounds with different targets (insecticides, herbicides, fungicides …) and different chemical compositions. They are largely used worldwide to protect crops and landscape or to control pest populations. Potential exposure of human populations occurs during professional use and from environmental contamination of air, food, and water. Persistence in the environment and bioaccumulation of pesticides used decades ago, such as DDT, are two factors responsible for chronic exposure, which has led to a shift towards use of compounds with shorter half-life.

We will limit our review to studies focused on specific chemical classes of pesticides, disregarding studies in which chemical classes of pesticides have not been assessed. Several pesticides have been identified as likely causes of the alterations of the reproductive process observed in wild animals, and these alterations have been attributed to the action of pesticides on the endocrine system. Compounds such as vinclozolin, linuron, DDT, and DDE (a metabolite of DDT) are known androgen receptor antagonists [74]. These compounds, and others with xenohormonal activity, are suspected of being responsible for a number of disorders of human reproductive health such as altered sex ratio, or adverse outcomes among males such as congenital anomalies of the reproductive tract [75].

## Organochlorine pesticides and TCDD-contaminated chlorophenoxy herbicides (2,4,5-T)

### Fetal loss

A prospective study conducted among textile workers in China [76] avoided most limitations of previous studies since it associated preconception serum total DDT with biological detection of early conceptions. Authors found a positive, monotonic, association between early pregnancy losses and DDT exposure. A number of small studies looking at the impact of maternal serum hexachlorobenzene (HCB) level on the risk of fetal loss have shown mostly negative (i.e. null) results [4].

Retrospective studies using indirect exposure assessment have suggested a role of preconceptional exposure to chlorophenoxy herbicides [77], mostly of paternal origin, on the risk of spontaneous abortion, but their results are not consistent.

## Fetal growth, gestational duration

Using data collected in an early pregnancy cohort set up in the USA in the 1960s, a dose–response relationship was demonstrated between maternal serum concentration of DDE (median, 25 µg/L), preterm birth and SGA [78]. An association with decreased birthweight was found in the Great Lakes studies (median DDE maternal serum, 2.2 µg/L) [79] and an increasing trend in the risk of preterm birth in a study in Mexico (median maternal serum DDE, 150 ng/g lipid) [80] and in Spain (median maternal serum DDE, 0.89 µg/L) [81]. Such associations were not reported in studies conducted in Ukraine (median DDE, 2457 ng/g milk fat) [82] or in a highly exposed agricultural community in California, mostly from Mexico (median maternal serum DDE, 1000 ng/g lipid) [83]. These discordant findings may be attributable to differences in the mixtures of persistent pesticides present in different settings.

In several of the studies previously mentioned, other organochlorine pesticide residues were measured such as hexachlorobenzene (HCB), β- or γ-hexachlorocyclohexane (HCH), dieldrin, heptachlor epoxide, oxychlordane, trans-nonachlor, or mirex. No consistent associations were found between maternal exposure to any of these compounds and fetal growth or gestational duration, except for a suggestion of a decreased gestational length in relation with β-HCH levels in Mexico [80], and with HCB in a Californian study [83].

## Congenital malformations

A study conducted in Granada (Spain) has found an increased risk of male genital anomalies (cryptorchidism, hypospadias) associated with a measure of xenoestrogenic activity in placenta called total effective xenoestrogen burden (TEXB). This TEXB index was correlated with presence of DDT, lindane, mirex, and endosulfan [84]. This result is in agreement with a report from Denmark in which combined exposure to eight persistent pesticides measured in breast milk was associated with the risk of cryptorchidism [85]. Within the US Collaborative Perinatal Project, a birth cohort study begun in 1959–1966, maternal levels of DDE were associated with slightly elevated odds-ratios of cryptorchidism, hypospadias, and polythelia (extra-nipples); the results were consistent with a modest to moderate association, but the estimates were not very precise [86]. In the same population, the serum levels of heptachlor epoxide (HCE), hexachlorobenzene (HCB), and β-hexachlorocyclohexane (β-HCH) tended to be higher among the mothers of cryptorchidism cases,

but, again, estimates were imprecise [87]. In a study of malaria control workers in Mexico, paternal exposure to DDT was associated with an increased risk of congenital malformations (all considered simultaneously) in the offspring [88]. In a cohort from Chiapas (Mexico), where DDT had been previously used for malaria control, DDE levels were not associated with ano-genital distance or penile dimension in newborns [89].

# Organophosphate insecticides

## Fetal loss

The Ontario Farm Family Health Study (FFHS) did not show any association between fetal loss and indirect assessment of pre- or post-conceptual exposure to organophosphates [77]. This does not confirm findings of studies conducted in California suggesting an increased risk of fetal deaths due to congenital anomalies following organophosphate applications near the family residence around the time of pregnancy [90].

## Fetal growth, gestational duration

A number of studies using biomarkers of exposure to organophosphate pesticides used indoors (chlorpyrifos, diazinon) or for agricultural purposes have been published. Several of them showed associations between prenatal maternal exposure and decreased birthweight, gestational age, or increased risk of intrauterine growth retardation [52,91]. It has been suggested that low genetic expression of paraoxonase 1 (PON1), an enzyme acting in the detoxifying system of organophosphate pesticides, may modify the effect of chlorpyrifos exposure of the mother on the child's head circumference at birth [92].

# Other insecticides

In California, an association between stillbirths and neonatal deaths from birth defects and agricultural pyrethroid insecticide application in early pregnancy near maternal residence has been reported [90]. Other publications have suggested an impact of indoor use of insecticides on the risk of stillbirth [4].

Few studies have evaluated the impact on fetal growth of exposure to pyrethroids [92] or carbamates [91]. One study suggested an impact of exposure to propoxur on birth length [91].

# Miscellaneous herbicides

## Fetal loss

In the Ontario FFHS, no association was found between first-trimester exposure to atrazine or glyphosate and fetal death, whereas risks were slightly increased when preconception exposure was considered. Preconception exposure to thiocarbamates was associated with an increased risk of late spontaneous abortions (occurring between 12 and 19 gestational weeks) whereas there was no indication of excess risk with postconception exposure [77]. A study in Minnesota reported a modification of spraying season on the effect measure of paternal use of herbicides (including sulfonylurea and imidizolinone) on the risk of fetal loss [93].

### Fetal growth

Ecological studies linking birth certificate information with measurements of herbicides such as atrazine, cyanazine, and metolachlor in drinking water at the place of residence at birth have suggested an association with SGA births [4].

## Fungicides

Weak associations have been found between exposure to pentachlorophenol and duration of gestation or birthweight [4].

## Pesticides and successful pregnancies: conclusion

Availability of biomarkers of exposure to pesticides has considerably improved exposure assessment of studies conducted in recent years. Despite that, evidence concerning the developmental impact of prenatal or pre-conceptional exposure to various pesticides remains equivocal. There is limited evidence that prenatal exposure to organochlorine pesticides might be responsible for an increased risk of fetal loss and that prenatal exposure to organophosphate results in alterations in fetal growth. Evidence concerning other developmental outcomes should at this point be considered inadequate [94]. Only a limited number of studies have been conducted on pesticides other than these two chemical classes. There are also suggestions of effects of pre-conceptional exposure, mainly of paternal origin, that need to be elucidated.

## Polychlorinated biphenyls, PCDDs (dioxin), and PCDFs

Polychlorinated biphenyls (PCBs), polychlorinated dibenzo-dioxin (PCDD, a family including 2,3,7,8 TCDD) and polychlorinated dibenzofurans (PCDFs) are three related classes of aromatic heterocyclic compounds. The PCBs consist of two benzene (phenyl) rings connected by a single carbon-to-carbon bond, in which one or several chlorine atoms are bound to the carbon backbone. In PCDFs, there is an additional oxygen atom linking the two phenyl rings; for PCDDs, the number of oxygen atoms is two (see Chapter 2).

### Fetal growth

Follow-up of women pregnant during the episodes of contamination of rice oil (Yu-Cheng in Taiwan, or Yu-Cho in Japan, for "oil disease") by PCBs and their heat-degradation products such as PCDFs indicated that these compounds could alter birthweight not adjusted for gestational age [95]. Such an effect might also exist at lower internal doses, such as those encountered among pregnant women in Western countries in the 1990s [96]. Head circumference may also be altered by PCBs, as indicated by a study of Californian women pregnant in the 1960s before the end of the production of PCBs [97]. In this study, an effect of PCBs on birthweight adjusted for gestational age was only observed for male newborns.

### Gestational duration

The above-mentioned Californian study suggested that maternal PCB levels may entail a decrease in gestational duration (considered as a continuous outcome); the effect size tended to be slightly greater for female than for male births, but sex-specific confidence intervals largely overlapped [97].

### Sex ratio

In the Italian population exposed after the Seveso accident in 1976, paternal exposure to 2,3,7,8-TCDD before the age of 19 years, as assayed from a blood sample drawn shortly after the explosion of the plant, has been associated with a decrease in the proportion of male births [98]. A study based on the California child health and development cohort, conducted in the 1960s, reported a decreased proportion of male births, this time in association with maternal PCB levels assayed during pregnancy [99].

### Congenital malformations

The concentrations of PCBs assayed after birth in colostrum of lactating women have been associated with an increased risk of cryptorchidism at birth in a case–control study in Côte d'Azur, France. PCB levels assessed in cord blood were not significantly different between cases and controls [100]. Children exposed to PCBs in utero during the Yu-Cheng episode have been reported to have increased frequencies of hyperpigmentation and dystrophic nails, compared with controls [101].

# Brominated flame retardants

Brominated flame retardants (BFR) have been routinely added to consumer products for decades to reduce fire-related damage. The major BFRs are tetrabromobisphenol-A (TBBPA), hexabromocyclododecane (HBCD), and mixtures of polybrominated diphenyl ethers (PBDEs). Like PCDFs, PBDEs consist of two benzene (phenyl) rings connected by an oxygen atom, but bromine (and not chlorine) atoms are bound to the carbon backbones. There is strong evidence of increasing contamination of the environment and people by these chemicals due to their persistence and bioaccumulation.

## Congenital malformations

Most BFRs are characterized by their potential for disrupting thyroid homeostasis and for endocrine disruption. Experimental data showed adverse effects on reproductive outcome in rats after gestational exposure to PBDE-99, including reduced ano-genital distance among male offspring [102]. One prospective Danish–Finnish study recently reported an association between prenatal exposure to PBDEs (as assessed from breast milk samples) and the risk of cryptorchidism [103].

# Perfluorinated compounds (PFOS, PFOA)

Perfluorinated compounds are used as industrial surfactants and emulsifiers and are present in consumer products such as non-stick pans, carpets, furniture, household cleaners, shampoos, clothing, and food packaging. They are persistent compounds. Within this family, perfluorooctanesulfonate (PFOS) and perfluorooctanoic acid (PFOA) have been investigated in relation with pregnancy outcomes.

Fei *et al.* [104] highlighted a decrease in mean birthweight in relation with maternal plasma levels of PFOA, and did not highlight an association between birthweight and PFOS. Within this population of 1400 mother–child pairs from the Danish birth cohort, biomarkers of exposure were assessed from maternal blood samples collected between gestational weeks 4 and 14. The PFOA levels were also associated with smaller abdominal circumference at birth and birth length, and a non-statistically significant trend was observed with head circumference, at birth [105]. Within a population of 293 newborns from Maryland, PFOS and PFOA were assessed at birth in cord blood and were both associated with gestational age-adjusted birthweight, head circumference, and ponderal index, which corresponds to the ratio between weight and the cubic value of height at birth [106]. A similar association was highlighted between PFOS and PFOA assessed from maternal serum taken during the third trimester of pregnancy and birthweight in a Japanese cohort including 447 newborns [107]. Associations between PFOS and head circumference did not reach the significance level chosen by the authors, but effect sizes were coherent with those reported by Apelberg *et al.* [106]. There is experimental support for an effect of PFOS and PFOA on fetal development (quoted for example in [104]).

# Diethylstilbestrol (DES)

Diethylstilbestrol (DES), a synthetic estrogen, was prescribed for pregnant women between 1947 and at least the end of the 1970s in some countries, under the wrong assumption that it would help to prevent abortions.

## Fetal loss and gestational duration in the first generation exposed in utero

Among the daughters of women who were prescribed DES as they were pregnant, in addition to an increased frequency of vaginal clear-cell adenocarcinoma, increases in the risk of adverse reproductive outcomes (ectopic pregnancy, fetal loss, premature delivery) have been reported [108].

## Congenital malformations in the first and second generations

Among the daughters of the women who were prescribed DES, an increased frequency of cervical and uterine abnormalities (including hypoplastic or "T-shaped" uterus) has been shown [108]. More recently, concerns have been raised about a possibly increased risk of a congenital malformation of the male genitalia, hypospadias, in the offspring of women exposed to DES in utero – that is, the grandsons of the women who were prescribed DES [109–112]. Such transgenerational studies faced numerous methodological challenges, both in terms of assessment of exposure to DES, which was retrospective in all but one study [111], and also in terms of assessment of hypospadias, which has minor forms that sometimes remain undetected. Figure 10.2 provides a summary of the published results, showing that the confidence intervals of most published studies overlap and that the meta-analytical odds-ratio of hypospadias associated with exposure to DES is in favor of an excess risk. There is evidence for heterogeneity among the

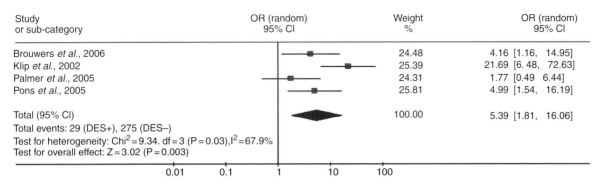

| Study or sub-category | OR (random) 95% CI | Weight % | OR (random) 95% CI |
|---|---|---|---|
| Brouwers et al., 2006 | | 24.48 | 4.16 [1.16, 14.95] |
| Klip et al., 2002 | | 25.39 | 21.69 [6.48, 72.63] |
| Palmer et al., 2005 | | 24.31 | 1.77 [0.49 6.44] |
| Pons et al., 2005 | | 25.81 | 4.99 [1.54, 16.19] |
| Total (95% CI) | | 100.00 | 5.39 [1.81, 16.06] |

Total events: 29 (DES+), 275 (DES–)
Test for heterogeneity: Chi$^2$=9.34. df=3 (P=0.03),I$^2$=67.9%
Test for overall effect: Z=3.02 (P=0.003)

0.01    0.1    1    10    100

**Fig. 10.2.** Maternal in utero exposure to DES and risk of hypospadias in the offspring. Meta-analysis of four publications [109–112]. The unadjusted odds-ratios (OR) of hypospadias associated with DES are indicated by the squares. The overall OR (as estimated from a random effect model, diamond) corresponds to 5.4 (95% CI, 1.8–16.1).

published studies, which is in line with the fact that the study that reported the highest odds-ratio [109] was conducted among a cohort of women undergoing in vitro fertilization. Other congenital malformations, and in particular esophageal anomalies [113], might also be more frequent in association with maternal intrauterine exposure to DES.

## Phthalates

Phthalates is the common designation of diesters of phthalic acids. These are a family of man-made chemicals with broad industrial uses, in particular as plasticizers in many consumer products and medical devices, as components of personal-care products such as perfumes and cosmetics or as solvents. Exposure in the general population is widespread [114]. Animal experiments showed that several phthalates act as endocrine disruptors and that exposure during fetal life can induce reproductive tract anomalies in males, such as hypospadias, cryptorchidism, and reduced ano-genital distance [115, 116]. Phthalates have a short half-life in the human body and urinary levels of phthalate metabolites exhibit relatively important day-to-day variability [114], which is a great challenge in epidemiologic studies, in particular when the focus is on congenital anomalies of the male genitalia, for which the time window of sensitivity to xenobiotics is probably very narrow.

### Gestational duration

Higher levels of di-(2-ethylhexyl)phthalate (DEHP), assessed in cord blood after delivery, have been measured for premature, compared with non-premature, births [117]. Three additional studies in which exposure has been assessed in prenatal urine samples have been published. One study (Meeker et al., Env. Health Perspect, 2009) also reported a decreased gestational duration with DEHP metabolites, whereas associations were in the opposite direction in two other studies (Wolff et al., Env. Health Perspect, 2008; Adibi et al., Am J Epidemiol, 2009).

### Congenital malformations

A reduced ano-genital distance (assessed on average 13 months after birth) has been reported in male newborns in relation to the concentration of phthalate monoester metabolites assayed in maternal urine collected during pregnancy [118]. In an update of this study, the concentrations of DEHP metabolites were also associated with an increased frequency of incomplete testicular descent, defined if one or both testicles were found not to be "normal" or "normal retractile" during the postnatal study visit taking place on average 13 months after delivery [119]. In a case–control study based on 471 cases of hypospadias referred to surgeons in south-east England and randomly selected birth controls, Ormond et al. reported an increased risk of hypospadias in association with maternal occupational exposure to phthalates [120]. Exposure to phthalates (14 mothers of cases, 4 mothers of controls) has been assessed from maternal occupation, using a job-exposure matrix, and was strongly correlated with occupational use of hairsprays since jobs with potential phthalate exposure include hairdressers and beauty therapists [120]. Experiments on rodents clearly support a role of phthalate exposure during pregnancy on incidence of hypospadias [115].

## Solvents

Organic solvents are ubiquitous in non-occupational settings and they also constitute one of the most frequent classes of chemicals in both female and male working environments. They are often present as mixtures that differ according to the type of industry and time period, and the detailed assessment of the toxicity of single chemicals has often been limited by this situation. However, in some industries, specific chemicals are preponderant, such as tetrachloroethylene in the dry cleaning industry or ethylene glycol ethers in the semiconductor industry. Episodes of contamination of drinking water by chlorinated solvents (a family of compounds that differs from the above-mentioned chlorination by-products) have also been the subject of a number of studies in the USA [53].

## Glycol ethers: effects on fetal loss and congenital malformations

There is currently sufficient evidence that maternal occupational exposure to ethylene glycol ethers entails increased risks of spontaneous abortion, and limited evidence concerning the risk of birth defects in the offspring [4, 121]. Although the specific agents involved have not been formally identified in epidemiologic studies, animal experiments provide strong support for developmental toxicity of short-chain ethylene glycol ethers, most of which have now restricted use.

## Tetrachloroethylene and trichloroethylene (chlorinated solvents)

### Fetal loss

Studies conducted in dry-cleaning shops in Scandinavian countries have consistently reported an association between exposure to tetrachloroethylene and the risk of fetal loss [122].

### Fetal growth and congenital malformations

The overall evidence summarized from five studies conducted in communities served by drinking water containing high levels of chlorinated solvents suggest increased risks of neural tube defects, oral clefts, and cardiac defects, and an impact on the risk of low birthweight especially among male births [53]. Because of uncertainties in exposure assessment in these last studies, the evidence should still be considered limited. Some experimental studies support a teratogenic effect of trichloroethylene in drinking water at relatively low levels of exposure (< 250 ppb) [123], but in some experiments, effects were observed only in the presence of marked maternal toxicity [121].

## Aromatic solvents (including benzene)

### Fetal loss

Work in the printing industry, the painting and maintenance trade and the petrochemical industry entails exposure to aromatic solvents such as toluene, xylene, benzene, and styrene. Epidemiologic studies conducted in these industries, where high exposure levels were present, have consistently shown an increased risk of spontaneous abortions after maternal exposure and also paternal exposure. It was not possible to attribute this excess to one type of solvent in particular [70].

### Fetal growth

There is experimental evidence in rodents for effects of airborne aromatic solvents such as benzene to impact on fetal growth [124]. There are currently too few epidemiologic studies with good exposure assessment to discuss the reality of such an effect in humans [125].

### Gestational duration

Two studies indicated a possibly shortened gestational duration in association with maternal occupational exposure to benzene [126] or solvents in general [127], differing across genotypes of the *CYP1A1* and *GSTT1* xenobiotic-metabolizing gene.

## Radiation

Concerns have been raised about a possible effect of electromagnetic (non-ionizing) radiation on pregnancy outcome. A review suggests that the overall epidemiologic evidence in favor of such an effect is very limited [128]. In this section, we will focus on ionizing radiation.

Ionizing radiations are heterogeneous in terms of energy, physical nature (they consist of electrons, corresponding to β-rays, alpha particles, made of two protons and two neutrons, neutrons, or, in the case of γ- or X-rays, photons), and ability to be absorbed by human tissues (with alpha radiation being absorbed very locally in case of ingestion, whereas γ-rays can cross the whole body). The situations of exposure include environmental exposure to cosmic rays, radon in the air, subsoil natural gamma radiation, occupational exposures, through some medical imaging devices, treatment of cancers by radiotherapy, discharge from civil nuclear facilities, fallout from military nuclear tests, and nuclear disasters such as the Hiroshima and Nagasaki bombings in 1945 or the Chernobyl accident (Ukraine) in April 1986.

## Fetal loss

Two large British studies documented the possible effects of paternal occupational exposure to γ ionizing radiation before the conception of a pregnancy on the risk of stillbirth. For an increase by 100 mSievert in paternal total exposure before conception, Parker *et al.* [129] reported an odds-ratio of stillbirth of 1.24 (95% confidence interval, 1.04, 1.45); Doyle *et al.* [130] reported a similar effect size, with overlapping confidence intervals. Taken together, these studies provide some evidence for an effect of paternal exposure to ionizing radiation before conception on the risk of stillbirth.

Concerning maternal occupational exposure, a study based on small numbers is inconclusive in terms of possible effects on fetal loss [130]. Finally, an ecological study reported a possibly differentially increased risk of stillbirth in eastern Europe in 1986, compared with central and western Europe; since the nuclear fallouts following the Chernobyl accident in 1986 were more important in eastern Europe, such trends raise the question of the consequence of this radioactive contamination on the stillbirth risk [131].

## Fetal growth

Maternal pelvis exposure to ionizing radiation before conception because of radiation therapy has also been associated with an increased risk of delivering a low birthweight baby [132]. One study suggested a possible decrease in birthweight following paternal preconceptional X-ray examinations [133].

## Congenital malformations

In humans, ionizing radiation constitute the first iatrogenic agent recognized as being able to cause congenital malformations (in particular, microcephaly or reduced head circumference, hypoplasia of the genitalia, hypospadias, palatoschisis, ocular malformations), with reports published as early as 1929 [134]. These effects are established for doses above 0.1 Gray; the literature is more limited for lower doses. Studies in occupational settings, which generally provide a prospective assessment of personal exposure, mostly focused on paternal exposure. In a case–control study conducted among workers from the Hanford nuclear site, an increased risk of neural tube defects has been reported in association with parental preconception exposure, on the basis of a small number of cases [135]. A similar association was not found in a cohort of nuclear industry workers [130]. Following the Chernobyl accident in Ukraine, time clusters of Down syndrome (trisomy 21) have been reported 9 months after the accident in neighboring Belarus [136] or in the more distant and less contaminated Berlin area [137]. Elevated mutation rates of germline cells of paternal origin at minisatellite loci have also been reported among children born in Belarus, compared with children born in the UK [138]. A study of 205 children exposed in the first half of pregnancy during the Hiroshima bombing has shown an increased frequency of microcephaly and mental retardation [139]. In a review, the weight of evidence for an effect of low doses of ionizing radiation on congenital malformations was considered limited [140].

## Sex ratio

Two studies have been conducted among nuclear industry workers in the UK. One study focused on exposure to γ radiation in the 3 months before conception and reported an increase in the proportion of male births in association with exposure [141]. Another study focused on total occupational exposure cumulated before conception and reported odds-ratios of male births associated with exposure close to unity [142]. In Czech regions, the proportion of male births significantly dropped in November 1986, about 6 months after the most radioactive cloud from Chernobyl passed over the Czech Republic; this reduction was strongest in the eastern regions, where the radioactive fallout was most elevated [143].

# Overview

The epidemiologic study of environmental impacts on healthy and successful pregnancies is a research field that emerged in the late 1970s and early 1980s, focusing initially on active smoking and occupational exposures; it experienced rapid development since the late 1990s, in parallel with the increasing availability and decreasing costs of analytical chemistry tools allowing assessment of exposure to environmental compounds in large-scale population-based studies. A lot of knowledge is probably yet to come from the use of these biomarkers of exposure, but also of biomarkers of effects, provided these are assayed on biological samples collected during the relevant time window, and not postnatally as has most often been the case so far. Knowledge about the modifications of effect measures of environmental exposures by other environmental, behavioral, or sociodemographic factors is still very

**Table 10.1.** Overview of considered reproductive outcomes and level of evidence for a possible sensitivity to specific environmental pollutants in humans*. Pat. indicates that the level of evidence relates to a possible effect of paternal exposures.

| Pollutant | Fetal loss Early (< 20 weeks) | Fetal loss Late | Fetal growth | Gestational length | Complications of pregnancy | Secondary sex-ratio | Congenital malformations |
|---|---|---|---|---|---|---|---|
| Atmospheric pollutants | | Limited | Limited/sufficient | Limited/sufficient | Limited (preeclampsia) | Inadequate | Limited (cardiac malformations) |
| Passive smoking (ETS) | Limited | Limited | Sufficient | Sufficient | Inadequate | Inadequate | Limited/sufficient |
| Water pollutants | | | | | | | |
| Disinfection by-products | Inadequate | Inadequate | Limited/sufficient | Inadequate | Inadequate | Inadequate | Limited |
| Nitrates | Inadequate | | Inadequate | Inadequate | | | Inadequate |
| *Other chemical compounds* | | | | | | | |
| Metals | | | | | | | |
| Lead | Sufficient | | Limited/sufficient | Limited/sufficient | Sufficient/Limited (gestational hypertension) | Limited/ sufficient (pat.) | Inadequate |
| Mercury | Limited (pat.) | | Limited (pat.) | Limited (pat.) | | | |
| Cadmium | Limited (pat.) | | Inadequate | Limited | | | Sufficient |
| Arsenic | Limited | | Inadequate | Inadequate | | | Limited |
| PCB, PCDD, PCDF | | | Limited (PCB) | Inadequate (PCB) | | Limited (pat. TCDD) | Limited (PCBs) |
| Flame retardants PBDE | | | Limited/ sufficient | Inadequate | | | Limited |
| Perfluorinated chemicals (PFOS, PFOA) | | | | Inadequate | | | |
| Organochlorine pesticides | | | | | | | |
| DDT, DDE | Limited | Inadequate (pat.) | Limited | Limited | | Inadequate (pat.) | Limited |
| Other organochlorines | | Inadequate | Inadequate | Limited | | | Limited (pat.) |
| Organophosphate pesticides | | Inadequate | Limited | Limited | | | Limited |
| Phthalates | | | | Inadequate | | | Inadequate |
| Solvents | | | | | | | |
| Glycol ethers | Sufficient | | | | | | |
| Chlorinated | Limited/sufficient | | | | | | Limited |
| Aromatic | Limited (pat.) | | Inadequate | Limited/sufficient | | | Limited |
| Radiations (low doses) | | | | | | | |
| ionizing | | Limited (pat.) | Limited/sufficient | | Inadequate | Limited | Limited/sufficient |
| non-ionizing | Inadequate | | | | | | |

* The level of evidence has been classified as *sufficient* (several good quality studies by different groups, or an expert panel already considered the level of proof as sufficient), *limited* (evidence is suggestive of an association, e.g. based on at least one good quality study, but remains limited), or *inadequate* (available studies are of insufficient quality, consistency or statistical power to permit a conclusion regarding the presence or absence of an association), as a modification of what has been suggested elsewhere [4]. See text for chemical name in full.

limited. This is also the case for effect modification by genetic or epigenetic factors, whose incorporation in epidemiologic studies might help document biological mechanisms and estimate subgroup-specific effects of environmental exposures.

## Effects of paternal exposures

Most of the evidence reviewed concerned maternal exposure. In coherence with animal studies, there is some evidence of a paternally mediated effect in humans for a few environmental factors [144]. This is in particular the case for male exposures to dioxin, inorganic lead (impact on sex ratio, fetal growth), for exposure to ionizing radiation (stillbirth and hereditary mutations), for mercury (fetal loss), and DDT (fetal growth, congenital malformations).

## Conclusion

The environmental factors for which effects on the course and outcome of pregnancy have been suggested are summarized in Table 10.1. Those for which a sufficient weight of evidence exist at the time of the writing of this review are passive smoking (effects on fetal growth, preterm birth, and possibly of congenital malformations), lead (pregnancy-induced hypertension, fetal loss, fetal growth), glycol ethers (effect on early fetal loss) and ionizing radiation effects on congenital malformations and fetal growth. Additionally, factors with a limited to sufficient evidence for an impact on pregnancy outcome are atmospheric pollutants (for effects on fetal growth and preterm birth), DBPs present in drinking water (effects on fetal growth), perfluorinated chemicals (effects on fetal growth), chlorinated solvents (effects on fetal loss), and aromatic solvents (effects on gestational length). Very few risk assessment studies quantified the impact of these pollutants on pregnancy outcome in terms of number of adverse outcomes at the population level; since exposure to most of these pollutants is widespread the impact at the population level could be large [145]. For most of the other environmental contaminants considered here, some toxicologic evidence indicative of a danger exists, and many challenges in exposure assessment in humans have not been overcome yet; the current lack of clear evidence for adverse effects on the course and outcome of pregnancy should certainly not be interpreted as evidence of a lack of effect.

## References

1. ChildInfo. UNICEF, 2008. http://www.childinfo.org/mortality_infantmortality.php

2. Saigal S, Doyle LW. An overview of mortality and sequelae of preterm birth from infancy to adulthood. *Lancet* 2008; **371**: 261–9.

3. Hanson MA, Gluckman PD. Developmental origins of health and disease: new insights. *Basic Clin Pharmacol Toxicol* 2008; **102**: 90–3.

4. Wigle DT, Arbuckle TE, Turner MC. et al. Epidemiologic evidence of relationships between reproductive and child health outcomes and environmental chemical contaminants. *J Toxicol Environ Health B Crit Rev* 2008; **11**: 373–517.

5. Poole C. Low P-values or narrow confidence intervals: which are more durable? *Epidemiology* 2001; **12**: 291–4.

6. Kortenkamp A. Ten years of mixing cocktails: a review of combination effects of endocrine-disrupting chemicals. *Environ Health Perspect* 2007; **115** (Suppl. 1): 98–105.

7. Kline J, Stein ZA, Susser M. et al. Smoking: a risk factor for spontaneous abortion. *New Engl J Med* 1977; **297**: 793–6.

8. Mitchell EA, Milerad J. Smoking and the sudden infant death syndrome. *Rev Environ Health* 2006; **21**: 81–103.

9. Burguet A, Kaminski M, Abraham-Lerat L. et al. The complex relationship between smoking in pregnancy and very preterm delivery. Results of the Epipage study. *Br J Obstet Gynaecol* 2004; **111**: 258–65.

10. Morales-Suarez-Varela MM, Bille C, Christensen K. et al. Smoking habits, nicotine use, and congenital malformations. *Obstet Gynecol* 2006; **107**: 51–7.

11. Engel SM, Janevic TM, Stein CR. et al. Maternal smoking, preeclampsia, and infant health outcomes in New York City, 1995–2003. *Am J Epidemiol* 2009; **169**: 33–40.

12. Pereira LA, Loomis D, Conceicao GM. et al. Association between air pollution and intrauterine mortality in Sao Paulo, Brazil. *Environ Health Perspect* 1998; **106**: 325–9.

13. de Medeiros APP, Gouveia N, Perez Machado RP. et al. Traffic related air pollution and perinatal mortality: a case-control study. *Environ Health Perspect* 2009; **117**: 127–32.

14. Mohallem SV, de Araujo Lobo DJ, Pesquero CR. et al. Decreased fertility in mice exposed to environmental air pollution in the city of Sao Paulo. *Environ Res* 2005; **98**: 196–202.

15. Glinianaia SV, Rankin J, Bell R. et al. Particulate air pollution and fetal health: a systematic review of the epidemiologic evidence. *Epidemiology* 2004; **15**: 36–45.

16. Lacasana M, Esplugues A, Ballester F. Exposure to ambient air pollution and prenatal and early childhood health effects. *Eur J Epidemiol* 2005; **20**: 183–99.

17. Slama R, Darrow LA, Parker JD. et al. Atmospheric pollution and human reproduction: report of the Munich International Workshop. *Environ Health Perspect* 2008; **116**: 791–8.

18. Sram RJ, Binkova B, Dejmek J. *et al.* Ambient air pollution and pregnancy outcomes: a review of the literature. *Environ Health Perspect* 2005; **113**: 375–82.

19. Slama R, Morgenstern V, Cyrys J. *et al.* Traffic-related atmospheric pollutants levels during pregnancy and offspring's term birth weight: a study relying on a land-use regression exposure model. *Environ Health Perspect* 2007; **115**: 1283–92.

20. Jedrychowski W, Bendkowska I, Flak E. *et al.* Estimated risk for altered fetal growth resulting from exposure to fine particles during pregnancy: an epidemiologic prospective cohort study in Poland. *Environ Health Perspect* 2004; **112**: 1398–402.

21. Choi H, Rauh V, Garfinkel R. *et al.* Prenatal exposure to airborne polycyclic aromatic hydrocarbons and risk of intrauterine growth restriction. *Environ Health Perspect* 2008; **116**: 658–65.

22. Parker JD, Woodruff TJ, Basu R. *et al.* Air pollution and birth weight among term infants in California. *Pediatrics* 2005; **115**: 121–8.

23. Ritz B, Yu F. The effect of ambient carbon monoxide on low birth weight among children born in southern California between 1989 and 1993. *Environ Health Perspect* 1999; **107**: 17–25.

24. Hansen CA, Barnett AG, Pritchard G. The effect of ambient air pollution during early pregnancy on fetal ultrasonic measurements during mid-pregnancy. *Environ Health Perspect* 2008; **116**: 362–9.

25. Rocha E Silva IR, Lichtenfels AJ, Amador Pereira LA. *et al.* Effects of ambient levels of air pollution generated by traffic on birth and placental weights in mice. *Fertil Steril* 2008; **90**(5): 1921–4.

26. Wilhelm M, Ritz B. Local variations in CO and particulate air pollution and adverse birth outcomes in Los Angeles County, California, USA. *Environ Health Perspect* 2005; **113**: 1212–21.

27. Huynh M, Woodruff TJ, Parker JD. *et al.* Relationships between air pollution and preterm birth in California. *Paediatr Perinat Epidemiol* 2006; **20**: 454–61.

28. Sagiv SK, Mendola P, Loomis D. *et al.* A time-series analysis of air pollution and preterm birth in Pennsylvania, 1997–2001. *Environ Health Perspect* 2005; **113**: 602–6.

29. Parker JD, Mendola P, Woodruff TJ. Preterm birth after the Utah Valley steel mill closure: a natural experiment. *Epidemiology* 2008; **19**: 820–3.

30. Ritz B, Yu F, Fruin S. *et al.* Ambient air pollution and risk of birth defects in Southern California. *Am J Epidemiol* 2002; **155**: 17–25.

31. Gilboa SM, Mendola P, Olshan AF. *et al.* Relation between ambient air quality and selected birth defects, seven county study, Texas, 1997–2000. *Am J Epidemiol* 2005; **162**: 238–52.

32. Cordier S, Chevrier C, Robert-Gnansia E. *et al.* Risk of congenital anomalies in the vicinity of municipal solid waste incinerators. *Occup Environ Med* 2004; **61**: 8–15.

33. Dummer TJ, Dickinson HO, Parker L. Adverse pregnancy outcomes around incinerators and crematoriums in Cumbria, north west England, 1956–93. *J Epidemiol Community Health* 2003; **57**: 456–61.

34. Hwang BF, Jaakkola JJ. Ozone and other air pollutants and the risk of oral clefts. *Environ Health Perspect* 2008; **116**: 1411–15.

35. Lichtenfels AJ, Gomes JB, Pieri PC. *et al.* Increased levels of air pollution and a decrease in the human and mouse male-to-female ratio in Sao Paulo, Brazil. *Fertil Steril* 2007; **87**: 230–2.

36. Dempsey D, Jacob P, 3rd, Benowitz NL. Accelerated metabolism of nicotine and cotinine in pregnant smokers. *J Pharmacol Exp Ther* 2002; **301**: 594–8.

37. California Environmental Protection Agency: Air Resources Board. *Proposed Identification of Environmental Tobacco Smoke as a Toxic Air Contaminant.* California Environmental Protection Agency, 2005.

38. Venners SA, Wang X, Chen C. *et al.* Paternal smoking and pregnancy loss: a prospective study using a biomarker of pregnancy. *Am J Epidemiol* 2004; **159**: 993–1001.

39. Windham GC, Von Behren J, Waller K. *et al.* Exposure to environmental and mainstream tobacco smoke and risk of spontaneous abortion. *Am J Epidemiol* 1999; **149**: 243–7.

40. George L, Granath F, Johansson AL. *et al.* Environmental tobacco smoke and risk of spontaneous abortion. *Epidemiology* 2006; **17**: 500–5.

41. Bracken MB. Cotinine and spontaneous abortion: might variations in metabolism play a role? *Epidemiology* 2006; **17**: 492–4.

42. Kharrazi M, DeLorenze GN, Kaufman FL. *et al.* Environmental tobacco smoke and pregnancy outcome. *Epidemiology* 2004; **15**: 660–70.

43. Lie RT, Wilcox AJ, Taylor J. *et al.* Maternal smoking and oral clefts: the role of detoxification pathway genes. *Epidemiology* 2008; **19**: 606–15.

44. Suarez L, Felkner M, Brender JD. *et al.* Maternal exposures to cigarette smoke, alcohol, and street drugs and neural tube defect occurrence in offspring. *Matern Child Health J* 2008; **12**: 394–401.

45. Fukuda M, Fukuda K, Shimizu T *et al.* Parental periconceptional smoking and male: female ratio of newborn infants. *Lancet* 2002; **359**: 1407–8.

46. Heron J, Ness A. Lack of association between smoking behavior and the sex ratio of offspring in the Avon longitudinal study of parents and children. *Fertil Steril* 2004; **81**: 700–2.

47. US EPA. *The Occurrence of Disinfection By-products of Health (DBPs) Concern in Drinking Water: Results of a Nationwide DBP Occurrence Study.* Athens, GA: US Environmental Protection Agency, National

Exposure Research Laboratory. EPA 2002 600/R-01/068, 2002.

48. Waller K, Swan SH, DeLorenze G. *et al.* Trihalomethanes in drinking water and spontaneous abortion. *Epidemiology* 1998; **9**: 134–40.

49. Savitz DA, Singer PC, Herring AH. *et al.* Exposure to drinking water disinfection by-products and pregnancy loss. *Am J Epidemiol* 2006; **164**: 1043–51.

50. Dodds L, King W, Allen AC. *et al.* Trihalomethanes in public water supplies and risk of stillbirth. *Epidemiology* 2004; **15**: 179–86.

51. Toledano MB, Nieuwenhuijsen MJ, Best N. *et al.* Relation of trihalomethane concentrations in public water supplies to stillbirth and birth weight in three water regions in England. *Environ Health Perspect* 2005; **113**: 225–32.

52. Windham G, Fenster L. Environmental contaminants and pregnancy outcomes. *Fertil Steril* 2008; **89**: e111–6; discussion e7.

53. Bove F, Shim Y, Zeitz P. Drinking water contaminants and adverse pregnancy outcomes: a review. *Environ Health Perspect* 2002; **110** (Suppl. 1): 61–74.

54. Nieuwenhuijsen MJ, Toledano MB, Eaton NE. *et al.* Chlorination disinfection byproducts in water and their association with adverse reproductive outcomes: a review. *Occup Environ Med* 2000; **57**: 73–85.

55. Savitz DA, Andrews KW, Pastore LM. Drinking water and pregnancy outcome in central North Carolina: source, amount, and trihalomethane levels. *Environ Health Perspect* 1995; **103**: 592–6.

56. Infante-Rivard C. Drinking water contaminants, gene polymorphisms, and fetal growth. *Environ Health Perspect* 2004; **112**: 1213–16.

57. Aggazzotti G, Righi E, Fantuzzi G. *et al.* Chlorination by-products (CBPs) in drinking water and adverse pregnancy outcomes in Italy. *J Water Health* 2004; **2**: 233–47.

58. Hoffman CS, Mendola P, Savitz DA. *et al.* Drinking water disinfection by-product exposure and fetal growth. *Epidemiology* 2008; **19**: 729–37.

59. Hwang BF, Jaakkola JJ. Water chlorination and birth defects: a systematic review and meta-analysis. *Arch Environ Health* 2003; **58**: 83–91.

60. Nieuwenhuijsen MJ, Toledano MB, Bennett J. *et al.* Chlorination disinfection by-products and risk of congenital anomalies in England and Wales. *Environ Health Perspect* 2008; **116**: 216–22.

61. Joyce SJ, Cook A, Newnham J. *et al.* Water disinfection by-products and pre-labor rupture of membranes. *Am J Epidemiol* 2008; **168**: 514–21.

62. Weselak M, Arbuckle TE, Walker MC. *et al.* The influence of the environment and other exogenous agents on spontaneous abortion risk. *J Toxicol Environ Health B Crit Rev* 2008; **11**: 221–41.

63. Bukowski J, Somers G, Bryanton J. Agricultural contamination of groundwater as a possible risk factor for growth restriction or prematurity. *J Occup Environ Med* 2001; **43**: 377–83.

64. Manassaram DM, Backer LC, Moll DM. A review of nitrates in drinking water: maternal exposure and adverse reproductive and developmental outcomes. *Environ Health Perspect* 2006; **114**: 320–7.

65. Borja-Aburto VH, Hertz-Picciotto I, Rojas Lopez M. *et al.* Blood lead levels measured prospectively and risk of spontaneous abortion. *Am J Epidemiol* 1999; **150**: 590–7.

66. Lindbohm ML, Sallmen M, Anttila A. *et al.* Paternal occupational lead exposure and spontaneous abortion. *Scand J Work Environ Health* 1991; **17**: 95–103.

67. Rothenberg SJ, Kondrashov V, Manalo M. *et al.* Increases in hypertension and blood pressure during pregnancy with increased bone lead levels. *Am J Epidemiol* 2002; **156**: 1079–87.

68. Bellinger DC. Teratogen update: lead and pregnancy. *Birth Defects Res A Clin Mol Teratol* 2005; **73**: 409–20.

69. Simonsen CR, Roge R, Christiansen U. *et al.* Effects of paternal blood lead levels on offspring sex ratio. *Reprod Toxicol* 2006; **22**: 3–4.

70. Savitz DA, Sonnenfeld NL, Olshan AF. Review of epidemiologic studies of paternal occupational exposure and spontaneous abortion. *Am J Ind Med* 1994; **25**: 361–83.

71. Xue F, Holzman C, Rahbar MH. *et al.* Maternal fish consumption, mercury levels, and risk of preterm delivery. *Environ Health Perspect* 2007; **115**: 42–7.

72. Marsh DO, Clarkson TW, Cox C. *et al.* Fetal methylmercury poisoning. Relationship between concentration in single strands of maternal hair and child effects. *Arch Neurol* 1987; **44**: 1017–22.

73. Vahter M. Health effects of early life exposure to arsenic. *Basic Clin Pharmacol Toxicol* 2008; **102**: 204–11.

74. Gray LE, Ostby J, Furr J. *et al.* Effects of environmental antiandrogens on reproductive development in experimental animals. *Hum Reprod Update* 2001; **7**: 248–64.

75. Woodruff TJ, Carlson A, Schwartz JM. *et al.* Proceedings of the Summit on Environmental Challenges to Reproductive Health and Fertility: executive summary. *Fertil Steril* 2008; **89**: e1–e20.

76. Venners SA, Korrick S, Xu X. *et al.* Preconception serum DDT and pregnancy loss: a prospective study using a biomarker of pregnancy. *Am J Epidemiol* 2005; **162**: 709–16.

77. Arbuckle TE, Lin Z, Mery LS. An exploratory analysis of the effect of pesticide exposure on the risk of spontaneous abortion in an Ontario farm population. *Environ Health Perspect* 2001; **109**: 851–7.

78. Longnecker MP, Klebanoff MA, Zhou H. *et al.* Association between maternal serum concentration

of the DDT metabolite DDE and preterm and small-for-gestational-age babies at birth. *Lancet* 2001; **358**: 110–14.

79. Weisskopf MG, Anderson HA, Hanrahan LP. *et al.* Maternal exposure to Great Lakes sport-caught fish and dichlorodiphenyl dichloroethylene, but not polychlorinated biphenyls, is associated with reduced birth weight. *Environ Res* 2005; **97**: 149–62.

80. Torres-Arreola L, Berkowitz G, Torres-Sanchez L. *et al.* Preterm birth in relation to maternal organochlorine serum levels. *Ann Epidemiol* 2003; **13**: 158–62.

81. Ribas-Fito N, Sala M, Cardo E. *et al.* Association of hexachlorobenzene and other organochlorine compounds with anthropometric measures at birth. *Pediatr Res* 2002; **52**: 163–7.

82. Gladen BC, Shkiryak-Nyzhnyk ZA, Chyslovska N. *et al.* Persistent organochlorine compounds and birth weight. *Ann Epidemiol* 2003; **13**: 151–7.

83. Fenster L, Eskenazi B, Anderson M. *et al.* Association of in utero organochlorine pesticide exposure and fetal growth and length of gestation in an agricultural population. *Environ Health Perspect* 2006; **114**: 597–602.

84. Fernandez MF, Olmos B, Granada A. *et al.* Human exposure to endocrine-disrupting chemicals and prenatal risk factors for cryptorchidism and hypospadias: a nested case-control study. *Environ Health Perspect* 2007; **115** (Suppl. 1): 8–14.

85. Damgaard IN, Skakkebaek NE, Toppari J. *et al.* Persistent pesticides in human breast milk and cryptorchidism. *Environ Health Perspect* 2006; **114**: 1133–8.

86. Longnecker MP, Klebanoff MA, Brock JW. *et al.* Maternal serum level of 1,1-dichloro-2,2-bis(p-chlorophenyl)ethylene and risk of cryptorchidism, hypospadias, and polythelia among male offspring. *Am J Epidemiol* 2002; **155**: 313–22.

87. Pierik FH, Klebanoff MA, Brock JW. *et al.* Maternal pregnancy serum level of heptachlor epoxide, hexachlorobenzene, and beta-hexachlorocyclohexane and risk of cryptorchidism in offspring. *Environ Res* 2007; **105**: 364–9.

88. Salazar-Garcia F, Gallardo-Diaz E, Ceron-Mireles P. *et al.* Reproductive effects of occupational DDT exposure among male malaria control workers. *Environ Health Perspect* 2004; **112**: 542–7.

89. Longnecker MP, Gladen BC, Cupul-Uicab LA. *et al.* In utero exposure to the antiandrogen 1,1-dichloro-2,2-bis(p-chlorophenyl)ethylene (DDE) in relation to anogenital distance in male newborns from Chiapas, Mexico. *Am J Epidemiol* 2007; **165**: 1015–22.

90. Bell EM, Hertz-Picciotto I, Beaumont JJ. A case-control study of pesticides and fetal death due to congenital anomalies. *Epidemiology* 2001; **12**: 148–56.

91. Whyatt RM, Rauh V, Barr DB. *et al.* Prenatal insecticide exposures and birth weight and length among an urban minority cohort. *Environ Health Perspect* 2004; **112**: 1125–32.

92. Berkowitz GS, Wetmur JG, Birman-Deych E. *et al.* In utero pesticide exposure, maternal paraoxonase activity, and head circumference. *Environ Health Perspect* 2004; **112**: 388–91.

93. Garry VF, Harkins M, Lyubimov A. *et al.* Reproductive outcomes in the women of the Red River Valley of the north. I. The spouses of pesticide applicators: pregnancy loss, age at menarche, and exposures to pesticides. *J Toxicol Environ Health A* 2002; **65**: 769–86.

94. Weselak M, Arbuckle TE, Foster W. Pesticide exposures and developmental outcomes: the epidemiological evidence. *J Toxicol Environ Health B Crit Rev* 2007; **10**: 41–80.

95. Rogan WJ, Gladen BC, Hung KL. *et al.* Congenital poisoning by polychlorinated biphenyls and their contaminants in Taiwan. *Science* 1988; **241**: 334–6.

96. Sagiv SK, Tolbert PE, Altshul LM. *et al.* Organochlorine exposures during pregnancy and infant size at birth. *Epidemiology* 2007; **18**: 120–9.

97. Hertz-Picciotto I, Charles MJ, James RA. *et al.* In utero polychlorinated biphenyl exposures in relation to fetal and early childhood growth. *Epidemiology* 2005; **16**: 648–56.

98. Mocarelli P, Gerthoux PM, Ferrari E. *et al.* Paternal concentrations of dioxin and sex ratio of offspring. *Lancet* 2000; **355**: 1858–63.

99. Hertz-Picciotto I, Jusko TA, Willman EJ. *et al.* A cohort study of in utero polychlorinated biphenyl (PCB) exposures in relation to secondary sex ratio. *Environ Health* 2008; **7**: 37.

100. Brucker-Davis F, Wagner-Mahler K, Delattre I. *et al.* Cryptorchidism at birth in Nice area (France) is associated with higher prenatal exposure to PCBs and DDE, as assessed by colostrum concentrations. *Hum Reprod* 2008; **23**: 1708–18.

101. Guo YL, Lambert GH, Hsu CC. Growth abnormalities in the population exposed in utero and early postnatally to polychlorinated biphenyls and dibenzofurans. *Environ Health Perspect* 1995; **103** (Suppl. 6): 117–22.

102. Lilienthal H, Hack A, Roth-Härer A. *et al.* Effects of developmental exposure to 2,2′,4,4′,5-pentabromodiphenyl ether (PBDE-99) on sex steroids, sexual development, and sexually dimorphic behavior in rats. *Environ Health Perspect* 2006; **114**: 194–201.

103. Main KM, Kiviranta H, Virtanen HE. *et al.* Flame retardants in placenta and breast milk and cryptorchidism in newborn boys. *Environ Health Perspect* 2007; **115**: 1519–26.

104. Fei C, McLaughlin JK, Tarone RE. *et al.* Perfluorinated chemicals and fetal growth: a study within the Danish

National Birth Cohort. *Environ Health Perspect* 2007; **115**: 1677–82.

105. Fei C, McLaughlin JK, Tarone RE. *et al.* Fetal growth indicators and perfluorinated chemicals: a study in the Danish National Birth Cohort. *Am J Epidemiol* 2008; **168**: 66–72.

106. Apelberg BJ, Witter FR, Herbstman JB. *et al.* Cord serum concentrations of perfluorooctane sulfonate (PFOS) and perfluorooctanoate (PFOA) in relation to weight and size at birth. *Environ Health Perspect* 2007; **115**: 1670–6.

107. Washino N, Saijo Y, Sasaki S. *et al.* Correlations between prenatal exposure to perfluorinated chemicals and reduced fetal growth. *Environ Health Perspect* 2009; **117**: 660–7.

108. Swan SH. Intrauterine exposure to diethylstilbestrol: long-term effects in humans. *APMIS* 2000; **108**: 793–804.

109. Klip H, Verloop J, van Gool JD. *et al.* Hypospadias in sons of women exposed to diethylstilbestrol in utero: a cohort study. *Lancet* 2002; **359**: 1102–7.

110. Brouwers MM, Feitz WF, Roelofs LA. *et al.* Hypospadias: a transgenerational effect of diethylstilbestrol? *Hum Reprod* 2006; **21**: 666–9.

111. Palmer JR, Wise LA, Robboy SJ. *et al.* Hypospadias in sons of women exposed to diethylstilbestrol in utero. *Epidemiology* 2005; **16**: 583–6.

112. Pons JC, Papiernik E, Billon A. *et al.* Hypospadias in sons of women exposed to diethylstilbestrol in utero. *Prenat Diagn* 2005; **25**: 418–19.

113. Felix JF, Steegers-Theunissen RP, de Walle HE. *et al.* Esophageal atresia and tracheoesophageal fistula in children of women exposed to diethylstilbestrol in utero. *Am J Obstet Gynecol* 2007; **197**: 38 e1–5.

114. Hauser R, Calafat AM. Phthalates and human health. *Occup Environ Med* 2005; **62**: 806–18.

115. Foster PM. Disruption of reproductive development in male rat offspring following in utero exposure to phthalate esters. *Int J Androl* 2006; **29**: 140–7; discussion 81–5.

116. Sharpe RM. "Additional" effects of phthalate mixtures on fetal testosterone production. *Toxicol Sci* 2008; **105**: 1–4.

117. Latini G, De Felice C, Presta G. *et al.* In utero exposure to di-(2-ethylhexyl)phthalate and duration of human pregnancy. *Environ Health Perspect* 2003; **111**: 1783–5.

118. Swan SH, Main KM, Liu F. *et al.* Decrease in anogenital distance among male infants with prenatal phthalate exposure. *Environ Health Perspect* 2005; **113**: 1056–61.

119. Swan SH. Environmental phthalate exposure in relation to reproductive outcomes and other health endpoints in humans. *Environ Res* 2008; **108**: 177–84.

120. Ormond G, Nieuwenhuijsen M, Nelson P. *et al.* Endocrine disruptors in the workplace, hair spray,

folate supplementation, and risk of hypospadias: case-control study. *Environ Health Perspect* 2009; **117**: 303–7.

121. Health Council of the Netherlands. *Occupational Exposure to Organic Solvents: Effects on Human Reproduction.* The Hague: Health Council of the Netherlands; publication n°2008/11OSH, 2008.

122. Olsen J, Hemminki K, Ahlborg G. *et al.* Low birthweight, congenital malformations, and spontaneous abortions among dry-cleaning workers in Scandinavia. *Scand J Work Environ Health* 1990; **16**: 163–8.

123. Johnson PD, Goldberg SJ, Mays MZ. *et al.* Threshold of trichloroethylene contamination in maternal drinking waters affecting fetal heart development in the rat. *Environ Health Perspect* 2003; **111**: 289–92.

124. Agency for Toxic Substances, and Disease Registry (ATSDR). *Toxicological Profile for Benzene (Draft).* Atlanta, GA: U.S. Public Health Service, U.S. Department of Health and Human Services, 2007.

125. Chen D, Cho SI, Chen C. *et al.* Exposure to benzene, occupational stress, and reduced birth weight. *Occup Environ Med* 2000; **57**: 661–7.

126. Wang X, Chen D, Niu T. *et al.* Genetic susceptibility to benzene and shortened gestation: evidence of gene-environment interaction. *Am J Epidemiol* 2000; **152**: 693–700.

127. Qin X, Wu Y, Wang W. *et al.* Low organic solvent exposure and combined maternal-infant gene polymorphisms affect gestational age. *Occup Environ Med* 2008; **65**: 482–7.

128. Shaw GM. Adverse human reproductive outcomes and electromagnetic fields: a brief summary of the epidemiologic literature. *Bioelectromagnetics* 2001; Suppl. 5: S5–18.

129. Parker L, Pearce MS, Dickinson HO. *et al.* Stillbirths among offspring of male radiation workers at Sellafield nuclear reprocessing plant. *Lancet* 1999; **354**: 1407–14.

130. Doyle P, Maconochie N, Roman E. *et al.* Fetal death and congenital malformation in babies born to nuclear industry employees: report from the nuclear industry family study. *Lancet* 2000; **356**: 1293–9.

131. Scherb H, Weigelt E, Bruske-Hohlfeld I. European stillbirth proportions before and after the Chernobyl accident. *Int J Epidemiol* 1999; **28**: 932–40.

132. Chiarelli AM, Marrett LD, Darlington GA. Pregnancy outcomes in females after treatment for childhood cancer. *Epidemiology* 2000; **11**: 161–6.

133. Shea KM, Little RE. Is there an association between preconception paternal x-ray exposure and birth outcome? The ALSPAC Study Team. Avon Longitudinal Study of Pregnancy and Childhood. *Am J Epidemiol* 1997; **145**: 546–51.

134. De Santis M, Di Gianantonio E, Straface G. *et al.* Ionizing radiations in pregnancy and teratogenesis: a review of literature. *Reprod Toxicol* 2005; **20**: 323–9.

135. Sever LE, Gilbert ES, Hessol NA. *et al.* A case-control study of congenital malformations and occupational exposure to low-level ionizing radiation. *Am J Epidemiol* 1988; **127**: 226–42.

136. Zatsepin I, Verger P, Robert-Gnansia E. *et al.* Down syndrome time-clustering in January 1987 in Belarus: link with the Chernobyl accident? *Reprod Toxicol* 2007; **24**: 289–95.

137. Sperling K, Pelz J, Wegner RD. *et al.* Significant increase in trisomy 21 in Berlin nine months after the Chernobyl reactor accident: temporal correlation or causal relation? *Br Med J* 1994; **309**: 158–62.

138. Dubrova YE, Nesterov VN, Krouchinsky NG. *et al.* Further evidence for elevated human minisatellite mutation rate in Belarus eight years after the Chernobyl accident. *Mutat Res* 1997; **381**: 267–78.

139. Plummer G. Anomalies occurring in children exposed in utero to the atomic bomb in Hiroshima. *Pediatrics* 1952; **10**: 687–93.

140. Committee on Medical Aspects of Radiation in the Environment(COMARE). *Eighth Report–Review of Pregnancy Outcomes Following Preconceptional Exposure to Radiation.* National Radiological Protection Board, 2004.

141. Dickinson HO, Parker L, Binks K. *et al.* The sex ratio of children in relation to paternal preconceptional radiation dose: a study in Cumbria, northern England. *J Epidemiol Community Health* 1996; **50**: 645–52.

142. Maconochie N, Roman E, Doyle P. *et al.* Sex ratio of nuclear industry employees' children. *Lancet* 2001; **357**: 1589–91.

143. Peterka M, Peterkova R, Likovsky Z. Chernobyl: relationship between the number of missing newborn boys and the level of radiation in the Czech regions. *Environ Health Perspect* 2007; **115**: 1801–6.

144. Cordier S. Evidence for a role of paternal exposures in developmental toxicity. *Basic Clin Pharmacol Toxicol* 2008; **102**: 176–81.

145. Wong EY, Gohlke J, Griffith WC. *et al.* Assessing the health benefits of air pollution reduction for children. *Environ Health Perspect* 2004; **112**: 226–32.

# Environmental contaminants and reproductive and fertility effects in the male

## 11.1 Introduction

Sarah J. Janssen

Male reproductive health is defined by both the proper development of the reproductive system and maintenance of function throughout adult life, including the capacity to reproduce. As described in Chapter 4, the development of male reproductive organs is an intricate and complex process that begins during fetal development and continues through puberty, resulting in the mature male reproductive tract which relies on hormonal control for maintenance of function.

Birth defects of male genitalia (cryptorchidism and hypospadias), alterations in male reproductive hormones, poor sperm quality, and testicular germ cell cancer adversely impact male reproductive health and can result in infertility.

Exposure to environmental contaminants and their association with these adverse endpoints and disease processes are the focus of this chapter. The first section examines the evidence for fetal exposure to environmental contaminants and the description of a unifying hypothesis for the inter-relatedness of adverse male reproductive health outcomes. This hypothesis is called testicular dysgenesis syndrome and describes how maldevelopment of the testis can result in multiple male reproductive outcomes. The second section of this chapter examines the evidence for adult exposures to environmental contaminants and male reproductive health. Both sections focus on human epidemiologic studies which have examined outcomes occurring at everyday levels of exposure.

As summarized in Table 11.1, there is extensive overlap between the chemicals found to impact fetal development and the chemicals found to interfere with adult male reproductive function. Many of these chemicals are endocrine disruptors which have been shown to interfere with the action of sex hormones important for both development and maintenance of male reproductive health. Some of these exposures are short-lived in the body (e.g. phthalates) while others can take decades to break down and be excreted (e.g. DDT and PCBs). Whether the mechanism of action for causing male reproductive toxicity is hormone receptor interference or a decrease in synthesis of sex hormones, the ultimate endpoint that is adversely impacted is the male reproductive system.

Therefore, when considering the toxicity of chemicals that impact male reproductive health, one must not consider the impact of a single chemical but rather the mixture of chemicals that an average male is exposed to on a daily basis. A recent report by the US National Research Council has recognized the importance of evaluating mixtures of chemicals from multiple exposures and has recommended that federal regulatory agencies, such as the US Environmental Protection Agency (EPA), consider common adverse outcomes (such as altered male reproductive development) and not mechanism of action (such as receptor binding) when conducting risk assessments of environmental contaminants. If adopted, future regulatory decisions of environmental contaminants will consider the cumulative risks of exposure to the chemicals listed in Table 11.1, instead of setting a standard for each individual chemical, which is the current practice.

Identifying environmental chemicals that can interfere with male reproductive tract development and adult functioning is critical for informing strategies to preventing harmful exposures and preserving male reproductive health. Insights from this collective science can inform the potential impact of other chemicals affecting development and function of the male reproductive tract.

*Environmental Impacts on Reproductive Health and Fertility*, ed. T. J. Woodruff, S. J. Janssen, L. J. Guillette, and L. C. Giudice. Published by Cambridge University Press. © Cambridge University Press 2010.

**Table 11.1.** Summary of environmental contaminants that impact male reproductive health.

| Study population | Chemical exposure and matrix | Main outcome | Reference* |
|---|---|---|---|
| Young men with prenatal exposure to tobacco smoke | Maternal questionnaire on tobacco use during pregnancy | Reduced sperm count and decreased testis size | [31] |
| Newborn males | PBDEs in placenta and breast milk as surrogate for prenatal exposure | Newborn males with cryptorchidism had significantly higher levels in breast milk, but not placenta | [35] |
| Newborn males | Chlorinated pesticides, breast milk as surrogate for prenatal exposure | Newborn males with cryptorchidism had significantly higher levels of mixture of eight chlorinated pesticides | [37] |
| Breast feeding, Infant boys, 3 months old | Phthalate metabolites in maternal breast milk | Alterations in hormone levels | [39] |
| Newborn males | Phthalate metabolites in mother's prenatal urine as surrogate for exposure | Decrease in ano-genital distance (AGD) with higher levels of phthalate exposure | [41] |
| Adult men being treated at infertility clinic | Phthalate metabolites in urine | Higher levels of exposure associated with poorer sperm quality | *[5]* |
| Adult male transcripts | Phthalate metabolites in urine | No association with semen quality | *[6]* |
| Adult men being treated at infertility clinic | Phthalate metabolites in urine | DNA damage to sperm | *[7]* |
| Adult male partners of pregnant women | Non-persistent pesticide metabolites in urine | Poor semen quality associated with higher levels of exposure | *[11]* |
| Adult men being treated at infertility clinic | Non-persistent pesticide metabolites in urine. | Decreased semen quality, sperm DNA damage and decreased testosterone associated with higher exposures | *[12–14]* |
| Adult men being treated at infertility clinic | Pyrethroid pesticide metabolites in urine | Decreased semen quality, sperm DNA damage and altered hormone levels associated with higher exposures | *[16]* |
| Adult men | PCBs measured in blood samples | Decreased sperm motility Increased sperm DNA damage Alterations in hormone levels associated with higher exposures | *[21, 23, 24]* *[25]* |
| Adult men | DDT measured in blood samples | Some studies demonstrate declines in semen quality and sperm DNA damage | *[10, 28]* |
| Adult men, occupational exposures | Solvents | Decrease in semen quality | *[29]* |
| Adult men, environmental exposures | Lead, measured in semen and blood | Decrease in semen quality | *[16, 37]* |
| Adult men, environmental exposures | Manganese measured in blood samples | Decrease in semen quality | *[38]* |
| Adult men, environmental exposures | Mercury, measured in blood, hair and semen | Altered hormone levels Decrease in semen quality | *[39, 40]* |
| Adult men, environmental exposures | Molybdenum measured in blood | Decrease in semen quality Altered hormone levels | *[9, 16]* |

* References in italics are from the second reference list in this chapter.

# 11.2 Possible role of fetal exposure

Jorma Toppari, Helena E. Virtanen, and Niels E. Skakkebaek

## Introduction

Fertility is always dependent on both male and female factors. Therefore it is often difficult to assess the sex-specific contribution to problems that may occur. However, it is estimated that infertility is caused by either only male or only female factors in one third of the cases for each, and in the remaining third both sexes influence. Worldwide it has become more and more common to seek help from assisted reproduction techniques (ART) and today at least 7% of Danish children have been conceived by ART [1] and a significant number of those include intracytoplasmic sperm injection (ICSI) which is used to overcome poor sperm function [2].

Male subfertility appears usually as impaired semen quality. Sperm number, motility, and morphology can be affected. Often all of these sperm characteristics are poor at the same time, i.e. a man with a low sperm number often also has a high percentage of structurally defective spermatozoa. Semen quality seems to have deteriorated over several decades and large regional variation is apparent [3–7]. Time to pregnancy studies have shown that fertility becomes compromised when sperm counts drop below 40 or 55 million sperm per ml [8–10]. Almost all studies on young men from the general population show that the median number of sperm per ml are close to these figures indicating that at least half of the men have suboptimal fertility [11]. The crucial question, of course, is: What is causing poor semen quality?

## Connection between impaired semen quality and other male reproductive health problems

Men with a history of cryptorchidism (undescended testes) or hypospadias tend to have poor semen quality and suffer from infertility more often than other men [12]. Both conditions are caused by fetal maldevelopment, the origin of which remains unknown in the vast majority of cases. However, in patients with different inactivating mutations of androgen receptor or defects in androgen biosynthesis, these are the typical outcomes. Androgen insensitivity is a rather rare diagnosis and defects in steroid biosynthesis are even more infrequent. There are several genetic defects that can cause either cryptorchidism or hypospadias (for review, see Kalfa *et al.* [13] and Virtanen *et al.* [14]), but these are present only in a small percentage of all cases. Studies in experimental animals and observations in wildlife suggest that it is very likely that environmental factors have a major impact on these congenital malformations.

Testicular germ cell cancers are preceded by local malignant cells in the seminiferous tubules called carcinoma *in situ* (CIS) [15–17]. These CIS cells share the properties of primordial germ cells or gonocytes that normally occur in fetal testis. This and the pattern of the cancer incidence, such as connection to birth cohorts [18], suggest that the origin of the disease occurs in the fetal period. Migration studies also support the idea that the fetal period is decisive for the occurrence of the cancer [19].

The incidence of testis cancer has two age periods of relatively high rate: the first months of life and young adulthood [20, 21]. Childhood, when the levels of both gonadotropins and sex steroids are low, is characterized by an extremely low rate of testicular cancer. The incidence starts to increase right after puberty and peaks around 25 years of age. Thus, there seems to be a clear connection between the development of cancer and hormonal activity. This is true also for the newborn period when boys have an active reproductive hormone production [22]. The testis cancer rate rapidly declines after 30 years of age, suggesting that most of the cases have been diagnosed by then.

Testis cancer patients have fewer children than other men already years before the diagnosis, suggesting that their fertility is not normal [23]. Indeed, in testis cancer patients one can find dysgenetic changes in the contralateral testis in 25% of cases [24]. These dysgenetic changes undoubtedly influence semen quality, too. The causes of testicular cancer are not known at all, but epidemiologic studies indicate that both genetic and environmental factors are important. The rapid increase in the incidence of testis cancer over the last century implies that our environment is causing most of the observed change.

Cryptorchidism is a well-known risk factor for testicular cancer. Men with a history of cryptorchidism

*Environmental Impacts on Reproductive Health and Fertility*, ed. T. J. Woodruff, S. J. Janssen, L. J. Guillette, and L. C. Giudice. Published by Cambridge University Press. ©Cambridge University Press 2010.

have an almost five-fold risk of developing testicular germ cell tumours compared with others [25, 26]. Hypospadias is also a risk factor for testis cancer as well as for cryptorchidism. Furthermore, these conditions have several common risk factors, such as small birthweight and being small for gestational age [12, 27]. Close similarity of risk factors, fetal origin, and frequent presentation of two or more of these conditions in the same patients strongly suggest a common etiology that is also influencing semen quality. The underlying reason appears to be maldevelopment of the testis, and this has given the name testicular dysgenesis syndrome (TDS) for these reproductive health problems [12]. This helps to illustrate the developmental concept that is important in searching for genetic and environmental causes for these problems. The possibility of male subfertility should therefore be kept in mind in connection with other forms of TDS. Poor semen quality may be a mild presentation of TDS, while malformations and tumorigenesis possibly represent the most serious end of the disease spectrum.

## Trends in the incidence of TDS and life style

The incidence of different TDS components has increased and regional variation is remarkable. Two Nordic countries Denmark and Finland show marked differences in semen quality and the incidence of testicular cancer, cryptorchidism, and hypospadias [5, 28, 29, 30], which has raised the obvious question: what could explain the differences? It is obvious that there is not one explanation that would give an answer, but there may be complex interactions of genetic and environmental factors that contribute to TDS.

Semen quality studies have shown that mothers smoking during pregnancy is associated with reduced sperm counts and decreased testis size in the adult sons [31]. This further shows the importance of fetal exposure to adult reproductive health. The effects of maternal smoking on the incidence of cryptorchidism are more equivocal: we have not found an association in our studies [32], but there are reports linking heavy smoking to an increased risk of cryptorchidism [33]. Instead of smoking, the use of nicotine substitution during pregnancy was associated with an increased prevalence of cryptorchidism [32]. Maternal alcohol consumption showed a dose-dependent association to cryptorchidism risk of the offspring [34]. These life-style factors can be easily addressed in epidemiologic studies,

but exposure to other environmental chemicals is more difficult to evaluate. We have analyzed chemicals both in the placenta and in breast milk from mothers who have given birth to cryptorchid or normal boys.

## Chemical exposures

Recent research has shown associations between chemical exposures and an increased risk of cryptorchidism. Thus, concentration of polybrominated diphenyl ethers in breast milk was higher in the group of cryptorchid boys as compared with controls [35]. Some of these compounds have been shown to be antiandrogenic, which could be the reason for the risk if there were a causal relationship [36].

Concentrations of chlorinated pesticides tended also to be higher in breast milk of cryptorchid boys' mothers than in controls, and combined statistical analysis showed that pesticide levels were significantly higher in cases than in controls [37]. Many of the measured pesticides, e.g. P.P′-DDE, had been identified as endocrine disrupters in animal or in vitro experiments [38]. Polychlorinated compounds are very persistent and these kind of exposures are easy to measure, whereas chemicals that do not bioaccumulate and are rapidly metabolized and secreted, such as phthalates, are more difficult to study.

We measured phthalates in milk samples and found no correlation to cryptorchidism, but they did correlate to hormone levels of the boys at 3 months [39]. Increased levels of the phthalate metabolites, mono-methyl phthalate, mono-ethyl phthalate, and mono-$n$-butyl phthalate were associated to an increased ratio of LH and free testosterone. The increased ratio indicates the possibility of primary hypogonadism, i.e. testicular malfunction. We noticed that Finnish cryptorchid boys as a group have an increased LH-testosterone ratio [40]. In an American study, the ano-genital index correlated to phthalate concentrations in mothers' urine [41]. Males have normally longer ano-genital distance than females, and impaired fetal androgen action should therefore lead to shortened ano-genital distance in exposed boys. Ano-genital index takes the size of the baby into account and it can be used to measure the androgen action in a newborn child.

All the above-mentioned studies give only exposure-outcome associations, but they do not indicate causal relationships. Experimental data are necessary to look for the mechanisms and possible cause–effect relationships.

# Experimental data of endocrine disrupters

Endocrine disrupters with antiandrogenic properties prevent normal masculinization of male fetuses, and androgenic compounds can masculinize female fetuses. Timing of the endocrine disruption is crucial. In an elegant series of experiments, Richard Sharpe's group demonstrated that exposure to an antiandrogen, flutamide, in an early time window, on rat embryonic days (ED) 15.5–17.5, caused the most severe demasculinizing effects, whereas exposure in a late time window on ED 19.5–21.5 had much less severe effects [42]. Androgen production peaks on ED 19.5, and one would intuitively assume that receptor blockage at that time point would be most harmful. However, it is obvious that androgens have earlier programming effects and sensitive exposure windows can be rather narrow.

The list of antiandrogenic chemicals keeps growing to include some pesticides that act mainly by receptor antagonism and phthalates that act mainly by interfering with androgen biosynthesis. DDT and its congeners are well-characterized endocrine disrupters. These are all discussed in Chapter 2.

The fungicides vinclozolin and procymidone are antiandrogens that act at the receptor level. Vinclozolin itself does not bind to the androgen receptor, but its two metabolites M1 and M2 do [43, 44]. Therefore, only test systems that allow conversion of vinclozolin to these metabolites can demonstrate antiandrogenic effects. Procymidone is an effective androgen receptor antagonist itself. Both fungicides cause typical antiandrogenic effects in developing animals: hypospadias, cleft phallus, vaginal pouch, reduced ano-genital distance, reduced accessory sex gland size, and induction of retained nipples in the male offspring [45]. These antiandrogens function dose-additively together and bring about adverse effects at their established no-adverse effect levels when administered together [38, 46, 47]. The mixture effects have received increasing attention and the whole risk-assessment procedure has to be reconsidered in light of chemical complexity of our environment [45].

Linuron is an antiandrogenic herbicide that was identified by Hershberger assay [48] which is an OECD standard method to test antiandrogenicity. In other reproductive and developmental toxicity tests linuron also caused antiandrogenic effects, e.g. nipple retention, reduced ano-genital distance, and alterations in androgen-dependent tissues [48–50].

Receptor antagonism is the mechanism of action of some antiandrogenic chemicals, whereas the synthesis and metabolism of androgens are influenced by many other chemicals. Furthermore, some compounds exert both effects, e.g. the fungicide prochloraz [51–53] and the herbicide linuron [48]. Antiandrogenic effects in the offspring have been described also after exposure of dams to 2,3,7,8-tetrachlorodibenzo-*p*-dioxin (TCDD), polychlorinated dibenzo-furans (PCDFs) and polychlorinated biphenyls (PCBs) [54–59]. The effects are mediated by aryl hydrocarbon receptors, the structure of which varies influencing the outcome in different species and rat strains [60, 61].

Several phthalate esters, such di-(2-ethylhexyl) phthalate (DEHP), di-*n*-butyl phthalate (DBP), and benzylbutyl phthalate, disturb androgen biosynthesis. These chemicals have numerous applications in plastics and are commonly present in our environment. Their metabolism is rather fast, but exposure peaks can be substantial. It is the monoester form of the phthalate that is usually causing the biological effects, e.g. in the case of DEHP, mono-(2-ethylhexyl) phthalate (MEHP) is responsible for many adverse effects. Neither DEHP nor MEHP bind to the androgen receptor [62], but they inhibit fetal Leydig cell function and testosterone production [62, 63]. Fetal exposure to DBP results in several antiandrogenic effects that have been described as a phthalate syndrome or a rat TDS comparable to human TDS [64, 65]. The exposed rats have malformations in the epididymis and vas deferens, hypospadias, cryptorchidism, reduced ano-genital distance, nipple retention, and structural abnormalities in the testis [66, 67]. In contrast to human TDS, testicular cancer does not manifest in the animal models, but some of the structural features in DBP-exposed rats resemble changes that occur in testes of men with TDS [68].

Estrogens were the primary concern when endocrine disrupters became the focus of reproductive toxicology [69], and only later antiandrogens received more of the attention. Antiandrogens affect only male fetuses, whereas estrogens can harm both sexes. Many of the estrogenic effects are similar to those of antiandrogens in male fetuses, and androgen–estrogen balance is important for normal development [70].

The sad experience with the use of diethylstilbestrol (DES) in the treatment of pregnant women alerted endocrinologists to endocrine-disrupting effects of estrogens in the 1970s. John McLachlan and coworkers showed that fetal exposure of male mice to DES caused multiple structural and functional adverse effects, e.g. epididymal cysts, distended seminal vesicles, retained müllerian ducts, undescended testes, and impaired spermatogenesis [71, 72]. Human effects were found to be very similar [73, 74], although fertility was assessed to be normal [75]. Testicular cancer risk was approximately doubled in prenatally DES-exposed men [69, 76].

Diethylstilbestrol is thus far the only estrogen that has been shown to affect the development of human male external genitalia, but in experimental animals ethinyl estradiol and estradiol benzoate have similar effects [77, 78]. Raman-Wilms *et al.* [79] made a meta-analysis of 14 studies on the first-trimester exposure of fetuses to sex hormones excluding DES, and did not find an association. The epidemiologic studies were based on accidental exposures, such as use of contraceptive pills during early pregnancy, and therefore many inherent problems created a lot of uncertainties, whereas some of the early DES studies were based on previous randomized, placebo-controlled studies [80] which gave them good power. In DES studies the adverse effects were clearly dose- and time-dependent. Exposure to synthetic estrogens in early pregnancy may cause adverse effects that are not yet apparent at birth, but influence later sexual development. Extensive lists of environmental estrogens have been published and they may have additive effects like the antiandrogens do. The low-dose effects have remained very controversial [78, 81], but it may even be irrelevant when the main problem is the big mixture that we are exposed to [82]. Genetic susceptibility is also an important factor, and studies on gene–environment interactions are currently rapidly producing new data on polymorphisms that influence hormonal effects [83, 84].

## Perspectives

Studies on environmental effects on fertility are challenging and there are no short-cuts to rapid advance in research. Long-term, multidisciplinary studies are necessary to identify harmful endocrine-disrupting agents in our environment. Only in this way can we start to prevent deterioration of reproductive health and safeguard future generations. However, to make real progress in this area of human reproductive health more involvement from clinical researchers is needed. Human studies taking the role of early fetal programming into consideration are particularly challenging and cannot be carried out unless more concerned clinicians will join in this endeavor.

## References

1. Nyboe Andersen A, Balen A, Platteau P. *et al.* Predicting the FSH threshold dose in women with WHO Group II anovulatory infertility failing to ovulate or conceive on clomiphene citrate. *Hum Reprod* 2008; **23**(6): 1424–30.

2. Skakkebaek NE, Jorgensen N, Main KM. *et al.* Is human fecundity declining? *Int J Androl* 2006; **29**: 2–11.

3. Carlsen E, Giwercman A, Keiding N, Skakkebaek NE. Evidence for decreasing quality of semen during past 50 years. *Bc Med J*, 1992; **305**(6854): 609–13.

4. Jorgensen N, Andersen AG, Eustache F. *et al.* Regional differences in semen quality in Europe. *Hum Reprod* 2001; **16**: 1012–19.

5. Jorgensen N, Carlsen E, Nermoen I. *et al.* East-West gradient in semen quality in the Nordic-Baltic area: a study of men from the general population in Denmark, Norway, Estonia and Finland. *Hum Reprod* 2002; **17**: 2199–208.

6. Paasch U, Salzbrunn A, Glander HJ. *et al.* Semen quality in sub-fertile range for a significant proportion of young men from the general German population: a co-ordinated, controlled study of 791 men from Hamburg and Leipzig. *Int J Androl* 2008; **31**: 93–102.

7. Swan SH. Semen quality in fertile US men in relation to geographical area and pesticide exposure. *Int J Androl* 2006; **29**: 62–8; discussion 105–8.

8. Bonde JP, Ernst E, Jensen TK. *et al.* Relation between semen quality and fertility: a population-based study of 430 first-pregnancy planners, *Lancet* 1998; **352**(9135): 1172–7.

9. Guzick DS, Overstreet JW, Factor-Litvak P. *et al.* Sperm morphology, motility, and concentration in fertile and infertile men. *New Engl J Med* 2001; **345**(19): 1388–93.

10. Slama R, Eustache F, Ducot B. *et al.* Time to pregnancy and semen parameters: a cross-sectional study among fertile couples from four European cities. *Hum Reprod* 2002; **17**: 503–15.

11. Andersson AM, Jorgensen N, Main KM. *et al.* Adverse trends in male reproductive health: we may have reached a crucial 'tipping point'. *Int J Androl* 2008; **31**: 74–80.

12. Skakkebaek NE, Rajpert-De Meyts E, Main KM. Testicular dysgenesis syndrome: an increasingly common developmental disorder with environmental aspects. *Hum Reprod* 2001; **16**: 972–8.

13. Kalfa N, Philibert P, Sultan, C. Is hypospadias a genetic, endocrine or environmental disease, or still an unexplained malformation? *Int J Androl* 2009; **32**(3): 187–97.

14. Virtanen HE, Cortes D, Rajpert-De Meyts E. *et al.* Development and descent of the testis in relation to cryptorchidism. *Acta Paediatr* 2007; **96**: 622–7.

15. Rajpert-De Meyts E. Developmental model for the pathogenesis of testicular carcinoma in situ: genetic

and environmental aspects. *Hum Reprod Update* 2006; **12**: 303–23.

16. Skakkebaek NE. Possible carcinoma-in-situ of the testis. *Lancet* 1972; **2**(7776): 516–17.

17. Skakkebaek NE, Berthelsen JG, Giwercman A, Muller J. Carcinoma-in-situ of the testis: possible origin from gonocytes and precursor of all types of germ cell tumours except spermatocytoma. *Int J Androl* 1987; **10**: 19–28.

18. Bergstrom R, Adami HO, Mohner M. *et al.* Increase in testicular cancer incidence in six European countries: a birth cohort phenomenon. *J Natl Cancer Inst* 1996; **88**: 727–33.

19. Hemminki K, Chen B. Familial risks in testicular cancer as aetiological clues. *Int J Androl* 2006; **29**(1): 205–10.

20. Ekbom A, Akre O. Increasing incidence of testicular cancer – birth cohort effects. *Apmis* 1998; **106**: 225–9; discussion 229–31.

21. Skakkebaek NE, Rajpert-De Meyts E, Jorgensen N. *et al.* Testicular cancer trends as 'whistle blowers' of testicular developmental problems in populations. *Int J Androl* 2007; **30**: 198–204; discussion 204–5.

22. Andersson AM, Toppari J, Haavisto AM. *et al.* Longitudinal reproductive hormone profiles in infants: peak of inhibin B levels in infant boys exceeds levels in adult men. *J Clin Endocrinol Metab* 1998; **83**: 675–81.

23. Moller H, Skakkebaek NE. Risk of testicular cancer in subfertile men: case-control study. *Br Med J*, 1999; **318**(7183): 559–62.

24. Hoei-Hansen CE, Holm M, Rajpert-De Meyts E, Skakkebaek NE. Histological evidence of testicular dysgenesis in contralateral biopsies from 218 patients with testicular germ cell cancer. *J Pathol* 2003; **200**: 370–4.

25. Dieckmann KP, Pichlmeier U. Clinical epidemiology of testicular germ cell tumors. *World J Urol* 2004; **22**: 2–14.

26. Giwercman A, Grindsted J, Hansen B, Jensen OM, Skakkebaek NE. Testicular cancer risk in boys with maldescended testis: a cohort study. *J Urol* 1987; **138**(5): 1214–16.

27. Virtanen HE, Toppari J. Epidemiology and pathogenesis of cryptorchidism. *Hum Reprod Update* 2008; **14**: 49–58.

28. Boisen KA, Chellakooty M, Schmidt IM. *et al.* Hypospadias in a cohort of 1072 Danish newborn boys: prevalence and relationship to placental weight, anthropometrical measurements at birth, and reproductive hormone levels at three months of age. *J Clin Endocrinol Metab* 2005; **90**: 4041–6.

29. Boisen KA, Kaleva M, Main KM. *et al.* Difference in prevalence of congenital cryptorchidism in infants between two Nordic countries, *Lancet* 2004; **363**(9417): 1264–9.

30. Jacobsen R, Moller H, Thoresen SO. *et al.* Trends in testicular cancer incidence in the Nordic countries, focusing on the recent decrease in Denmark. *Int J Androl* 2006; **29**: 199–204.

31. Jensen TK, Jorgensen N, Punab M. *et al.* Association of in utero exposure to maternal smoking with reduced semen quality and testis size in adulthood: a cross-sectional study of 1,770 young men from the general population in five European countries. *Am J Epidemiol* 2004; **159**: 49–58.

32. Damgaard IN, Jensen TK, Petersen JH. *et al.* Risk factors for congenital cryptorchidism in a prospective birth cohort study. *PLoS ONE* 2008; **3**(8): e3051.

33. Thorup J, Cortes D, Petersen BL. The incidence of bilateral cryptorchidism is increased and the fertility potential is reduced in sons born to mothers who have smoked during pregnancy. *J Urol* 2006; **176**: 734–7.

34. Damgaard IN, Jensen TK, Petersen JH. *et al.* Cryptorchidism and maternal alcohol consumption during pregnancy. *Environ Health Perspect* 2007; **115**: 272–7.

35. Main KM, Kiviranta H, Virtanen HE. *et al.* Flame retardants in placenta and breast milk and cryptorchidism in newborn boys. *Environ Health Perspect* 2007; **115**: 1519–26.

36. Darnerud PO. Brominated flame retardants as possible endocrine disrupters. *Int J Androl* 2008; **31**: 152–60.

37. Damgaard IN, Skakkebaek NE, Toppari J. *et al.* Persistent pesticides in human breast milk and cryptorchidism. *Environ Health Perspect* 2006; **114**: 1133–8.

38. Rider CV, Furr J, Wilson VS, Gray LE Jr. A mixture of seven antiandrogens induces reproductive malformations in rats. *Int J Androl* 2008; **31**: 249–62.

39. Main KM, Mortensen GK, Kaleva MM. *et al.* Human breast milk contamination with phthalates and alterations of endogenous reproductive hormones in infants three months of age, *Environ Health Perspect* 2006; **114**: 270–6.

40. Suomi AM, Main KM, Kaleva M. *et al.* Hormonal changes in 3-month-old cryptorchid boys. *J Clin Endocrinol Metab* 2006; **91**: 953–8.

41. Swan SH, Main KM, Liu F. *et al.* Decrease in anogenital distance among male infants with prenatal phthalate exposure. *Environ Health Perspect* 2005; **113**: 1056–61.

42. Welsh M, Saunders PT, Fisken M. *et al.* Identification in rats of a programming window for reproductive tract masculinization, disruption of which leads to hypospadias and cryptorchidism. *J Clin Invest* 2008; **118**: 1479–90.

43. Kelce WR, Monosson E, Gamcsik MP, Laws SC, Gray LE Jr. Environmental hormone disruptors: evidence that vinclozolin developmental toxicity is mediated by antiandrogenic metabolites. *Toxicol Appl Pharmacol* 1994; **126**: 276–85.

44. Wolf CJ, LeBlanc GA, Ostby JS, Gray LE Jr. Characterization of the period of sensitivity of fetal

male sexual development to vinclozolin. *Toxicol Sci* 2000; **55**: 152–61.

45. Ostby J, Kelce WR, Lambright C. *et al.* The fungicide procymidone alters sexual differentiation in the male rat by acting as an androgen-receptor antagonist in vivo and in vitro. *Toxicol Ind Health* 1999; **15**(1–2): 80–93.

46. Christiansen S, Scholze M, Axelstad M. *et al.* Combined exposure to anti-androgens causes markedly increased frequencies of hypospadias in the rat, *Int J Androl* 2008; **31**: 241–8.

47. Wilson VS, Blystone CR, Hotchkiss AK, Rider CV. Gray LE Jr. Diverse mechanisms of anti-androgen action: impact on male rat reproductive tract development. *Int J Androl* 2008; **31**: 178–87.

48. Lambright ES, Kang EH, Force S. *et al.* Effect of preexisting anti-herpes immunity on the efficacy of herpes simplex viral therapy in a murine intraperitoneal tumor model. *Mol Ther* 2000; **2**: 387–93.

49. Gray LE Jr, Wolf C, Lambright C. *et al.* Administration of potentially antiandrogenic pesticides (procymidone, linuron, iprodione, chlozolinate, p,p'-DDE, and ketoconazole) and toxic substances (dibutyl- and diethylhexyl phthalate, PCB 169, and ethane dimethane sulphonate) during sexual differentiation produces diverse profiles of reproductive malformations in the male rat. *Toxicol Ind Health* 1999; **15**(1–2): 94–118.

50. McIntyre BS, Barlow NJ, Wallace DG. *et al.* Effects of in utero exposure to linuron on androgen-dependent reproductive development in the male Crl:CD(SD)BR rat. *Toxicol Appl Pharmacol* 2000; **167**: 87–99.

51. Noriega NC, Ostby J, Lambright C, Wilson VS, Gray LE Jr. Late gestational exposure to the fungicide prochloraz delays the onset of parturition and causes reproductive malformations in male but not female rat offspring. *Biol Reprod* 2005; **72**: 1324–35.

52. Vinggaard AM, Christiansen S, Laier P. *et al.* Perinatal exposure to the fungicide prochloraz feminizes the male rat offspring. *Toxicol Sci* 2005; **85**: 886–97.

53. Vinggaard AM, Nellemann C, Dalgaard M, Jorgensen EB, Andersen HR. Antiandrogenic effects in vitro and in vivo of the fungicide prochloraz. *Toxicol Sci* 2002; **69**: 344–53.

54. Gray LE, Ostby J, Furr J. *et al.* Effects of environmental antiandrogens on reproductive development in experimental animals. *Hum Reprod Update* 2001; **7**: 248–64.

55. Gray LE, Wolf C, Mann P, Ostby JS. In utero exposure to low doses of 2,3,7,8-tetrachlorodibenzo-p-dioxin alters reproductive development of female Long Evans hooded rat offspring. *Toxicol Appl Pharmacol* 1997; **146**: 237–44.

56. Mably TA, Bjerke DL, Moore RW, Gendron-Fitzpatrick A, Peterson RE. In utero and lactational exposure of male rats to 2,3,7,8-tetrachlorodibenzo-p-dioxin. 3. Effects on spermatogenesis and reproductive capability. *Toxicol Appl Pharmacol* 1992; **114**: 118–26.

57. Mably TA, Moore RW, Goy RW, Peterson RE. In utero and lactational exposure of male rats to 2,3,7,8-tetrachlorodibenzo-p-dioxin. 2. Effects on sexual behavior and the regulation of luteinizing hormone secretion in adulthood. *Toxicol Appl Pharmacol* 1992; **114**: 108–17.

58. Mably TA, Moore RW, Peterson RE. In utero and lactational exposure of male rats to 2,3,7,8-tetrachlorodibenzo-p-dioxin. 1. Effects on androgenic status. *Toxicol Appl Pharmacol* 1992; **114**: 97–107.

59. Theobald HM, Peterson RE. In utero and lactational exposure to 2,3,7,8-tetrachlorodibenzo-$\rho$-dioxin: effects on development of the male and female reproductive system of the mouse. *Toxicol Appl Pharmacol* 1997; **145**: 124–35.

60. Simanainen U, Adamsson A, Tuomisto JT. *et al.* Adult 2,3,7,8-tetrachlorodibenzo-p-dioxin (TCDD) exposure and effects on male reproductive organs in three differentially TCDD-susceptible rat lines. *Toxicol Sci* 2004; **81**: 401–7.

61. Simanainen U, Haavisto T, Tuomisto JT. *et al.* Pattern of male reproductive system effects after in utero and lactational 2,3,7,8-tetrachlorodibenzo-p-dioxin (TCDD) exposure in three differentially TCDD-sensitive rat lines. *Toxicol Sci* 2004; **80**: 101–8.

62. Parks LG, Ostby JS, Lambright CR. *et al.* The plasticizer diethylhexyl phthalate induces malformations by decreasing fetal testosterone synthesis during sexual differentiation in the male rat. *Toxicol Sci* 2000; **58**: 339–49.

63. Arcadi FA, Costa C, Imperatore C. *et al.* Oral toxicity of bis(2-ethylhexyl) phthalate during pregnancy and suckling in the Long-Evans rat. *Food Chem Toxicol* 1998; **36**: 963–70.

64. Fisher JS, Macpherson S, Marchetti N, Sharpe RM. Human 'testicular dysgenesis syndrome': a possible model using in-utero exposure of the rat to dibutyl phthalate. *Hum Reprod* 2003; **18**: 1383–94.

65. Foster PM. Disruption of reproductive development in male rat offspring following in utero exposure to phthalate esters. *Int J Androl* 2006; **29**: 140–7; discussion 181–5.

66. Foster PM, Mylchreest E, Gaido KW, Sar M. Effects of phthalate esters on the developing reproductive tract of male rats. *Hum Reprod Update* 2001; **7**: 231–5.

67. Hutchison GR, Sharpe RM, Mahood IK. *et al.* (2008) The origins and time of appearance of focal testicular dysgenesis in an animal model of testicular dysgenesis syndrome: evidence for delayed testis development? *Int J Androl* 2008; **31**: 103–11.

68. Sharpe RM, Skakkebaek NE. Testicular dysgenesis syndrome: mechanistic insights and potential new downstream effects. *Fertil Steril* 2008; **89** (Suppl. 2): e33–8.

69. Toppari J, Larsen JC, Christiansen P. *et al.* Male reproductive health and environmental xenoestrogens. *Environ Health Perspect* 1996; **104** (Suppl. 4): 741–803.

70. Williams K, McKinnell C, Saunders PT. *et al.* Neonatal exposure to potent and environmental oestrogens and abnormalities of the male reproductive system in the rat: evidence for importance of the androgen-oestrogen balance and assessment of the relevance to man. *Hum Reprod Update* 2001; **7**: 236–47.

71. McLachlan JA, Newbold RR, Bullock, B. Reproductive tract lesions in male mice exposed prenatally to diethylstilbestrol. *Science* 1975; **190**: 991–2.

72. McLachlan JA, Newbold RR, Burow ME, Li SF. From malformations to molecular mechanisms in the male: three decades of research on endocrine disrupters. *Apmis* 2001; **109**: 263–72.

73. Gill WB, Schumacher GF, Bibbo M. Pathological semen and anatomical abnormalities of the genital tract in human male subjects exposed to diethylstilbestrol in utero. *J Urol* 1977; **117**: 477–80.

74. Gill WB, Schumacher GF, Bibbo M, Straus FH 2nd, Schoenberg HW. Association of diethylstilbestrol exposure in utero with cryptorchidism, testicular hypoplasia and semen abnormalities. *J Urol* 1979; **122**: 36–9.

75. Wilcox AJ, Baird DD, Weinberg CR, Hornsby PP, Herbst AL. Fertility in men exposed prenatally to diethylstilbestrol. *New Engl J Med* 1995; **332**(21): 1411–16.

76. Strohsnitter WC, Noller KL, Hoover RN. *et al.* Cancer risk in men exposed in utero to diethylstilbestrol. *J Natl Cancer Inst* 2001; **93**(7): 545–51.

77. Arai Y, Mori T, Suzuki Y, Bern HA. Long-term effects of perinatal exposure to sex steroids and diethylstilbestrol on the reproductive system of male mammals. *Int Rev Cytol* 1983; **84**: 235–68.

78. Thayer KA, Ruhlen RL, Howdeshell KL. *et al.* Altered prostate growth and daily sperm production in male mice exposed prenatally to subclinical doses of 17alpha-ethinyl oestradiol, *Hum Reprod* 2001; **16**: 988–96.

79. Raman-Wilms L, Tseng AL, Wighardt S, Einarson TR, Koren G. Fetal genital effects of first-trimester sex hormone exposure: a meta-analysis. *Obstet Gynecol* 1995; **85**: 141–9.

80. Dieckmann WJ, Davis ME, Rynkiewicz LM, Pottinger RE. Does the administration of diethylstilbestrol during pregnancy have therapeutic value? *Am J Obstet Gynecol* 1953; **66**(5): 1062–81.

81. Ashby J. Testing for endocrine disruption post-EDSTAC: extrapolation of low dose rodent effects to humans. *Toxicol Lett* 2001; **120**: 233–42.

82. Kortenkamp A. Low dose mixture effects of endocrine disrupters: implications for risk assessment and epidemiology. *Int J Androl* 2008; **31**: 233–40.

83. Spearow JL, Doemeny P, Sera R, Leffler R, Barkley M. Genetic variation in susceptibility to endocrine disruption by estrogen in mice. *Science* 1999; **285**(5431): 1259–61.

84. Watanabe M, Yoshida R, Ueoka K. *et al.* Haplotype analysis of the estrogen receptor 1 gene in male genital and reproductive abnormalities. *Hum Reprod* 2007; **22**(5): 1279–84.

# 11.3 Adult exposure and effects on fertility

John D. Meeker and Russ Hauser

## Introduction

Recent reports of temporal downward trends in semen quality [1] and testosterone levels [2] among human populations has increased scientific and public concern regarding the potential risk of environmental chemicals to male reproductive health. These observations, in addition to recent findings of high geographic variability in semen quality [3], raise the possibility that human exposure to environmental chemicals may play a role.

The assessment of semen quality (i.e. sperm concentration, motility, and morphology) is used not only clinically to assess fertility, but also in epidemiologic studies as a biomarker for the potential effects of toxicants on the male reproductive system. Semen quality may be altered through toxicant effects on the neuroendocrine system (i.e. the hypothalamic–pituitary–testis axis), the testis (which includes Sertoli and Leydig cells as well as the spermatogenic cells), and on post-testicular sites such as the epididymis. Toxicants may affect reproductive function by interacting with or disturbing one or more of these targets. Recent advances in the measurement of sperm cell DNA integrity (e.g. DNA damage or chromatin fragmentation) and circulating reproductive hormone levels have also led to increased use of these indices in research and clinical practice.

The present chapter focuses on the human data generated to date on the relationship between adulthood exposures to environmental chemicals and male reproductive health. The agents discussed here – phthalates, pesticides, organochlorines, solvents, and metals – were chosen based on their exposure prevalence and the presence of existing human data. Further detailed information for many of these contaminants can be found in Chapter 2.

## Human evidence for adverse male reproductive effects in relation to environmental contaminants

We focus here on epidemiologic studies of environmental exposures and male reproductive function as measured by declines in semen quality parameters, increased sperm DNA damage/fragmentation, or altered reproductive hormone levels. Studies included in this chapter were chosen based on quality and relevance, where larger and more recent studies using sensitive markers of exposure and outcome were given preference. For a more detailed discussion, the reader is directed to the referenced articles.

## Phthalates

Despite animal data demonstrating that some phthalates are male reproductive toxicants and endocrine disruptors, human studies remain limited. Duty and colleagues [4] recently reported inverse associations between urinary phthalate metabolites and semen quality, with a follow-up analysis reported by Hauser et al. [5]. Study subjects consisted of male partners of subfertile couples that presented to an infertility clinic in Massachusetts, USA. In the initial report there were dose–response relationships (after adjusting for age, abstinence time, and smoking status) between mono-$n$-butyl phthalate (MBP) (a metabolite of di-$n$-butylphthalate (DBP)) and below-reference sperm motility and sperm concentration among 168 men [4]. In the recent follow-up report including these 168 men, plus an additional 295 men newly recruited into the study, Hauser and colleagues [5] confirmed the associations between MBP and increased odds of below-reference sperm concentration and motility. In a recently published study from Sweden, Jonsson and colleagues [6] recruited 234 young Swedish men at the time of their medical conscript examination. In contrast to the US study, in the Swedish study there were no relationships of MBP with any of the semen parameters, but men in the highest quartile for MEP had fewer motile sperm and more immotile sperm than men in the lowest MEP (a metabolite of DEP) quartile. Although the Swedish study had some similarities to the US study, in that they were both cross-sectional studies, there were also many important differences including the age range of the study population, infertility patients as compared with young men from the general population, and differences in the analytical methods used to measure phthalates.

In the Massachusetts study, semen samples from 379 men were also analyzed for sperm DNA damage

*Environmental Impacts on Reproductive Health and Fertility*, ed. T. J. Woodruff, S. J. Janssen, L. J. Guillette, and L. C. Giudice. Published by Cambridge University Press. © Cambridge University Press 2010.

using the neutral comet assay [7]. After adjustment for age and smoking status, positive associations were found for at least one of the three sperm DNA damage measures with MEP, MBP, MBzP (a metabolite of butyl benzyl phthalate), and MEHP (a metabolite of DEHP). Another interesting finding was that MEHP was strongly associated with all three DNA damage measures after adjustment for the oxidized DEHP metabolites, which may serve as phenotypic markers of DEHP metabolism to "less toxic" metabolites and lower susceptibility to exposure-related effects compared with those individuals with low concentrations of oxidized DEHP metabolites relative to MEHP concentration. Since the monoester metabolite may be the more bioactive and toxic form of the phthalate, individuals who have lower metabolism of MEHP to the oxidized metabolites may have increased sensitivity to phthalate exposure.

Three human studies have investigated associations between exposure to phthalates and circulating reproductive hormone levels in men. In a study of workers producing PVC flooring with high exposure to DEHP and DBP, urinary concentrations of metabolites of these phthalates were inversely associated with free testosterone levels [8]. Likewise, a report on 425 men from the Massachusetts infertility clinic study found that MEHP was inversely associated with testosterone and estradiol [9]. On the other hand, the study of 234 young Swedish men found an inverse association between urinary MEP and LH but no association between MEP, MBP, MEHP, or other phthalate metabolites in urine and FSH, testosterone, estradiol, or inhibin B [6].

In summary, the epidemiologic data on semen quality, sperm cell DNA integrity, and altered reproductive hormone levels in relation to phthalate exposure among men remains limited. Additional studies are critically needed to help elucidate possible explanations for differences across studies, and most importantly to address whether phthalate exposure alters semen quality, sperm function, and male fertility.

## Non-persistent pesticides

Some common classes of non-persistent pesticides in use today include organophosphates, carbamates, and pyrethroids. Though environmentally non-persistent, due to the extensive use of pest control in various settings, a majority of the general population is exposed to some of the more widely used pesticides at low levels.

A number of studies have reported alterations in male reproductive health markers in relation to non-persistent pesticide exposure in agricultural and industrial (e.g. pesticide manufacture and packaging) settings [10], the majority of which relied on non-specific assessment of exposure and thus limited the interpretation of findings. More recently, researchers have utilized urinary and serum biomarkers of pesticide exposure to explore associations between low-level exposure, representative of exposures among the general population, and reduced semen quality. In a US study on the male partners of pregnant women, Swan and coworkers [11] compared urinary levels of pesticide biomarkers in 34 men with sperm concentration, motility, and morphology below the median (defined as cases) with 52 men with above median semen parameters (defined as controls). They found elevated odds-ratios for alachlor mercapturate, 2-isopropoxy-4-methyl-pyrimidinol (IMPY; diazinon metabolite), atrazine mercapturate, 1-naphthol (carbaryl and naphthalene metabolite), and 3,5,6-trichloro-2-pyridinol (TCPY; chlorpyrifos metabolite). However, a small study size led to wide confidence intervals that restrict interpretation of the study results.

Using urinary biomarker data representative of low environmental levels of pesticides commonly encountered among the US general population, Meeker et al. [12] studied 272 men from the Massachusetts infertility clinic study. They found inverse associations between urinary levels of 1-naphthol, a metabolite of both carbaryl and naphthalene, with sperm concentration and motility. They also found a suggestive inverse relationship between the urinary metabolite of chlorpyrifos (TCPY) and sperm motility. Within the same study population, statistically significant positive associations between TCPY and 1N and sperm DNA damage were also reported [13], as were significant inverse associations between the insecticide metabolites and serum testosterone levels [14].

New restrictions have been placed on chlorpyrifos and other common organophosphate insecticides in many countries, which have resulted in the increased availability and usage of synthetic pyrethroid insecticides [15]. Meeker and colleagues [16] recently reported inverse associations between urinary pyrethroid metabolites and sperm concentration, motility, and morphology, and a positive association between pyrethroid metabolites and sperm DNA damage, in men from the Massachusetts study. The findings for sperm concentration were consistent with results from a study of 376 Chinese men with no occupational pesticide exposure [17]. There is also recent evidence for altered hormone levels in relation to environmental pyrethroid exposure. Among men in the Massachusetts study, pyrethroid metabolites were positively associated with FSH and LH, and inversely associated with inhibin B and testosterone [18].

In summary, in addition to evidence from occupational studies, there are limited human studies suggesting male reproductive toxicity in relation to non-occupational exposure to non-persistent pesticides, specifically some herbicides and insecticides. However, more research is clearly needed.

## Polychlorinated biphenyls and organochlorine pesticides

Compared to other known or suspected endocrine disruptors, PCBs have been relatively well studied in relation to male reproductive health, especially measures of semen quality [19, 20]. Among 305 young men undergoing a conscript examination for military service, Richthoff and coworkers [21] reported inverse associations between PCB 153 and percent motile sperm, but not sperm concentration or total sperm count, when considering potential confounding variables. Rignell-Hydbom *et al.* [22, 23] reported on the associations between PCBs with semen parameters and sperm chromatin integrity in Swedish fishermen from two regions. When PCB 153 was categorized into quintiles, the highest quintile had decreased sperm motility compared with men in the lowest quintile. There were no consistent associations of PCB 153 with sperm concentration. Among men with sperm chromatin integrity results, there was a positive association between PCB 153 and the percentage of sperm showing DNA fragmentation. This study population was part of a large 4-center study of 2269 men from European and Inuit populations, which found that PCB 153 was positively associated with DNA fragmentation in an analysis of all European men in the study, and inversely associated with percentage of progressive sperm in an analysis of all men (European and Inuit) who participated in the study [24]. Hauser and colleagues [25] conducted a study of PCB levels in blood and semen quality parameters among 212 of the men in the Massachusetts infertility clinic study. After adjusting for confounders there were significant dose–response relationships between PCB 138 and below-reference sperm motility and sperm morphology. Associations between semen parameters and PCB 153 were not consistent. Hauser *et al.* [26] also studied the relationship between PCBs with DNA integrity in sperm using the neutral comet assay, but did not find any strong or consistent associations.

Several studies have assessed associations between PCB exposure and circulating reproductive hormone levels in men. A recent US study of men that were sport-caught fish consumers found significant inverse associations between serum PCB concentrations and sex hormone binding globulin (SHBG)-bound testosterone but not total or free testosterone, suggesting PCB exposure may affect steroid binding [27]. On the other hand, a Swedish study of military conscripts reported an inverse association between PCB 153 and free testosterone [21], which was also reported in European men from the study of European and Inuit men mentioned earlier [24]. A positive association between PCB 153 and LH was also found among the Inuit population in the study [24].

Although the organochlorine pesticide DDT was banned for use in most industrialized nations, it is currently used for malaria control in several countries. DDT or its metabolites (e.g. DDE) have been associated with significant or suggestive declines in semen quality in a number of studies from multiple continents [10, 19, 28]. There is also evidence that DDT and/or DDE is positively associated with sperm DNA damage, though results between studies have been inconsistent [10, 24, 26]. A number of recent studies have also assessed reproductive hormone levels in relation to DDT or its metabolites, but the majority of the studies were small in size and results have been inconsistent.

In summary, the data on the relationship between PCBs and measures of semen quality support an inverse association of PCBs with reduced sperm motility. The associations found were generally consistent across studies performed in different countries (India, Netherlands, Taiwan, Sweden, and USA) that used different methods to measure semen quality and PCBs. Furthermore, associations were consistently found despite a range of PCB levels; that is, there did not appear to be a threshold. The data for DDT or its metabolites in relation to semen quality are less consistent.

## Solvents

Organic solvents are widely used for cleaning in industrial production processes and are also found in paint systems. Traditional solvents have long been used for the degreasing of metal, glass or plastic work pieces in electroplating facilities, paint shops, and assembly plants, while new solvents have been introduced over the last few decades for specialized applications in the military, aerospace, biotechnology, and computer/semiconductor industries. Human studies of specific occupational solvent exposure and negative impacts on male reproduction are limited but have been reviewed previously [29]. Inverse associations between solvent exposure and semen quality have been reported for ethylene glycol ethers, trichloroethylene, styrene, benzene, toluene, and xylene. However, because new chemical formulations continue to be introduced in industry to fit specific process requirements, reproductive toxicology and epidemiology data are not extensive for many solvents currently in use. Several other human studies of solvent exposure and semen quality involve occupational exposure to broad classes of solvents as opposed to specific chemicals [30, 31]. Additional human studies investigating occupational exposure to specific solvents which are suspected male reproductive toxicants, such as 2-bromopropane, are greatly needed. For solvents that are commonly used in households and consumer products, studies of low-level (non-occupational) solvent exposure and male reproduction are also needed.

## Metals

Some metals, such as cadmium, lead, arsenic, and mercury, are non-essential xenobiotics that are known to be harmful to human health, while others (e.g. chromium, copper, manganese, molybdenum, selenium, and zinc) are essential for good health at low levels but may be harmful above certain doses. A number of metals are reproductive toxicants and suspected endocrine disruptors, but the biological mechanisms involved remain largely unclear. Cadmium and lead have been the most studied metals in relation to male reproduction, and both have been reported to be associated with adverse effects on male reproductive function in occupational studies [32]. Recent studies have focused on exposure outside the workplace. The general population is exposed to metals at trace concentrations either voluntarily through supplementation or involuntarily through intake of contaminated food and water or contact with contaminated soil, dust, or air. Among Croatian men with no specific occupational exposure to metals, researchers have reported that blood cadmium concentrations were associated with increased serum testosterone, FSH and estradiol, and declined testis size, after adjusting for several potential confounders [33, 34]. However, these studies, as well as a recent US study [35], did not find associations between cadmium and semen quality parameters. In agreement with the Croatian findings involving hormone levels, a recent study of 1262 men participating in the third US National Health and Nutrition Examination Survey (NHANES) reported positive associations between urinary cadmium and testosterone, estradiol, and SHBG that were confounded by smoking status [36].

Although environmental lead exposure levels have been declining in industrialized nations for the past few decades, health effects from low exposure levels remain a concern. Among men with no known occupational exposure, studies of Croatian men have reported that blood lead concentrations were positively associated with testosterone and estradiol levels, as well as increased immature sperm and percentage of pathologic, wide, and round sperm [33, 34]. Another study in Mexico found that lead measured in spermatozoa or seminal fluid, but not in blood, was associated with decreased semen quality [37]. A recent US study also reported only weak, inconsistent inverse associations between low concentrations of lead in blood and semen quality [35].

Studies of exposure to metals other than cadmium or lead in relation to male reproductive function are more limited but suggest that several of them may be male reproductive toxicants. Most studies to date have been among occupationally exposed men (e.g. welders) and results have been conflicting. Among 200 non-occupationally exposed men, manganese levels in blood were inversely associated with sperm concentration and motility [38]. Mercury, a transition metal and common environmental contaminant, was recently found to be associated with increased estradiol levels in men (as well as in women) from a small residential population in Cambodia [39]. Mercury concentrations in semen were also associated with abnormalities in sperm morphology and sperm motion in a study of men in Hong Kong [40]. Molybdenum, a metal commonly found in drinking water and in multi-mineral supplements, was inversely associated with semen quality parameters and testosterone levels in two recent reports from a US study [35, 41]. Finally, a recent study of exposure to arsenic, a metalloid with both man-made and natural environmental sources of contamination, and erectile dysfunction suggested that arsenic may impart increased risk through a reduction of circulating testosterone levels [42]. Based on these findings, more research is needed on the potential male reproductive toxicity metals following environmental exposure.

## Other emerging contaminants of concern

In addition to the environmental chemicals discussed in this chapter, there are other classes of chemicals that require further study as to their relation with human reproductive health. These chemicals include, among others, alkylphenols, such as 4-nonylphenol, bisphenol-A (BPA), brominated flame retardants, such as polybrominated diphenyl ethers (PBDEs), and fluorinated organic compounds such as perfluorooctanoic acid (PFOA) and perfluorooctanesulfonate (PFOS). Alkylphenols are used as surface active agents in cleaning/washing agents, paints, and cosmetics, while BPA is used in the manufacture of polycarbonate plastics and epoxy resins. The PBDEs have been added to textiles, polyurethane foams (e.g. in mattresses and furniture), and plastics used in electronics to prevent them from burning. The perfluorinated compounds are used to make fabrics stain-resistant/water repellent and in coatings on cookware and other products. Although human exposure to these chemicals has been demonstrated, as have adverse reproductive effects in animals in relation to exposure to these chemicals, the epidemiologic evidence on potential health effects remains very limited.

## Conclusions and future research needs

The epidemiologic data on environmental chemicals described here suggest that there may be associations with altered endocrine and reproductive function. However, the limited human data, and in certain instances inconsistent data across studies, highlight the need for further epidemiologic research on these chemicals. Most studies to date have been cross sectional in nature. Future longitudinal studies are needed to explore the temporal relationship between exposure to environmental chemicals and adverse reproductive outcomes to provide more information on whether these relationships may be causal in nature.

Researchers face a number of challenges that need to be addressed to further our understanding of the relationship between environmental chemicals and male reproductive function. One future challenge includes shifts in exposure levels among populations over time due to the ever-changing patterns of production and use of these compounds. Another challenge is to understand how simultaneous co-exposures to these chemicals may affect endocrine and reproductive function. It is well known that humans are exposed to all of these compounds simultaneously, as well as to many other chemicals. However, most studies to date have only addressed single chemicals or classes of chemicals, and there are limited data on the interactions between chemicals within a class or across classes. Chemicals may interact additively, multiplicatively, or antagonistically. For example, greater than additive interactions of phthalate metabolites MBP and MBzP with PCB 153 in relation to sperm motility have recently been reported [43]. However, the human health risks of exposure to chemical mixtures remains highly understudied.

Despite the challenges listed here, evolving and innovative technologies designed to improve the assessment of human exposure and intermediate biological markers of effect should provide enhanced opportunities for improving our understanding of the relationship between these environmental chemicals and reproductive health. Innovations include improved biomarkers of exposure, more sophisticated statistical methods that deal with multiple exposures simultaneously, sensitive new measures of intermediate alterations in human endocrine function and reproductive health, and methods for pinpointing important windows of exposure whether they are in utero, during childhood or adolescence, as an adult, or a combination of these life stages.

## References

1. Swan SH, Elkin EP, Fenster L. The question of declining sperm density revisited: an analysis of 101 studies published 1934–1996. *Environ Health Perspect* 2000; **108**: 961–6.

2. Travison TG, Araujo AB, O'Donnell AB, Kupelian V, McKinlay JB. A population-level decline in serum testosterone levels in American men. *J Clin Endocrinol Metab* 2007; **92**: 196–202.

3. Jorgensen N, Andersen AG, Eustache F. *et al.* Regional differences in semen quality in Europe. *Hum Reprod* 2001; **16**: 1012–9.

4. Duty SM, Silva MJ, Barr DB. *et al.* Phthalate exposure and human semen parameters. *Epidemiology* 2003; **14**: 269–77.

5. Hauser R, Meeker JD, Duty S, Silva MJ, Calafat AM. Altered semen quality in relation to urinary concentrations of phthalate monoester and oxidative metabolites. *Epidemiology* 2006; **17**: 682–91.

6. Jonsson BA, Richthoff J, Rylander L, Giwercman A, Hagmar L. Urinary phthalate metabolites and biomarkers of reproductive function in young men. *Epidemiology* 2005; **16**: 487–93.

7. Hauser R, Meeker JD, Singh NP. *et al.* DNA damage in human sperm is related to urinary levels of phthalate monoester and oxidative metabolites. *Hum Reprod* 2007; **22**: 688–95.

8. Pan G, Hanaoka T, Yoshimura M. *et al.* Decreased serum free testosterone in workers exposed to high levels of di-n-butyl phthalate (DBP) and di-2-ethylhexyl phthalate (DEHP): a cross-sectional study in China. *Environ Health Perspect* 2006; **114**: 1643–8.

9. Meeker JD, Calafat AM, Hauser R. Urinary metabolites of di(2-ethylhexyl) phthalate are associated with decreased steroid hormone levels in adult men. *J Androl* 2009; **30**: 287–97.

10. Perry MJ. Effects of environmental and occupational pesticide exposure on human sperm: a systematic review. *Hum Reprod Update* 2008; **14**: 233–42.

11. Swan SH, Kruse RL, Liu F. *et al.* Semen quality in relation to biomarkers of pesticide exposure. *Environ Health Perspect* 2003; **111**: 1478–84.

12. Meeker JD, Ryan L, Barr DB. *et al.* The relationship of urinary metabolites of carbaryl/naphthalene and chlorpyrifos with human semen quality. *Environ Health Perspect* 2004; **112**: 1665–70.

13. Meeker JD, Singh NP, Ryan L. *et al.* Urinary levels of insecticide metabolites and DNA damage in human sperm. *Hum Reprod* 2004; **19**: 2573–80.

14. Meeker JD, Ryan L, Barr DB, Hauser R. Exposure to nonpersistent insecticides and male reproductive hormones. *Epidemiology* 2006; **17**: 61–8.

15. Williams MK, Rundle A, Holmes D. *et al.* Changes in pest infestation levels, self-reported pesticide use, and permethrin exposure during pregnancy after the 2000–2001 U.S. Environmental Protection Agency restriction of organophosphates. *Environ Health Perspect* 2008; **116**: 1681–8.

16. Meeker JD, Barr DB, Hauser R. Human semen quality and sperm DNA damage in relation to urinary metabolites of pyrethroid insecticides. *Hum Reprod* 2008; **23**: 1932–40.

17. Xia Y, Han Y, Wu B. *et al.* The relation between urinary metabolite of pyrethroid insecticides and semen quality in humans. *Fertil Steril* 2008; **89**: 1743–50.

18. Meeker JD, Barr DB, Hauser R. Pyrethroid insecticide metabolites are associated with serum hormone levels in adult men. *Reprod Toxicol* 2009; **27**: 155–60.

19. Phillips KP, Tanphaichitr N. Human exposure to endocrine disrupters and semen quality. *J Toxicol Environ Health B Crit Rev* 2008; **11**: 188–220.

20. Hauser R. The environment and male fertility: recent research on emerging chemicals and semen quality. *Semin Reprod Med* 2006; **24**: 156–67.

21. Richthoff J, Rylander L, Jonsson BA. *et al.* Serum levels of 2,2',4,4',5,5'-hexachlorobiphenyl (CB-153) in relation to markers of reproductive function in young males from the general Swedish population. *Environ Health Perspect* 2003; **111**: 409–13.

22. Rignell-Hydbom A, Rylander L, Giwercman A. *et al.* Exposure to CB-153 and p,p'-DDE and male reproductive function. *Hum Reprod* 2004; **19**: 2066–75.

23. Rignell-Hydbom A, Rylander L, Giwercman A. *et al.* Exposure to PCBs and p,p'-DDE and human sperm chromatin integrity. *Environ Health Perspect* 2005; **113**: 175–9.

24. Bonde JP, Toft G, Rylander L. *et al.* Fertility and markers of male reproductive function in Inuit and European populations spanning large contrasts in blood levels of persistent organochlorines. *Environ Health Perspect* 2008; **116**: 269–77.

25. Hauser R, Chen Z, Pothier L, Ryan L, Altshul L. The relationship between human semen parameters and environmental exposure to polychlorinated biphenyls and p,p'-DDE. *Environ Health Perspect* 2003; **111**: 1505–11.

26. Hauser R, Singh NP, Chen Z, Pothier L, Altshul L. Lack of an association between environmental exposure to polychlorinated biphenyls and p,p'-DDE and DNA damage in human sperm measured using the neutral comet assay. *Hum Reprod* 2003; **18**: 2525–33.

27. Turyk ME, Anderson HA, Freels S. *et al.* Associations of organochlorines with endogenous hormones in male Great Lakes fish consumers and nonconsumers. *Environ Res* 2006; **102**: 299–307.

28. Aneck-Hahn NH, Schulenburg GW, Bornman MS, Farias P, de Jager C. Impaired semen quality associated with environmental DDT exposure in young men living in a malaria area in the Limpopo Province, South Africa. *J Androl* 2007; **28**: 423–34.

29. Figa-Talamanca I, Traina ME, Urbani E. Occupational exposures to metals, solvents and pesticides: recent evidence on male reproductive effects and biological markers. *Occup Med (Lond)* 2001; **51**: 174–88.

30. Tielemans E, Burdorf A, te Velde ER. *et al.* Occupationally related exposures and reduced semen quality: a case-control study. *Fertil Steril* 1999; **71**: 690–6.

31. Cherry N, Labreche F, Collins J, Tulandi T. Occupational exposure to solvents and male infertility. *Occup Environ Med* 2001; **58**: 635–40.

32. Benoff S, Jacob A, Hurley IR. Male infertility and environmental exposure to lead and cadmium. *Hum Reprod Update* 2000; **6**:107–21.

33. Jurasovic J, Cvitkovic P, Pizent A, Colak B, Telisman S. Semen quality and reproductive endocrine function with regard to blood cadmium in Croatian male subjects. *Biometals* 2004; **17**: 735–43.

34. Telisman S, Colak B, Pizent A, Jurasovic J, Cvitkovic P. Reproductive toxicity of low-level lead exposure in men. *Environ Res* 2007; **105**: 256–66.

35. Meeker JD, Rossano MG, Protas B. *et al.* Cadmium, lead and other metals in relation to semen quality: human evidence for molybdenum as a male reproductive toxicant. *Environ Health Perspect* 2008; **116**: 1473–9.

36. Menke A, Guallar E, Shiels MS. *et al*. The association of urinary cadmium with sex steroid hormone concentrations in a general population sample of US adult men. *BMC Public Health* 2008; **8**: 72.

37. Hernandez-Ochoa I, Garcia-Vargas G, Lopez-Carrillo L. *et al*. Low lead environmental exposure alters semen quality and sperm chromatin condensation in northern Mexico. *Reprod Toxicol* 2005; **20**: 221–8.

38. Wirth JJ, Rossano MG, Daly DC. *et al*. Ambient manganese exposure is negatively associated with human sperm motility and concentration. *Epidemiology* 2007; **18**: 270–3.

39. Agusa T, Kunito T, Iwata H. *et al*. Mercury in hair and blood from residents of Phnom Penh (Cambodia) and possible effect on serum hormone levels. *Chemosphere* 2007; **68**: 590–6.

40. Choy CM, Yeung QS, Briton-Jones CM. *et al*. Relationship between semen parameters and mercury concentrations in blood and in seminal fluid from subfertile males in Hong Kong. *Fertil Steril* 2002; **78**: 426–8.

41. Meeker JD, Rossano MG, Protas B. *et al*. Environmental exposure to metals and male reproductive hormones: Circulating testosterone is inversely associated with blood molybdenum. *Fertil Steril* Epulo Nov. 4, 2008.

42. Hsieh FI, Hwang TS, Hsieh YC. *et al*. Risk of erectile dysfunction induced by arsenic exposure through well water consumption in Taiwan. *Environ Health Perspect* 2008; **116**: 532–6.

43. Hauser R, Williams P, Altshul L, Calafat AM. Evidence of interaction between polychlorinated biphenyls and phthalates in relation to human sperm motility. *Environ Health Perspect* 2005; **113**: 425–30.

# Chapter

# 12

# Environmental contaminants, female reproductive health and fertility

Pauline Mendola and Germaine M. Buck Louis

## Introduction

Evidence continues to accumulate suggesting that environmental exposures adversely impact human reproductive function. Chemical exposures in the workplace, home, and ambient environment have demonstrated effects on women's reproductive health [1] and concerns have been raised about a broad spectrum of factors that influence women's health including the social, biological, and physical environment [2].

The current body of scientific evidence often relies on either a proxy of exposure such as consumption of polychlorinated biphenyl (PCB)-contaminated fish [3] or a single blood measurement [4] to assess the risk for an individual reproductive or developmental outcome such as time-to-pregnancy [4] or menstruation [5]. Epidemiologists have long articulated that research should be designed to capture the highly timed and interrelated nature of human reproduction and development [6]. Recognition of the need to consider life-course approaches in research design [7] is growing, particularly given the testicular dysgenesis [8] or ovarian dysgenesis [9] hypotheses that suggest an in utero origin for fecundity- and fertility-related disorders.

We define the environment to be inclusive of all non-genetic factors, but restrict our review to focus on chemical and pollutant exposure while recognizing the importance of other excluded factors (e.g. social, physical, and medical iatrogenic). A key premise underlying this chapter is that exposure to environmental chemicals and pollutants is ubiquitous and includes exposures of which women are not aware. The ability of epidemiologists to design studies in which these exposure(s) and sensitive outcomes can be measured is limited, especially during critical or sensitive windows [10], underscoring the importance of experimental animal studies for defining critical windows. Extrapolating to humans requires consideration of species-specific differences with respect to differentiation of structure, function, and physiology and a lack of common endpoints and milestones [11]. For many contaminants, there is no known "safe" threshold and there may be no "unexposed" individuals. Much of the available literature comprises samples of individuals with unique exposures from work (e.g. farmers) or following disasters (e.g. Seveso).

The strongest evidence that environmental contaminant exposures interfere with healthy reproductive function in women is for heavy metals, particularly lead. In addition, compounds that can influence the normal balance of hormones, including many pesticides and persistent pollutants, appear to increase risk for adverse reproductive outcomes among women. These endocrine-active compounds are a heterogeneous group of substances that include naturally occurring compounds as well as environmental contaminants. They may act directly on the reproductive system, indirectly through the immunological or nervous system, and may have transgenerational effects through epigenetic modifications [12, 13]. For the most part, the compounds of greatest concern interfere with hormone homeostasis rather than leading to biologic system failures or frank structural organ damage. Resulting changes in hormone formation, receptor status, function, and regulatory processes, interfere with the healthy foundation of women's reproductive function and can cause adverse events, particularly among susceptible women.

The findings and conclusions expressed in this chapter are those of the authors and do not necessarily represent the official position of the Centers for Disease Control and Prevention or the National Institutes of Health.

*Environmental Impacts on Reproductive Health and Fertility*, ed. T. J. Woodruff, S. J. Janssen, L. J. Guillette, and L. C. Giudice. Published by Cambridge University Press. © Cambridge University Press 2010.

Environmental health threats deserve more intense scrutiny because they are potentially modifiable. To the extent that hazards are known or suspected, women can minimize exposure by following label instructions when using chemicals or avoiding exposure to the extent that is possible. Precaution is generally prudent, especially where the evidence for risk is strongest, but it is also important to keep in mind that the research base is actually quite limited. While there is a great deal of concern that chemical exposures are increasing in the developed world and women are encountering more difficulties with fertility and reproductive function than previous generations, the causal ordering of these two phenomena has not been fully established.

In this chapter, we focus on women and how a variety of chemical and pollutant exposures throughout the life course can influence women's reproductive health and fertility. Wherever possible, our discussion is organized by life stage in recognition that achieving a functional level of biologic competence in early life (e.g. healthy ovarian function) is essential for outcomes at later stages (e.g. fertility) in keeping with an ovarian dysgenesis hypothesis. After considering the early life exposures that limit fertility, we move to the evidence for the influence of adult women's environmental exposures on ovarian and menstrual function and fertility.

Attempting to cover a dynamic life course of women's environmental exposures and a variety of reproductive health measures is bound to suffer from the limitations inherent in such a broad-scope exercise. First, many important and inter-related topics are covered elsewhere in this text including the development and maturation of the female reproductive system (Chapter 3), the impact of environmental exposures on puberty (Chapter 9) and pregnancy outcomes (Chapter 10). We also recognize that many outcomes used to assess "reproductive health" are, in fact, couple-dependent and male development and outcomes are also covered elsewhere (Chapters 4 and 11). Second, women play a unique role as mothers. Their bodies and the body burden of environmental contaminants that they bring to pregnancy serve as the biologic foundation for fetal development, and exposures during pregnancy can also influence the reproductive capacity of their children. Women also exercise a great deal of control over the environments experienced by infants and young children. Women's exposures are particularly important for transgenerational effects, since an adult woman's reproductive health as well as her response to environmental exposures are modified by her own in utero exposures or early childhood influences.

# In utero exposures and implications for reproductive health and later onset disease

Reproductive health denotes pregnancy or childbearing in the minds of many, but such a definition is unnecessarily restrictive and overly simplistic in that it fails to consider reproductive health in a non-pregnant state. We define reproductive health to include the biologic ability of women for reproduction irrespective of her pregnancy intentions or contraception practices. This paradigm includes the development and programming of fetuses through reproductive senescence, given the importance of exposures during critical and sensitive windows for reproductive health. Table 12.1 lists the spectrum of interrelated outcomes that comprise our definition of reproductive health across a woman's lifespan. The importance of reproductive health in the context of overall health status as well as for economic and social well-being have been previously discussed [14].

The longstanding premise that most females are born with the eventual capacity for delivering a healthy live-born infant is being revisited in recognition of the rapidly evolving body of evidence supporting an in utero origin of reproductive health and later-onset adult diseases. The impetus for this rethinking has been credited to the early origins of disease hypothesis first postulated for interpreting the relation between diminished birth size and adult cardiovascular disease [15], as discussed in detail in Chapter 7. This hypothesis stimulated thinking about other physiologic systems including the male reproductive system, eventually giving rise to the testicular dysgenesis syndrome (TDS) hypothesis, which posits a relation between intrauterine hormonal disturbances and a spectrum of adverse male fecundity endpoints such as genital–urinary malformations, decreased sperm counts, and testicular cancer [8]. While less well developed than TDS, an ovarian dysgenesis syndrome (ODS) has been proposed given the evidence suggesting an in utero origin for endometriosis, fibroids, and polycystic ovarian syndrome, which in turn have been associated with both gravid and later adult diseases such as pre-eclampsia, autoimmune disorders, and reproductive site cancers [9].

A model compound for the study of the reproductive effects of endocrine-active chemicals during

**Table 12.1.** Examples of the spectrum and interrelatedness of adverse reproductive health outcomes across the female lifespan.

| | Time frame for measurement of adverse reproductive outcomes | | | |
| --- | --- | --- | --- | --- |
| | In utero | Infancy and childhood | Adolescence | Adulthood |
| Reproductive endpoints | Reduction or destruction of follicles Epigenetic changes | Alterations in secondary sex ratios Malformations Primary chromosomal disorders | Pubertal disturbances | Gynecologic disorders Gynecologic malignancies |
| Examples | Reduced complement of follicles | Female excess of live births XXY | Precocious puberty Delayed onset and/or progression | Endometriosis, fibroids, premature ovarian insufficiency, polycystic ovarian syndrome |
| Implications for later-onset adult health | Primary ovarian insufficiency; impaired adult fecundity Possible transgenerational effects | Impaired adult fecundity | Primary ovarian insufficiency; impaired adult fecundity | Higher risk of gynecologic disorders (e.g., endometriosis, fibroids), gravid diseases (e.g. pre-eclampsia, gestational diabetes), reproductive cancers and autoimmune disorders |

critical windows of human development is diethyl-stilbestrol (DES). Diethylstilbestrol is a non-steroidal compound synthesized in the 1930s with a structure similar to estrogen. It is often used as the prototype compound for what is now known to include a spectrum of structural and functional changes throughout the reproductive track of men and women with an in utero exposure [16] including possible transgenerational effects [17].

Biologic plausibility for an in utero environmental origin of reproductive health is supported by a vast toxicologic literature that underscores the importance of quantifying exposures in relation to critical windows of human development, which are defined as time-sensitive periods for cellular, tissue or organ growth and development [18]. The prevalence of congenital uterine anomalies in relation to female fecundity was recently reviewed and reported to be higher for infertile women with recurrent pregnancy losses in comparison with either infertile women without recurrent losses or the general female population [19]. This suggests interrelated outcomes "diagnosed" over the lifespan that may have a similar in utero etiology. This evidence coupled with other work supports the need to move towards studies of sensitive windows to identify both structural and non-structural (e.g. functional or behavioral) effects associated with early exposures [7]. The increasing popularity of life-course epidemiologic inquiry, defined as the long-term study of biological,

behavioral, and psychosocial processes over sensitive windows of human development (in utero through adolescence) and adult health, may be responsive to this data gap [20].

In utero exposure to endocrine-active compounds has the potential to adversely affect women's eventual reproductive health either directly by affecting steroid hormone production (ovary) or interfering with control and/or action of ovarian hormones (HPG axis), or indirectly via immunologic or neurologic pathways. The rapidly dividing primordial germ cells and oogonia characterizing the fetal period may be extremely vulnerable to exposure to endocrine-active compounds. Exposure may affect the synthesis, secretion, transport, metabolism, binding, and/or elimination of the body's hormones. This is likely to be true for naturally occurring (e.g. phytoestrogens) or man-made chemicals that act like hormones or interfere with hormone function (e.g. persistent organic pollutants and heavy metals). Effects may manifest as an abnormal follicular development and an ensuing deficiency of a competent number of follicles clinically presenting as primary ovarian insufficiency. Folliculogenesis, the progression of an ovarian follicle from its primordial to pre-ovulatory state, is necessary for eventual fecundity or biologic capacity for reproduction. The timing of exposures during follicular growth may impact the type of effect seen, ranging from the complete destruction of primordial and primary follicles resulting in sexual

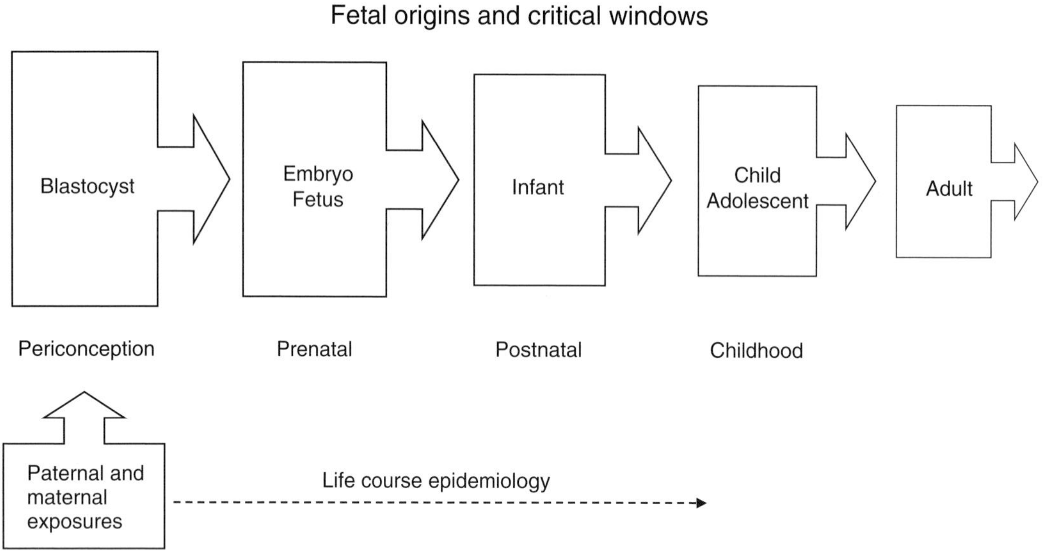

Fetal origins and critical windows

**Fig. 12.1.** Illustration of sensitive windows of female environmental exposures.

infantilism and/or sterility, to a reduction in number or quality clinically manifesting as impaired fecundity (e.g. primary ovarian insufficiency, premature ovarian failure, anovulation, or conception delays). Oocyte exposures may occur while in their arrested prophase of the first meiotic division or subsequently following the resumption of meiosis in response to the preovulatory gonadotropin surge. Oocyte maturation occurs in the follicle making them vulnerable to exposures that adversely affect steroid production. A number of environmental chemicals have been isolated from follicular fluid suggestive of exposure [21], but data on their effect on oocyte quality or ovulatory disorders possibly by increasing the rate of atresia is lacking.

## Evidence for an ovarian dysgenesis syndrome

For the purposes of this chapter, we define ODS as a constellation of adverse health outcomes including genital–urinary malformations, gynecologic disorders (e.g. endometriosis, fibroids, polycystic ovarian syndrome, premature ovarian insufficiency (POI)), gravid diseases (pre-eclampsia, gestational diabetes), fecundity and fertility impairments (conception delays, infecundity, altered secondary ratios), and other adult-onset diseases (e.g. autoimmune and reproductive site cancers) possibly attributed to periconceptional or in utero environmental exposures including those that are transgenerational in origin. Evidence for an ODS is still

somewhat dispersed in the literature by various reproductive endpoints ranging from pubertal onset and progression to gynecologic disorders such as endometriosis, polycystic ovaries to (premature) reproductive senescence. As such, the weight of evidence is currently insufficient for suggesting a shared etiology for the spectrum of endpoints. We provide examples of research supporting ODS by various endpoints below.

Figure 12.1 illustrates a paradigm for considering early exposures across sensitive windows of human development from periconception through adolescence. By design, the figure emphasizes the interrelatedness of sensitive windows and the potential for parentally mediated effects to be manifested across the lifespan.

Perhaps, the two reproductive endpoints most consistent with an intrauterine origin based upon available evidence to date are abnormal pubertal timing and polycystic ovarian syndrome (PCOS). A brief review of the evidence supporting a role for environmental factors and reproductive health follows.

### Puberty

Puberty represents that period of life during which children transition to adolescence, and is accompanied by the onset of secondary sexual characteristics along with overall physical and physiologic growth and development in the pathway to becoming fecund adults biologically capable of reproduction. Blank and colleagues [22] were among the first to report a possible adverse relation between in utero exposure to brominated flame retardants and puberty. Since that time, numerous other studies have found similar findings for various persistent halogenated organic chemicals such as PCBs, dichlorodiphenyltrichloroethane (DDT), dichlorophenyldichloroethylene (DDE) and, to a lesser extent, dioxin, hexachlorobenzene, endosulfan, and heavy metals as recently summarized [23]. Alterations in the onset and/or progression of puberty need to be considered when evaluating in utero exposures and, possibly, in the context of later gynecologic disorders to fully understand the implications of such early exposures.

## Polycystic ovary syndrome

Polycystic ovary syndrome is a common heterogeneous disorder whose prevalence varies by choice of diagnostic criteria. A leading definition established in 1990 required chronic anovulation and hyperandrogenism (including acne, hirsutism, and male pattern baldness) in the absence of known pathology such as congenital adrenal hyperplasia, hypercortisolism, thyroid dysfunction, and hyperprolactinemia [24]. A more recent definition requires only two of the following three criteria: (1) clinical or biochemical evidence of hyperandrogenism; (2) intermittent or absent menstrual cycles; and (3) polycystic ovary morphology as visualized by ultrasound [25]. The relation between PCOS and adult-onset diseases is now recognized. For example, girls and women with PCOS are at increased risk of developing impaired glucose tolerance and type II diabetes mellitus in comparison with unaffected women [26]. These disorders impair metabolic activity and, thereby, suppress insulin-mediated glucose uptake and lipolysis with ensuing hyperinsulinemia. Various pathways have been postulated including a primary ovarian abnormality [27], in utero environmental exposures leading to fetal reprogramming [28] or dysregulation of fat metabolism. Much of the evidence for in utero fetal reprogramming of gonadotropin secretory dynamics comes from female primates with intrauterine androgen exposure at sensitive windows of development being associated with PCOS [28].

Other evidence supporting an in utero origin for PCOS includes higher risk associated with increased birthweight and gestation [29]. The authors speculated that two forms of PCOS may arise in utero suggesting the importance of hormonal milieu on female reproductive and adult health. While a few authors have reported associations between PCOS and environmental chemicals such as bisphenol-A (BPA) [30],

we are unaware of any research where exposure was obtained during sensitive windows of development. Interestingly, the relation between PCOS and gravid health conditions is now emerging as affected women are reported to be at greater risk than unaffected women of developing pre-eclampsia, hypertension, and gestational diabetes [31].

## Endometriosis

Endometriosis is characterized by the growth of endometrial glands and stroma outside the uterine cavity. These endometriotic implants can be found anywhere in the pelvic, abdominal, or thoracic cavity and eventually produce vesicles or hemorrhages that visually appear as blue, brown, or black lesions. Approximately 10–15% of reproductive-age women are estimated to have endometriosis [32] but prevalence estimates vary greatly depending on the study sample; for example, prevalence increases to 20–40% among infertile women, and the estimates range from 4–65% among women with chronic pelvic pain and 1–22% among women undergoing gynecologic surgical procedures [33]. The absence of physical signs or definitive biomarkers necessitates the reliance on visualization with or without histologic confirmation for diagnosis. Retrograde menstruation remains the most commonly cited etiologic theory [34], yet implies that women acquire endometriosis through menstruation rather than from a point source such as in utero exposures.

The impact of environmental factors in the development of endometriosis is now recognized, particularly the role of polyhalogenated aromatic hydrocarbon chemicals: polychlorinated dibenzo-dioxins, dibenzofurans, PCBs, and naphthalenes. As endocrine-active compounds, these chemicals are postulated to affect development of endometriosis via a number of pathways: (1) alterations in the synthesis and metabolism of estradiol; (2) alterations in the production of proinflammatory growth factors or cytokines; and (3) misexpression of remodeling enzymes [35].

Recognition of a purported relation between dioxin and endometriosis first emerged in 1993 when Rier and colleagues reported a significant dose-dependent increase in the incidence and severity of endometriosis in exposed rhesus monkeys [36]. Subsequently, Yang *et al.* investigated the effects of dioxin on survival and growth of ectopic endometrium in monkeys following auto transplantation [37]. Human evidence is mixed, but five studies have reported significantly increased

165

risk of endometriosis in relation to exposure to PCBs and dioxin-like compounds [38–42].

An environmental in utero origin for endometriosis is now being considered given evidence suggesting women with in utero DES exposure are at greater risk than unexposed women [43]. Conversely, women exposed in utero to cigarette smoke are reported to be at reduced risk of developing endometriosis [44]. Women with endometriosis are reported to have lower body mass indices up to diagnosis in comparison with women without disease, suggestive of early programming [45]. In contrast to women with PCOS, women with endometriosis-associated infertility have recently been reported to have a lower incidence of pre-eclampsia and pregnancy-induced hypertension than women with male-factor infertility undergoing in vitro fertilization [46]. Affected women also are reported to be at increased risk of later-onset autoimmune diseases [47] and malignancies [48] in comparison with women without endometriosis.

### Leiomyoma

There is a very limited body of research focusing on a possible environmental origin for uterine leiomyomas (fibroids) despite their widespread prevalence among women of reproductive age, i.e. 70–80% lifetime cumulative incidence [49]. While its etiology is speculative, these tumors of smooth muscle origin are believed to be associated with ovarian hormones, prompting some authors to speculate about a role for exogenous estrogens [50]. A few such reports have been published including a positive association between in utero DES exposure [51], adult dioxin exposure [52], and risk of uterine leiomyoma.

### Menopause

While the research in this area is extremely limited, women with in utero DES exposure attained natural menopause earlier than unexposed women [53]. Additionally, low weight gain during infancy has been associated with early menopause, possibly suggesting a low rate of in utero linear growth [54]. An in utero origin for POI regardless of women's age has not been explored to our knowledge.

## Implications for fecundity and fertility beyond the ovarian dysgenesis syndrome

### Puberty

As Fig. 12.1 illustrates, the postnatal environment remains a possible sensitive window for children and adolescents whether as the result of earlier in utero programming coupled with subsequent exposures to which young girls may be exposed or from de novo exposures arising after birth through the attainment of puberty. Puberty has implications for female fecundity as its onset represents the lower bound of the reproductive age with menopause representing the upper bound. Precocious or delayed puberty, thereby, have implications for women's fecundity and the occurrence of gynecologic disorders tied to this window.

### Fecundity and fertility

There has been limited study of the effect of intrauterine exposures on female fecundity and fertility, and most that has been conducted relies upon the women's (rather than that of the mothers') self-reports. Some data have been discussed above in the ODS section, but other suggestive data include in utero exposure to cigarette smoke, which has been associated with diminished female fecundity as measured by a longer time-to-pregnancy [55]. In utero exposures to endocrine-active compounds are postulated to affect fertility by altering secondary sex ratios resulting in a higher than expected number of female to male live births [56]. Other than ovulation induction agents, few environmental exposures have been assessed in relation to other fertility endpoints such as multiple births.

## Adult exposures and adverse reproductive health effects

### Menstrual and ovarian function

Regular menstrual cycling is dependent on a pattern of hormone changes to support the development of a dominant ovarian follicle, thickening of the endometrium in preparation for implantation, rupture of the follicle and release of the ovum into the fallopian tube, and the sloughing of the uterine lining (menses) in the absence of a viable implantation. The "normal" menstrual cycle varies within and between women, and disturbances or menstrual disorders are typically measured by cycle length, duration of bleeding, and/or pain.

Amenorrhea is the cessation of menses and can be "primary" or the complete absence of menarche by 16 years of age, or "secondary" when menstruation ceases for an interval comparable to three times the typical length of a cycle. Oligomenorrhea is the absence of menstruation for shorter intervals ranging from 35 to 90 days, whereas, polymenorrhea is frequent menstruation or cycles less than 21 days. Anovulation is the absence of ovulation. Luteal phase defects occur when the corpus luteum fails to develop adequately or when progesterone production is compromised in the second half of the cycle. Lastly, dysmenorrhea refers to painful menstruation and is typically reliant on self-report or sometimes pain scales.

When adult women's exposure to environmental contaminants leads to disruption of menstrual or ovarian function, generally the variations observed (long or short cycles, changes in luteal or follicular phase) indicate an underlying perturbation of hormones rather than the development of clinical menstrual or ovarian disorders [1]. Many of the implicated compounds are known to be endocrine-active compounds.

Variations in cycle length are a common cross-sectional endpoint but the data on environmental exposure impact is equivocal with respect to the nature and strength of the associations. Shorter cycles have been observed among lead-battery plant workers [57] as well as among women exposed to chlordibromomethane in drinking water [58] and DDT [59]. In contrast, longer cycles have also been observed in association with dioxin [60], hormonally active pesticides [61], serum PCBs [62], and working in the semiconductor industry [63]. Many of these studies also observed associations with other menstrual disorders such as missed periods and abnormal bleeding [57, 61, 62]. No relation between menstrual abnormalities, cycle length, or other characteristics has been reported in studies of PCBs, metal exposure, DDE, and DDT [64, 65].

In studies with biomarker data, follicle-stimulating hormone was decreased in women exposed to pentachlorophenol [66]. Progesterone and estrogens have been reduced in women exposed to DDT and DDE, but no differences were observed in hormone profiles related to PCB level [67, 68].

Reproductive senescence or menopause is the final life stage related to menstrual and ovarian function, and is characterized by changes in hormonal milieu along with cessation of ovulation and menstruation. While evidence suggests a relation between endocrine-active compounds and ovarian function, the effect on menopause is suggestive though equivocal. Exposure to compounds such as DDT/DDE and dioxin has been associated with earlier and later ages at menopause [69, 70], while negative relations have been reported for PCB or PBB exposure [71]. A cancer case–control study that examined plasma levels of persistent pollutants suggested that DDE has a weak association with earlier age at menopause, but PCBs had no effect [72].

In contrast, DDT exposure in the Agricultural Health Study was associated with slightly older age at menopause [73]. Being a current smoker also appears to lower the age at menopause, while past or passive smoking does not [74]. These equivocal data may reflect the reliance on cross-sectional data and the inability of many researchers to collect exposure during critical and sensitive windows of development to establish a temporal ordering of exposure and outcomes.

## Gynecologic disorders

### Endometriosis

In addition to developmental effects discussed earlier in this chapter, there appears to be a role for persistent endocrine-active pollutants in the risk for endometriosis among adults. Some authors reported no difference in serum dioxin levels between women with and without endometriosis [53–56, 75, 76], though important methodologic limitations impact interpretation including restrictions to specific disease or exposed populations [55, 56]. On the other hand, there is some consistency in the evidence for increased risk of endometriosis associated with increased serum PCB and urinary phthalate ester concentrations in comparison to unaffected women [41, 42, 77–82].

## Fecundity and fertility

The bulk of the literature on environmental threats to adult female reproductive health is focused on the area of fecundity and fertility. For our purposes, fecundity and fertility studies include time-to-pregnancy (inclusive of conception delays and infecundity) and spontaneous abortion. Some of the strongest evidence implicating an environmental etiology is for pesticide application, primarily in agricultural and horticultural settings. Pesticide exposures have consistently been associated with reduced fecundity and fertility [83–88], although this effect was not observed in an adjusted analysis of greenhouse workers in Italy [89]. Increased time-to-pregnancy was the most common outcome observed in association with exposure [83, 85, 88, 89] as well as infertility [87] spontaneous abortion [84] and other pregnancy loss [86]. Preconception exposure appears to be most critical in elevating risk for spontaneous abortion [90] rather than exposure during pregnancy [91]. Lead, a key reproductive toxicant, has been associated with spontaneous abortion [57] and infertility [92].

**167**

Exposure to most persistent organochlorines reduces fecundity and fertility in several studies, though findings are equivocal in others, particularly for PCB exposure. Polychlorinated biphenyl-contaminated fish consumption from the Baltic Sea had no impact on fertility except in a subgroup analysis of heavy smokers [93, 94]; studies of serum PCB measures in the same populations also observed no effect [95]. In contrast, a longer time-to-pregnancy was associated with maternal consumption of Great Lakes sport fish [96], although in another angler cohort, maternal exposure disappeared after adjusting for male partner fish consumption [97]. No differences were observed for several outcomes (taking longer than one year to get pregnant, diagnosed fertility problems, and spontaneous abortion) in association with exposure to PCB-contaminated cooking oil [64]. However, maternal serum PCB and DDE concentrations were suggestive of a longer time-to-pregnancy in the Collaborative Perinatal Project [4] as was risk for a prior spontaneous abortion in relation to maternal serum DDT and DDE levels [98]. Spontaneous abortion risk was not associated with dioxin exposure in Seveso [99], but was found to be associated with living in petroleum hydrocarbon-contaminated areas in Ecuador [100].

The literature continues to be inconsistent with respect to studies based on biological measures of exposure and markers of early pregnancy. Early pregnancy losses identified using biomarkers to determine implantation were associated with serum DDT and metabolites but no association was observed for clinical losses [101]. Studies of solvent exposure in a variety of settings [102–104] suggest a relation between exposure and subfertility, including increased time-to-pregnancy. Other environmental exposures, including BPA, air quality, radiation, and other compounds have been associated with decrements in female fertility, but the literature is generally limited or inconclusive.

## Discussion

There is growing evidence from various scientific disciplines supporting a role for environmental influences including those occurring in utero in relation to female reproductive health. What is especially exciting is the recognition that such effects may manifest across a woman's lifespan, challenging researchers to embrace novel methodologies such as life-course epidemiologic methods for understanding these interrelated processes.

The weight of evidence to date, while suggestive, needs to be considered in relation to important methodologic limitations, many of which are expected when moving into a novel area of study and before the availability of concerted funding to support the conduct of population-based definitive research. These include reliance on convenience samples, incomplete exposure characterization irrespective of critical or sensitive windows, reliance on self-reported health outcomes, and limited data collection regarding other relevant time-varying covariates. Statistical models often do not address the mixtures of environmental chemicals to which women are exposed or the causal assumptions inherent when entering toxicologic concentrations that have been automatically adjusted for lipids or values below the limits of detection raising concern about potential biases [105, 106]. The importance of defining etiologic models that incorporate women's past reproductive history given the widely recognized clustering of reproductive endpoints will facilitate investigators' ability to assess weaker signals (e.g. chemical exposure) in the context of strong biological determinants (e.g. prior history of an adverse outcome) that may reflect genetic predisposition.

## Clinical and public health implications

Establishing causal links between reproductive endpoints across the lifespan is essential for understanding the implications of reproductive disorders with respect to women's health status. Gynecologic disorders may have important implications for other clinical disciplines such as internal medicine and the host of specialties. For example, in utero exposures may influence the timing of puberty and girls who enter puberty earlier may be at increased risk of developing PCOS, pre-eclampsia and gestational diabetes and, eventually, cardiovascular disease and type II diabetes. To some extent, the origin of all disease manifestation is determined or modified by intrauterine life.

If the early origins of disease hypothesis becomes mainstream, public health officials will be faced with the design and delivery of a new way of thinking about health. Individuals will need to be informed about current risks as well as advised how to minimize adverse effects and potentially improve the implications for their health in later life. More complex models and understanding of the problems faced across the lifespan will require moving beyond the current compartmentalization of health research and health care by clinical disciplines to embrace a more integrated global focus on the origins of exposure–outcome relationships and potential interventions to improve population health.

## Future research directions

Most public opinion polls reflect the public's concern about the role of the environment and health. In fact, public perception and behavior affects the market place as evidenced by the recent removal of infant bottles and cups containing BPA after consumer pressure and concern about exposure. Despite high levels of concern over many environmental pollutants and chemical exposures, there is still considerable uncertainty about the relation between most routinely encountered environmental contaminants and risk, underscoring the importance of researchers to devise effective strategies for communicating risk and uncertainty.

Our knowledge base is incomplete, particularly with regard to a life-course approach including the in utero period. This will require researchers to formally synthesize the available evidence and generate national research agendas such as that recently articulated for puberty and fecundity and fertility in the special supplements of *Pediatrics* (2008, **12**) and *Fertility and Sterility* (2008, **89**). Deciding which chemical or other environmental exposures to study is difficult and concerted thinking on the strategy for selection is needed, but might benefit from other paradigms including that used by the Center for the Evaluation of Risks to Human Reproduction, National Toxicology Program. We encourage these and other efforts to support the fledgling attempts at developing interdisciplinary approaches to investigating the dynamic interplay of exposures and outcomes across the lifespan.

## References

1. Mendola P, Messer LC, Rappazzo K. Review IV: Science linking environmental contaminant exposures with fertility and reproductive health impacts in the adult female. *Fertil Steril* 2008; **89**: e81–94.

2. Silbergeld EK. The environment and women's health: an overview. In Goldman MB, Hatch MC, eds. *Women & Health.* San Diego: Academic Press, 2000; 601–6.

3. Buck GM, Vena JE, Schisterman EF. *et al.* Parental consumption of contaminated sport fish from Lake Ontario and predicted fecundability. *Epidemiology* 2000; **11**: 388–93.

4. Gesnick Law DC, Klebanoff MA, Brock JW. *et al.* Maternal serum levels of polychlorinated biphenyls and 1,1-dichloro-2,2-bis(p-chlorophenyl)ethylene (DDE) and time to pregnancy. *Am J Epidemiol* 2005; **162**: 523–32.

5. Mendola P, Buck, GM, Sever LE. *et al.* Consumption of PCB-contaminated fresh water fish and shortened menstrual cycle. *Am J Epidemiol* 1997; **146**: 955–60.

6. Buck GM, Lynch CD, Stanford JB. *et al.* Prospective pregnancy study designs for assessing reproductive and developmental toxicants. *Environ Health Perspect* 2004; **112**: 79–86.

7. Ben-Schlomo Y, Kuh D. A life course approach to chronic disease epidemiology: conceptual models, empirical challenges and interdisciplinary perspectives. *Int J Epidemiol* 2002; **31**: 285–93.

8. Skakkebaek NE, Rajpert-De ME, Main KM. Testicular dysgenesis syndrome: an increasingly common developmental disorder with environmental aspects: Opinion. *Hum Reprod* 2001; **16**: 972–8.

9. Buck Louis GM, Cooney MA. Effects of environmental contaminants on ovarian function and fertility. In Gonzalez-Bulnes A, ed. *Novel Concepts in Ovarian Endocrinology.* Research Signpost. 2007; 249–68.

10. Selevan SG, Kimmel CA, Mendola P. Identifying critical windows of exposure for children's health. *Environ Health Perspect* 2000; **108** (Suppl 3): 451–5.

11. Morford LL, Henck JW, Breslin WJ. *et al.* Hazard identification and predictability of children's health risk from animal data. *Environ Health Perspect* 2004; **112**: 266–71.

12. Anway MD, Cupp AS. Uzumcu M. *et al.* Epigenetic transgenerational actions of endocrine disruptors and male fertility. *Science* 2005; **308**: 1466–9.

13. Crews D, McLachlan JA. Epigenetics, evolution, endocrine disruption, health and disease. *Endocrinology* 2006; **147**: S4–10.

14. Diczfalusy E. Reproductive health: a rendezvous with human dignity. *Contraception* 1995; **52**: 1–12.

15. Barker, DJ. Fetal origins of coronary heart disease. *Br Med J* 1995; **311**: 171–4.

16. Herbst AL, Bern HA. *Developmental Effects of Diethylstilbestrol (DES) in Pregnancy.* New York: Thieme-Stratton, 1981.

17. Titus-Ernstoff L, Troisi R, Hatch EE. *et al.* Offspring of women exposed in utero to diethylstilbestrol (DES): a preliminary report of benign and malignant pathology in the third generation. *Epidemiology* 2008; **19**: 251–7.

18. Wilson JG. Embryological considerations in teratology. In Wilson JG, Warkany J. eds. *Teratology: Principles and Techniques.* Chicago: The University of Chicago Press, 1965.

19. Saravelos SH, Cocksedge KA, Li TC. Prevalance and diagnosis of congenital uterine anomalies in women with reproductive failure: A critical appraisal. *Hum Reprod Update* 2008; **14**: 415–29.

20. Kuh D, Ben-Shlomo Y. *A Life Course Approach to Chronic Disease Epidemiology*, 2nd Edition. New York: Oxford University Press, 2005.

21. Pauwels A, Covaci A, Delbeke L. *et al.* The relation between levels of selected PCB congeners in human

serum and follicular fluid. *Chemosphere* 1999; **39**: 2433–41.

22. Blanck HM, Marcus M, Tolbert PE. *et al.* Age at menarche and Tanner stage in girls exposed in utero and postnatally to polybrominated biphenyl. *Epidemiology* 2000; **11**: 641–7.

23. Buck Louis GM, Gray LE Jr., Marcus M, *et al.* Environmental factors and puberty timing: expert panel research needs. *Pediatrics* 2008; **121**: S172–91.

24. Zawadski J, Dunaif A. Diagnostic criteria for polycystic ovary syndrome: towards a rational approach. In Dunaif A, Givens JR, Haseltine F, eds. *Polycystic Ovary Syndrome*. Oxford: Blackwell Science, 1992: 377–84.

25. The Rotterdam Eshre/Asrm-Sponsored Pcos consensus workshop group. Revised 2003 consensus on diagnostic criteria and long-term health risks related to polycystic ovary syndrome (PCOS). *Hum Reprod* 2004; **19**: 41–7.

26. Lewy VD, Danadian K, Witchel SF. *et al.* Early metabolic abnormalities in adolescent girls with polycystic ovarian syndrome. *J Pediatr* 2001; **138**: 38–44.

27. Wickenheisser JK, Nelson-DeGrave VL, McAllister JM. Human ovarian theca cells in culture. *Trends Endocrinol Metab* 2006; **17**: 65–71.

28. Abbott DH, Barnett DK, Bruns CM. *et al.* Androgen excess fetal programming of female reproduction: a developmental aetiology for polycystic ovary syndrome? *Hum Reprod Update* 2005; **11**: 357–74.

29. Cresswell JL, Barker DJP, Osmond C. *et al.* Fetal growth, length of gestation, and polycystic ovaries in adult life. *Lancet* 1997; **350**: 1131–5.

30. Takeuchi T, Tsutsumi O, Ikezuki Y. *et al.* Positive relationship between androgen and the endocrine disruptor, bisphenol A, in normal women and women with ovarian dysfunction. *Endocr J* 2004; **51**: 165–9.

31. Boomsma CM, Eijkemans MJ, Huges EG. *et al.* A meta analysis of pregnancy outcomes in women with polycystic ovarian syndrome. *Hum Reprod Update* 2006; **12**: 673–83.

32. Houston DE. Evidence for the risk of pelvic endometriosis by age, race and socioeconomic status. *Epidemiol Rev* 1984; **6**: 167–91.

33. Mahmood TA, Templeton A. Prevalence and genesis of endometriosis. *Hum Reprod* 1991; **6**: 544–9.

34. Sampson JA. Peritoneal endometriosis due to menstrual dissemination of endometrial tissue into the pelvic cavity. *Am J Obstet Gynecol* 1927; **14**: 422–69.

35. Rier SE, Foster WG. Environmental dioxins and endometriosis. *Toxicol Sci* 2002; **70**: 161–70.

36. Rier SE, Martin DC, Bowman RE. *et al.* Endometriosis in rhesus monkeys (*Macaca mulatta*) following chronic exposure to 2,3,7,8-tertrachlorodibenzo-*p*-dioxin. *Fundam Appl Toxicol* 1993; **21**: 433–41.

37. Yang JZ, Agarwal SK, Foster WG. Subchronic exposure to 2,3,7,8-tetrachlorodibenzo-*p*-dioxin

38. Gerhard I, Runnebaum B. The limits of hormone substitution in pollutant exposure and fertility disorders. *Zentralbl Gynakol* 1992; **114**: 593–602.

39. Mayani A, Barel S, Soback S. *et al.* Dioxin concentrations in women with endometriosis. *Hum Reprod* 1997; **12**: 373–5.

40. Heilier J, Ha AT, Lison D. *et al.* Increased serum polychlorinated biphenyl levels in Belgian women with adenomyotic nodules of the rectovaginal septum. *Fertil Steril* 2004; **81**: 456–8.

41. Buck Louis GM, Weiner JM, Whitcomb BW. *et al.* Environmental PCB exposure and risk of endometriosis. *Hum Reprod* 2005; **20**: 279–85.

42. Porpora MG, Ingelido AM, di Domenico A. *et al.* Increased levels of polychlorinated biphenyls in Italian women with endometriosis. *Chemosphere* 2006; **63**: 1361–7.

43. Missmer SA, Hankinson SE, Spiegelman D. *et al.* Reproductive history and endometriosis among premenopausal women. *Fertil Steril* 2004; **82**: 1501–8.

44. Buck Louis GM, Hediger ML, Pena JB. Intrauterine exposures and risk of endometriosis. *Hum Reprod* 2007; **22**: 3232–6.

45. Hediger ML, Hartnett HJ, Louis GM. Association of endometriosis with body size and figure. *Fertil Steril* 2005; **84**: 1366–74.

46. Brosens IA, De Sutter P, Hamerlynck T. *et al.* Endometriosis is associated with a decreased risk of pre-eclampsia. *Hum Reprod* 2007; **22**: 1725–9.

47. Sinaii N, Cleary SD, Ballweg ML. *et al.* High rates of autoimmune and endocrine disorders, fibromyalgia, chronic fatigue syndrome and atopic disease among women with endometriosis: a survey analysis. *Hum Reprod* 2002; **17**: 2715–24.

48. Brinton LA, Gridley G, Persson I. *et al.* Cancer risk after a hospital diagnosis of endometriosis. *Am J Obstet Gynecol* 1997; **176**: 572–9.

49. Baird DD, Dunson DB, Hill MC. *et al.* High cumulative incidence of uterine leiomyoma in black and white women: ultrasound evidence. *Am J Obstet Gynecol* 2003; **288**: 100–7.

50. Hunter DS, Hodges LC, Eagon PK. *et al.* Influence of exogenous estrogen receptor ligands on uterine leiomyoma: evidence from an in vitro/in vivo animal model for uterine fibroids. *Environ Health Perspect* 2000; **108** (Suppl. 5): 829–34.

51. Baird DD, Newbold R. Prenatal diethylstilbesterol (DES) exposure is associated with uterine leiomyoma development. *Reprod Toxicol* 2005; **20**: 81–4.

52. Eskenazi B, Warner M, Samuels S. *et al.* Serum dioxin concentrations and risk of uterine leiomyoma in the

Seveso Women's Health Study. *Am J Epidemiol* 2007; **166**: 79–87.

53. Hatch EE, Troisi R, Wise LA. *et al.* Age at natural menopause in women exposed to diethylstilbestrol in utero. *Am J Epidemiol* 2006; **164**: 682–8.

54. Cresswell JL, Egger P, Fall CHD. *et al.* Is the age of menopause determined in-utero? *Early Hum Develop* 1997; **49**: 143–8.

55. Jensen TK, Joffe M, Scheike T. *et al.* Early exposure to smoking and future fecundity among Danish twins. *Int J Androl* 2006; **29**: 603–13.

56. Taylor KC, Jackson LW, Lynch CD. *et al.* Preconception maternal polychlorinated biphenyl concentrations and the secondary sex ratio. *Environ Res* 2007; **103**: 99–105.

57. Tang N, Zhu ZQ. Adverse reproductive effects in female workers of lead battery plants. *Int J Occup Med Environ Health* 2003; **16**: 359–61.

58. Windham GC, Waller K, Anderson M. *et al.* Chlorination by-products in drinking water and menstrual cycle function. *Environ Health Perspect* 2003; **111**: 935–41; discussion A409.

59. Ouyang F, Perry MJ, Venners SA. *et al.* Serum DDT, age at menarche, and abnormal menstrual cycle length. *Occup Environ Med* 2005; **62**: 878–84.

60. Eskenazi B, Warner M, Mocarelli P. *et al.* Serum dioxin concentrations and menstrual cycle characteristics. *Am J Epidemiol* 2002; **156**: 383–92.

61. Farr SL, Cooper GS, Cai J. *et al.* Pesticide use and menstrual cycle characteristics among premenopausal women in the Agricultural Health Study. *Am J Epidemiol* 2004; **160**: 1194–204.

62. Cooper GS, Klebanoff MA, Promislow J. *et al.* Polychlorinated biphenyls and menstrual cycle characteristics. *Epidemiology* 2005; **16**: 191–200.

63. Hsieh GY, Wang JD, Cheng TJ, *et al.* Prolonged menstrual cycles in female workers exposed to ethylene glycol ethers in the semiconductor manufacturing industry. *Occup Environ Med* 2005; **62**: 510–16.

64. Yu ML, Guo YL, Hsu CC. *et al.* Menstruation and reproduction in women with polychlorinated biphenyl (PCB) poisoning: long-term follow-up interviews of the women from the Taiwan Yucheng cohort. *Int J Epidemiol* 2000; **29**: 672–7.

65. Chen A, Zhang J, Zhou L. *et al.* DDT serum concentration and menstruation among young Chinese women. *Environ Res* 2005; **99**: 397–402.

66. Gerhard I, Frick A, Monga B. *et al.* Pentachlorophenol exposure in women with gynecological and endocrine dysfunction. *Environ Res* 1999; **80**: 383–8.

67. Perry MJ, Ouyang F, Korrick SA. *et al.* A prospective study of serum DDT and progesterone and estrogen levels across the menstrual cycle in nulliparous women of reproductive age. *Am J Epidemiol* 2006; **164**: 1056–64.

68. Windham GC, Lee D, Mitchell P. *et al.* Exposure to organochlorine compounds and effects on ovarian function. *Epidemiology* 2005; **16**: 182–90.

69. Eskenazi B, Warner M, Marks AR. *et al.* Serum dioxin concentrations and age at menopause. *Environ Health Perspect* 2005; **113**: 858–62.

70. Akkina J, Reif J, Keefe T. *et al.* Age at natural menopause and exposure to organochlorine pesticides in Hispanic women. *J Toxicol Environ Health* 2004; **67**: 1407–22.

71. Blanck HM, Marcus M, Tolbert PE. *et al.* Time to menopause in relation to PBBs, PCBs, and smoking. *Maturitas* 2004; **49** 97–106.

72. Cooper GS, Savitz DA, Millikan R. *et al.* Organochlorine exposure and age at natural menopause. *Epidemiology* 2002; **13**: 729–33.

73. Farr SL, Cai J, Savitz DA, *et al.* Pesticide exposure and timing of menopause: the Agricultural Health Study. *Am J Epidemiol* 2006; **163**: 731–42.

74. Cooper GS, Sandler DP, Bohlig M. Active and passive smoking and the occurrence of natural menopause. *Epidemiology* 1999; **10**: 771–3.

75. Yoshida K, Ikeda S, Nakanishi J. Assessment of human health risk of dioxins in Japan. *Chemosphere* 2000; **40**: 177–85.

76. Lim Y, Yang J, Kim Y. *et al.* Assessment of human health risk of dioxin in Korea. *Environ Monitor Assess* 2004; **92**: 211–28.

77. Quaranta MG, Porpora MG, Mattioli B. *et al.* Impaired NK-cell-mediated cytotoxic activity and cytokine production in patients with endometriosis: a possible role for PCBs and DDE. *Life Sci* 2006; **79**: 491–8.

78. Rier SE. The potential role of exposure to environmental toxicants in the pathophysiology of endometriosis. *Ann NY Acad Sci* 2002; **955**: 201–12; discussion 30–2, 396–406.

79. Gerhard I, Monga B, Krahe J. *et al.* Chlorinated hydrocarbons in infertile women. *Environ Res* 1999; **80**: 299–310.

80. Reddy BS, Rozati R, Reddy S. *et al.* High plasma concentrations of polychlorinated biphenyls and phthalate esters in women with endometriosis: a prospective case control study. *Fertil Steril* 2006; **85**: 775–9.

81. Cobellis L, Latini G, De Felice C. *et al.* High plasma concentrations of di-(2-ethylhexyl)-phthalate in women with endometriosis. *Hum Reprod* 2003; **18**: 1512–15.

82. Reddy BS, Rozati R, Reddy BV. *et al.* Association of phthalate esters with endometriosis in Indian women. *Br J Obst Gynaecol.* 2006; **113**: 515–20.

83. Abell A, Juul S, Bonde JP. Time to pregnancy among female greenhouse workers. *Scand J Work Environ Health* 2000; **26**: 131–6.

84. Crisostomo L, Molina VV. Pregnancy outcomes among farming households of Nueva Ecija with conventional pesticide use versus integrated pest

management. *Int J Occup Environ Health* 2002;
**8**: 232–42.

85. Curtis KM, Savitz DA, Weinberg CR, *et al.* The effect of pesticide exposure on time to pregnancy. *Epidemiology* 1999; **10**: 112–17.

86. Garry VF, Harkins M, Lyubimov A. *et al.* Reproductive outcomes in the women of the Red River Valley of the north. I. The spouses of pesticide applicators: pregnancy loss, age at menarche, and exposures to pesticides. *J Toxicol Environ Health* 2002; **65**: 769–86.

87. Greenlee AR, Arbuckle TE, Chyou PH. Risk factors for female infertility in an agricultural region. *Epidemiology* 2003; **14**: 429–36.

88. Idrovo AJ, Sanin LH, Cole D. *et al.* Time to first pregnancy among women working in agricultural production. *Intl Arch Occup Environ Health* 2005; **78**: 493–500.

89. Lauria L, Settimi L, Spinelli A. *et al.* Exposure to pesticides and time to pregnancy among female greenhouse workers. *Reprod Toxicol* 2006; **22**: 425–30.

90. Arbuckle TE, Lin Z, Mery LS. An exploratory analysis of the effect of pesticide exposure on the risk of spontaneous abortion in an Ontario farm population. *Environ Health Perspect* 2001; **109**: 851–7.

91. Arbuckle TE, Savitz DA, Mery LS, Curtis KM. Exposure to phenoxy herbicides and the risk of spontaneous abortion. *Epidemiology* 1999; **10**: 752–60.

92. Chang SH, Cheng BH, Lee SL. *et al.* Low blood lead concentration in association with infertility in women. *Environ Res* 2006; **101**: 380–6.

93. Axmon A, Rylander L, Stromberg U. *et al.* Miscarriages and stillbirths in women with a high intake of fish contaminated with persistent organochlorine compounds. *Intl Arch Occup Environ Health* 2000; **73**: 204–8.

94. Axmon A, Rylander L, Stromberg U. *et al.* Female fertility in relation to the consumption of fish contaminated with persistent organochlorine compounds. *Scand J Work Environ Health* 2002; **28**: 124–32.

95. Axmon A, Rylander L, Stromberg U. *et al.* Polychlorinated biphenyls in blood plasma among Swedish female fish consumers in relation to time to pregnancy. *J Toxicol Environ Health* 2001; **64**: 485–98.

96. Buck Louis GM, Dmochowski J, Lynch CD. *et al.* Polychlorinated biphenyl serum concentrations, lifestyle and time-to-pregnancy. *Human Reprod* 2009; **24**: 451–8.

97. Courval JM, DeHoog JV, Stein AD. *et al.* Sport-caught fish consumption and conception delay in licensed Michigan anglers. *Environ Res* 1999; **80**: S183–8.

98. Longnecker MP, Klebanoff MA, Dunson DB. *et al.* Maternal serum level of the DDT metabolite DDE in relation to fetal loss in previous pregnancies. *Environ Res* 2005; **97**: 127–33.

99. Eskenazi B, Mocarelli P, Warner M. *et al.* Maternal serum dioxin levels and birth outcomes in women of Seveso, Italy. *Environ Health Perspect* 2003; **111**: 947–53.

100. San Sebastian M, Armstrong B, Stephens C. Outcomes of pregnancy among women living in the proximity of oil fields in the Amazon basin of Ecuador. *Int J Occup Environ Health* 2002; **8**: 312–19.

101. Venners SA, Korrick S, Xu X. *et al.* Preconception serum DDT and pregnancy loss: a prospective study using a biomarker of pregnancy. *Am J Epidemiol* 2005; **162**: 709–16.

102. Plenge-Bonig A, Karmaus W. Exposure to toluene in the printing industry is associated with subfecundity in women but not in men. *Occup Environ Med* 1999; **56**: 443–8.

103. Sallmen M, Baird DD, Hoppin JA. *et al.* Fertility and exposure to solvents among families in the Agricultural Health Study. *Occup Environ Med* 2006; **63**: 469–75.

104. Wennborg H, Bodin L, Vainio H. *et al.* Solvent use and time to pregnancy among female personnel in biomedical laboratories in Sweden. *Occup Environ Med* 2001; **58**: 225–31.

105. Schisterman EF, Whitcomb BW, Buck Louis GM, Louis TA. Lipid adjustment in the analysis of environmental contaminants and human health risks. *Environ Health Perspect* 2005; **113**: 853–7.

106. Schisterman EF, Vexler A, Whitcomb BW, Liu A. The limitations due to exposure detection limits for regression models. *Am J Epidemiol* 2006; **163**: 374–83.

# Chapter 3

# Environmental contaminants and related systems that have implications for reproduction

## 13.1 The neuroendocrine system

Andrea C. Gore

All vertebrates possess three major communication networks that allow detection of, and responses to, the external and internal environment. These three systems, the nervous, endocrine, and immune, play unique roles in enabling the organism to adapt to diverse stimuli. The nervous system mounts the most rapid responses, with neural signals transmitted on the order of milliseconds; the endocrine system is next fastest, responding in minutes to hours with hormonal signals that can endure for hours to days; and the immune system is the slowest to respond but the longest to act, with immune responses lasting for days or even years. Clearly, these communication systems of the body must interact with one another, and the nervous–endocrine, or neuroendocrine linkages enable rapid neural responses to be translated into more enduring endocrine responses [1]. Here, I will provide evidence that neuroendocrine systems of the brain are targets of environmental endocrine-disrupting chemicals (EDCs), the consequences of exposure to which are dysfunctions in endocrinology and reproduction.

## Introduction to neuroendocrine systems

Neuroendocrine cells have properties of both neurons and endocrine secretory cells. They are located in neural tissues and express specific cellular markers of neurons. They also exhibit typical properties of neurons such as electrical excitability, the ability to generate action potentials, and very rapid responses to stimuli. Rather than affecting their targets through the release of a classical neurotransmitter acting at a synapse, they instead release their neurotransmitter directly into a blood system. As endocrinology involves the release of a chemical into a vascular target, neuroendocrine cells are endocrine in nature. Thus, one may consider that neuroendocrine cells start out at their cell body (soma) as neurons, but end up at their terminals as endocrine cells. With respect to their hormonal signals, neuroendocrine cells of the brain produce monoamine or peptide hormones that are packaged into secretory vesicles and released from the termini of the neuroendocrine cells into a blood system. These shared features of neurons and endocrine cells enable these systems to respond rapidly and to result in a more sustained response from the body.

The brain's neuroendocrine tissues are found in the hypothalamus, a small region located at the base of the brain at the most anterior aspect of the brainstem. The hypothalamus is heterogeneous in morphology, function, and neurochemistry, but its general role is to maintain homeostasis. Of relevance to neuroendocrinology, there are two classes of hypothalamic regulatory cells. The first class, which will only be mentioned in passing here, are the two groups of large "magnocellular" neurosecretory cells that produce the neuropeptides vasopressin and oxytocin. These neurons have their cell bodies in the supraoptic nucleus and paraventricular nucleus subregions of the hypothalamus, and extend axonal projections directly into the posterior pituitary gland, or neurohypophysis. The neurohypophysis is highly vascularized by the general circulation, and thus, by releasing oxytocin or vasopressin into the bloodstream, the magnocellular hypothalamic neurons directly control the functions of milk ejection (oxytocin) and osmotic balance (vasopressin) among others [1].

The second class of neuroendocrine cells in the hypothalamus produces the hypothalamic-releasing

*Environmental Impacts on Reproductive Health and Fertility*, ed. T. J. Woodruff, S. J. Janssen, L. J. Guillette, and L. C. Giudice. Published by Cambridge University Press. © Cambridge University Press 2010.

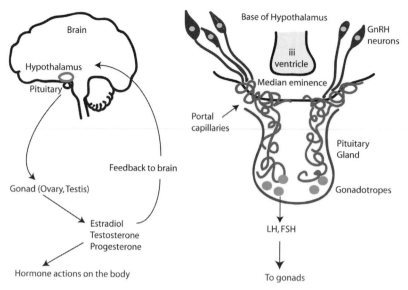

**Fig. 13.1.** Left: The hypothalamic–pituitary–gonadal (HPG) axis is depicted schematically. The hypothalamus (gray) is located at the base of the brain, immediately above the pituitary gland. Hypothalamic release of gonadotropin-releasing hormone (GnRH) causes the stimulation of anterior pituitary reproductive hormones, luteinizing hormone (LH) and follicle-stimulating hormone (FSH). These hormones cause subsequent actions upon the gonads, ovary or testis, to synthesize and release steroid hormones, particularly estradiol, progesterone, and testosterone, which act upon hormone-sensitive targets in the body. Sex steroid hormones also feed back to the brain to control reproductive function and behaviors. Right: The hypothalamic and pituitary level of the HPG axis is shown schematically at higher magnification. The base of the hypothalamus contains the median eminence, a region where hypothalamic-releasing hormones such as GnRH are released from nerve terminals into the portal capillary bed. These capillaries transport GnRH to the anterior pituitary, where GnRH binds to its receptors on a group of cells called gonadotropes (gray) to stimulate LH and FSH release. The LH and FSH in turn travel through the general circulation to act upon their target cells in the gonads.

or hypothalamic-inhibiting hormones. These neurons all have small "parvicellular" cell bodies in the anterior hypothalamus, periventricular regions, arcuate nucleus, and/or preoptic areas of the hypothalamus. Unlike the magnocellular neurons, these parvicellular neurons do not innervate the neurohypophysis. Instead, the parvicellular secretory cells project an axon to the base of the hypothalamus, called the median eminence, an area that is richly vascularized by the portal capillary vasculature (Fig. 13.1). This small blood system transports hypothalamic hormones to the anterior pituitary, or adenohypophysis. At the adenohypophysis, each hypothalamic hormone binds to a specific receptor, thereby stimulating (in the case of hypothalamic-releasing hormones) or inhibiting (in the case of hypothalamic-inhibiting hormones) release of a specific adenohypophysial hormone. These anterior pituitary hormones are then released into the general circulation where they target a tertiary organ, often to stimulate release of yet another hormone. This three-tier system of organization of the hypothalamic–adenohypophysial–target

organ neuroendocrine systems enables an amplication of signals from the brain to the body [1].

## Neuroendocrine control of reproduction

The hypothalamic neurons controlling reproduction have their cell somata in hypothalamic-preoptic regions of the brain. These cells are referred to as GnRH (gonadotropin-releasing hormone) neurons because they synthesize and release the ten amino acid neuropeptide, GnRH [2]. Only about 1000 neurons in the mammalian brain have the capacity to produce GnRH, a remarkably small number considering that in the absence of GnRH, reproduction cannot occur [3]. The GnRH neurons project a long axon to the median eminence, where the neuropeptide is released into the portal capillary vasculature. From there, the GnRH peptide travels through the capillaries to the anterior pituitary gland, where GnRH binds to its receptor that is expressed on specific cells called gonadotropes. In response to the GnRH signal, gonadotropes synthesize and release two hormones: luteinizing hormone (LH) and follicle-stimulating hormone (FSH). These two small proteins are released from the anterior pituitary gland into general circulation, where they target the gonads, ovary, or testis. In females, binding of LH and FSH to their receptors causes ovulation and follicular development, respectively. In males, LH and FSH are responsible for steroidogenesis and spermatogenesis.

The gonad is the third level of regulation of the hypothalamic–pituitary–gonadal (HPG) axis, and along with producing ova and sperm, the ovary and testis produce both steroid and non-steroid hormones. Of relevance to the current chapter, the three classes of sex steroid hormones, estrogens, progestins, and androgens, their primary members in mammals being estradiol-17β, progesterone, and testosterone, respectively, are produced in the gonads of both males and females, albeit in amounts that differ substantially between the sexes. These sex steroid hormones exert masculinizing and feminizing effects on the body and brain, and are important for normal sexual development, puberty, and adult reproductive functions.

Thus, there are three hormonal levels of organization of the reproductive system: the hypothalamic neuroendocrine GnRH cells; the pituitary gonadotropes and their hormones, LH and FSH; and the gonadal steroid hormones (Fig. 13.1). Importantly, while all three levels of the HPG axis are critical for normal reproduction, the primary drive upon this system is provided by the group of hypothalamic GnRH cells. This feed-forward input to pituitary, and subsequently gonad, must occur for reproductive functions to be initiated and maintained. In addition, the hypothalamus and pituitary are sensitive to feedback regulation from sex steroid hormones, exerted through actions of circulating steroids on their receptors, which are widely and densely distributed in the hypothalamus as well as other brain regions of male and female mammals [4, 5].

## Endocrine disruption of the hypothalamic–pituitary–gonadal axis

Endocrine-disrupting chemicals (EDCs) are substances that can perturb endocrine or reproductive systems through a variety of potential mechanisms including, but not limited to, actions on steroid hormone receptors, steroidogenic enzymes, metabolic pathways involved in synthesis or degradation of hormones, other cellular mechanisms involved in steroid

hormone signal transduction, and even non-steroid-mediated mechanisms such as neurotransmitter receptor systems [6, 7]. Any or all of these pathways may be exerted on the HPG axis, which is sensitive to disruptions of endogenous steroid signaling, administration of exogenous steroids, as well as perturbations of neurotransmitter pathways that regulate the GnRH neurons in the brain.

## GnRH neurons as targets for endocrine disruption: in vitro models

GnRH neurons can be direct targets of EDCs. The GT1 cell line is a homogeneous population of immortalized cells that has many properties of GnRH neurons, including synthesis and release of the decapeptide [8]. Endocrine-disrupting chemicals have been shown to alter GnRH gene expression, release, and cellular morphology of the GT1 cells. For example, polychlorinated biphenyls (PCBs) administered at levels estimated to be comparable to environmental exposures to humans and wildlife exerted significant effects on GnRH gene expression, GnRH peptide release, and the morphology of the GT1–7 cells [9]. More specifically, two mixtures of PCBs, Aroclor 1221 and Aroclor 1254, stimulated GnRH gene expression at low doses but had little effect at high doses, suggesting an inverted U-shaped dose–response curve. Such curves tend to be characteristic of EDCs [10, 11], because these compounds act through multiple mechanisms that may be activated/inactivated at very different ranges of doses. In that GnRH GT1 cell study, Aroclor 1221, but not Aroclor 1254, also stimulated GnRH release at low doses, an effect that was blocked by an estrogen-receptor antagonist, ICI 182,780 [9]. Thus, there are direct actions of PCBs on a GnRH cell line that is at least partially mediated by the estrogen receptor. Notably, whereas GT1 cells express the two major nuclear estrogen receptors, ER-α and ER-β [12, 13], GnRH neurons in the mammalian brain express ER-β [14] but not ER-α [15], so some of these results need to be extrapolated cautiously to the in vivo model. In addition, in interpreting these results, it should be considered that PCBs have effects on neurotransmitter systems [16], receptors for some of which are expressed on GnRH cells and GT1 cell lines, so this is another plausible mechanism of action of PCBs.

Organochlorine pesticides thought to be estrogenic in action have also been tested for effects on GnRH cell lines. When methoxychlor or chlorpyrifos were applied to GT1–7 cells, GnRH gene expression was significantly and robustly enhanced at low doses, and expression was significantly inhibited at high dosages [17]. Again, such an inverted U-shaped dose–response curve is characteristic of EDCs. Together, these data on the GT1 GnRH cell line, along with evidence that low-level toxicants do not kill the GT1 cells, suggest that environmental contaminants at low doses are not overtly toxic, but in many cases may actually be *stimulatory* to the GnRH response.

## GnRH neurons as targets for endocrine disruption: in vivo models

### Adult EDC exposures

Although the literature on effects of EDCs on GnRH neurons in vivo is relatively small, it is consistent with the in vitro data showing that GnRH cells are targets of EDCs. McGarvey *et al.* [18] used ovariectomized adult rats to show that the phytoestrogen, coumestrol, suppressed hypothalamic multi-unit activity thought to represent GnRH neuronal firing, concomitantly with a suppression of serum LH levels. Another phytoestrogen, genistein, did not have such an effect, indicating that different classes of phytoestrogens may act through differential mechanisms.

In fish, treatment with PCBs has significant effects on the HPG axis. The laboratories of Khan and Thomas have used the Atlantic croaker fish to demonstrate that PCBs decreased peptide content of GnRH in the hypothalamus, along with diminished pituitary GnRH receptors, and a reduced LH response to GnRH challenge [19]. Their laboratories have provided further evidence that the mechanism for this effect may occur through the serotonin system, a neurotransmitter affected by PCBs which itself modulates GnRH function. Indeed, considering that the GnRH neuroendocrine cells are in the brain and are highly interconnected with numerous other neurons that act through a variety of neurotransmitters and receptors, it is not surprising that EDCs, which can cause perturbations in these same neurotransmitters [16], have effects on GnRH functional properties.

### Developmental EDC exposures

In evaluating consequences of EDCs on neuroendocrine systems, it is important to consider the timing of exposure. There is consensus in the field of endocrine disruption that exposures during critical developmental time points are more likely to have detrimental consequences than adult exposures ([20]; reviewed by Gore [21]). Furthermore, the lag time between exposure and the onset of disease could be quite long. Nevertheless, this concept is particularly important when considering reproductive neuroendocrine systems. The developing hypothalamus is highly sensitive to even exquisitely low levels of endogenous hormones such as estradiol and testosterone, which play critical roles in the sexual differentiation of reproductive physiology and behavior (reviewed by Gore [21]). Thus, exposures to environmental EDCs during these early developmental periods may permanently alter this biological process, resulting in females that are masculinized or defeminized, and males that are feminized or demasculinized, with permanent repercussions on reproductive success.

There is mounting evidence that developmental exposures to EDCs disrupt HPG systems at the level of GnRH neurons. Following early postnatal treatment with genistein, female rats exhibited aberrations in the timing of puberty, accelerated reproductive senescence, and an attenuation of the estradiol-induced up-regulation of a marker of GnRH activity, assayed through co-expression of the immediate early gene *Fos* in GnRH cells [22]. Thus, early life exposure has permanent effects on the GnRH system as well as reproductive physiology. A preliminary study showed that GnRH mRNA levels were permanently elevated in female rats exposed perinatally to PCBs or organochlorine pesticides [23]. Tobet's laboratory showed that vinclozolin treatment to pregnant rabbits (vinclozolin is an endocrine-disrupting fungicide that acts at least in part through an antiandrogenic mechanism) decreased numbers of GnRH neurons in selected brain regions [24]. As a whole, these studies show that early life exposures to low levels of EDCs can have long-lasting effects on the hypothalamic GnRH system.

## Effects of EDCs on brain sexual differentiation and behavior

The concept of hormones influencing sexual development at critical periods, and subsequent consequences on the exhibition of male- or female-typical mating behaviors in adulthood, was proposed over a half century ago (reviewed by Gore [21]). Since then, it has become appreciated that both endogenous and exogenous hormones can permanently alter neural circuits and behaviors. In particular, testosterone and its metabolite estradiol influence the size and neurochemistry of hypothalamic brain regions that control reproductive physiology and behavior. This concept can be extrapolated to understanding why hormonally active EDCs given during critical developmental periods can profoundly affect brain sexual differentiation.

There are a number of hypothalamic subregions that differ significantly in size and cellular phenotype between male and female rats, and these differences are due in large part to early life exposures to endogenous steroid hormones. Under normal circumstances, the fetal testes of male mammals produce high levels of testosterone, which act in the brain through androgen receptors. In addition, some of this testosterone is converted into estradiol by the enzyme aromatase, thereby acting upon estrogen receptors in the brain [21]. By contrast, the fetal female ovary is relatively quiescent and produces lower levels of hormones. In addition, the female brain is protected from masculinizing effects of estradiol by the binding protein, alpha-fetoprotein [25]. Therefore, exogenous EDCs that may not bind well to alpha-fetoprotein and thereby get into the brain, or which elevate estrogens to supraphysiological levels, may masculinize the brain of females. This is evidenced by the loss of sexual dimorphisms in the morphology of hypothalamic brain regions and in the phenotype of cells within those regions, in rats that were exposed to EDCs during fetal development (reviewed in Dickerson and Gore [6]).

The effects of early life exposures to EDCs on brain morphology and neurochemistry would not be very meaningful were there not a functional consequence. This appears to be the case, as low doses of PCBs [26, 27] or soy [28] significantly attenuated aspects of mating behavior in female rats. Postnatal treatment with coumestrol, another phytoestrogen, diminished masculine [29] and feminine sexual behaviors [30]. Thus, early EDC exposures result in reproductive behavioral outcomes in adulthood.

## Transgenerational effects of EDCs on neuroendocrine systems

Reproductive neuroendocrinologists are beginning to investigate effects of early life exposures to EDCs not only on the exposed individuals, but also on subsequent generations. Further, the mechanisms for transmission seem to go beyond simple mutation and inheritance. Rather, at least some effects of EDCs on reproductive systems appear to involve epigenetic alterations to the DNA such as histone acetylation and DNA methylation [31, 32]. Importantly, Skinner and colleagues showed transgenerational effects of the endocrine disruptor, vinclozolin, on the male reproductive system

in a manner that was transmitted for up to at least four generations [33]. This finding broke new ground as to how a fetal exposure could cause an imprint on the male germline of the exposed individuals as well as their progeny. Since then, it was demonstrated that the third-generational male descendants of rats exposed prenatally to vinclozolin were less attractive to females than control (vehicle) descendant rats, suggesting transmission of a trait (presumably pheromonal, olfactory, or behavioral) several generations removed from the original vinclozolin exposure [34].

Work on reproductive physiologic systems is also revealing multigenerational effects of EDCs. Gore's laboratory recently published evidence that prenatal exposure to PCBs resulted in long-term changes in reproductive behavior in the adult female $F_1$ offspring [27]. In addition, when these adult females were allowed to give birth, their offspring (the $F_2$ generation) had significantly aberrant hormone profiles across the reproductive cycle [35]. Although we do not know the mechanism for this transmission, it is consistent with the persistence of effects of EDCs across several generations.

## Summary and conclusions

Reproductive processes require the careful coordination of hormones released from the hypothalamus, pituitary, and gonad. Although previous work has shown detrimental effects of EDCs on reproductive systems, most of these reports have focused on the reproductive tract, genitalia, and indices of fertility. These are clearly important endpoints, but it is also important to consider the neuroendocrine side of reproductive systems as a potential target for endocrine disruption. In fact, considering that the hypothalamus drives the pituitary and gonad, it is surprising that there has not been more research on effects of EDCs on the hypothalamic cells that control reproduction. This is an important future direction for endocrine disruption research.

## References

1. Gore AC. Neuroendocrine systems. In Bloom F, Berg D, Du Lac S. *et al.* eds. *Fundamental Neuroscience.* New York: Academic Press, 2008; 905–30.

2. Gore AC. *GnRH: The Master Molecule of Reproduction.* Norwell, MA: Kluwer Academic Publishers, 2002.

3. Krieger DT, Perlow MJ, Gibson MJ. *et al.* Brain grafts reverse hypogonadism of gonadotropin releasing hormone deficiency. *Nature* 1982; **298**: 468–71.

4. Simerly RB, Chang C, Muramatsu M, Swanson LW. Distribution of androgen and estrogen receptor mRNA-containing cells in the rat brain: an in situ hybridization study. *J Comp Neurol* 1990; **294**: 76–95.

5. Chakraborty TR, Gore AC. Aging-related changes in ovarian hormones, their receptors, and neuroendocrine function. *Exp Biol Med* 2004; **229**: 977–87.

6. Dickerson SM, Gore AC. Estrogenic environmental endocrine-disrupting chemical effects on reproductive neuroendocrine function and dysfunction across the life cycle. *Rev Endocrine Metab Disorders* 2007; **8**: 143–59.

7. Gore AC. *Endocrine-Disrupting Chemicals: From Basic Research to Clinical Practice.* Totowa, NJ: Humana Press, 2007.

8. Mellon PL, Windle JJ, Goldsmith PC. *et al.* Immortalization of hypothalamic GnRH neurons by genetically targeted tumorigenesis. *Neuron* 1990; **5**: 1–10.

9. Gore AC, Wu TJ, Oung T, Lee JB, Woller MJ. A novel mechanism for endocrine-disrupting effects of polychlorinated biphenyls: direct effects on gonadotropin-releasing hormone (GnRH) neurons. *J Neuroendocrinol* 2002; **14**: 814–23.

10. Cook R, Calabrese EJ. The importance of hormesis to public health. *Environ Health Perspect* 2006; **114**: 1631–5.

11. Gore AC, Heindel JJ, Zoeller RT. Endocrine disruption for endocrinologists (and others). *Endocrinology* 2006; **147**: S1–3.

12. Belsham DD, Evangelou A, Roy D, Le DV, Brown TJ. Regulation of gonadotropin-releasing hormone (GnRH) gene expression by 5-alpha dihydrotestosterone in GnRH-secreting GT1–7 hypothalamic neurons. *Endocrinology* 1998; **139**: 1108–14.

13. Roy D, Angelini NL, Belsham DD. Estrogen directly represses gonadotropin-releasing hormone (GnRH) gene expression in estrogen receptor-alpha (ERalpha) and ERbeta-expressing GT1–7 GnRH neurons. *Endocrinology* 1999; **140**: 5045–53.

14. Hrabovszky E, Steinhauser A, Barabás K, *et al.* Estrogen receptor-β immunoreactivity in luteinizing hormone-releasing hormone neurons of the rat brain. *Endocrinology* 2001; **142**(7): 3261–4.

15. Wintermantel TM, Campbell RE, Porteous R. *et al.* Definition of estrogen receptor pathway critical for estrogen positive feedback to gonadotropin-releasing hormone neurons and fertility. *Neuron* 2006; **52**: 271–80.

16. Seegal RF, Schantz SL. Neurochemical and behavioral sequelae of exposure to dioxins and PCBs. In Schechter A, ed. *Dioxins and Health.* New York: Plenum Press, 1994; 409–47.

17. Gore AC. Organochlorine pesticides directly regulate gonadotropin-releasing hormone gene expression and biosynthesis in the GT1–7 hypothalamic cell line. *Mol Cell Endocrinol* 2002; **192**: 157–70.

18. McGarvey C, Cates PS, Brooks NA. *et al.* Phytoestrogens and gonadotropin-releasing hormone pulse generator activity and pituitary luteinizing hormone release in the rat. *Endocrinology* 2001; **142**(3): 1202–8.

19. Khan IA, Thomas P. Disruption of neuroendocrine control of luteinizing hormone secretion by aroclor 1254 involves inhibition of hypothalamic tryptophan hydroxylase activity. *Biol Reprod* 2001; **64**: 955–64.

20. Barker DJP. The developmental origins of adult disease. *Eur J Epidemiol* 2003; **18**: 733–6.

21. Gore AC. Developmental exposures and imprinting on reproductive neuroendocrine systems. *Front Neuroendocrinol* 2008; **29**: 358–74.

22. Bateman HL, Patisaul HB. Disrupted female reproductive physiology following neonatal exposure to phytoestrogens or estrogen specific ligands is associated with decreased GnRH activation and kisspeptin fiber density in the hypothalamus. *Neurotoxicol* 2008; **29**: 988–97.

23. Gore AC. Environmental toxicant effects on neuroendocrine function. *Endocrine* 2001; **14**: 235–46.

24. Bisenius ES, Veeramachaneni, DN, Sammonds GE Tobet S. Sex differences and the development of the rabbit brain: effects of vinclozolin. *Biol Reprod* 2006; **75**: 469–76.

25. Bakker J, DeMees C, Douhard Q. *et al.* Alpha-fetoprotein protects the developing female mouse brain from masculinization and defeminization by estrogens. *Nat Neurosci* 2006; **9**: 220–6.

26. Chung YW, Nunez AA, Clemens LG. Effects of neonatal polychlorinated biphenyl exposure on female sexual behavior. *Physiol Behav* 2001; **74**: 363–70.

27. Steinberg RM, Juenger TE, Gore AC. The effects of prenatal PCBs on adult female paced mating reproductive behaviors in rats. *Horm Behav* 2007; **51**: 364–72.

28. Patisaul HB, Luskin JR, Wilson ME. A soy supplement and tamoxifen inhibit sexual behavior in female rats. *Horm Behav* 2004; **45**: 270–7.

29. Whitten PL, Lewis C, Russell E, Naftolin F. Phytoestrogen influences on the development of behavior and gonadotropin function. *Proc Soc Exp Biol Med* 1995; **208**: 82–6.

30. Kouki T, Okamoto M, Wada S, Kishitake M, Yamanouchi K. Suppressive effect of neonatal treatment

with a phytoestrogen, coumestrol, on lordosis and estrous cycle in female rats. *Brain Res Bull* 2005; **64**: 449–54.

31. Skinner MK. What is an epigenetic transgenerational phenotype? *Reprod Toxicol* 2008; **25**: 2–6.

32. Anway MD, Skinner MK. Epigenetic transgenerational actions of endocrine disruptors. *Endocrinology* 2006; **147**: S43–9.

33. Anway MD, Cupp AS, Uzumcu M, Skinner MK. Epigenetic transgenerational actions of endocrine

disruptors and male fertility. *Science* 2005; **308**: 1466–9.

34. Crews D, Gore AC, Hsu TS. *et al.* Transgenerational epigenetic imprints on mate preference. *Proc Natl Acad Sci USA* 2007; **104**: 5942–6.

35. Steinberg RM, Walker DM, Juenger TE, Woller MJ, Gore AC. The effects of prenatal PCBs on adult female rat reproduction. Development, reproductive physiology, and transgenerational effects. *Biol Reprod* 2008; **78**: 1091–101.

# 13.2 The thyroid system

R. Thomas Zoeller and John D. Meeker

Thyroid hormone is well known to be essential for development of many tissues, including the brain [1–3] and heart [4]. Less well understood is the potential role of thyroid hormone in the development of reproductive tissues that could impact adult fertility. However, important new information is appearing concerning the association between thyroid hormone and fertility in humans, as well as new experimental work in animals that may explain this association. Therefore, thyroid disruption may be an important route by which environmental chemicals could affect fertility in humans and wildlife. A large number of contaminants commonly found in human tissues are known to be thyroid toxicants [5, 6]. These toxicants were identified by their ability to alter serum concentrations of the thyroid hormone. However, recent evidence also indicates that some chemicals – polyhalogenated aryl hydrocarbons – can interfere directly with thyroid hormone receptors (TRs), and perhaps in a TR isoform-specific manner [7–9]. In addition, environmental chemicals could interact with proteins responsible for "activating" thyroid hormone or delivering thyroid hormone to important target tissues at the appropriate development time. These kinds of chemicals can affect fertility in unpredictable ways. The goal of this chapter is to provide a description of the thyroid hormone signaling system and its regulation, and the potential impact on reproduction of environmental endocrine disruptors.

## Thyroid hormone signaling

Thyroid hormones (thyroxine or tetraiodothyronine $(T_4)$ and triiodothyronine $(T_3)$) are hydroxylated, iodinated diphenyl ether molecules with an amino terminus. These compounds are produced by the condensation of two iodo-tyrosyl residues of thyroglobulin [10]. They have limited solubility in water, but are not lipophilic enough to easily pass through cell membranes without active transport. Thyroid hormones exert their action, largely, through nuclear proteins that act as ligand-regulated transcription factors [11]. There are two types of thyroid hormone receptors (TRs) – alpha (TR-α) and beta (TR-β) – that reside on different chromosomes. By a variety of mechanisms, these genes differentially express several isoforms including TR-α1, TR-α2, ΔTR-α1, and ΔTR-α2, TR-β1, TR-β2, TR-β3, ΔTR-β3[12]. These different TR isoforms are selectively expressed both spatially and temporally during development [13,14], and could play an important role in mediating the various actions of thyroid hormone during development. Thus, an important perspective driving research in this field is that thyroid hormone exerts its action on genes important for development through a diversity of receptor isoforms [15].

An important – but by no means exclusive – mechanism controlling thyroid hormone signaling is by controlling serum concentrations of thyroid hormones (see Fig. 13.2). Tetraiodothyronine $(T_4)$ is synthesized in and released from the thyroid gland in response to stimulation by the pituitary glycoprotein hormone, thyrotropin (TSH)[10, 16]. Because $T_4$ exerts a negative feedback on pituitary TSH secretion, the levels of these two hormones in the blood are inversely related [16, 17]. Total serum $T_4$, measured by radioimmunoassay, comprises $T_4$ dissolved in serum (i.e. "free") and $T_4$ bound to various serum binding proteins [18]. In principle, changes in serum binding proteins can cause changes in total $T_4$ without concomitant changes in thyroid function (e.g. during pregnancy [19]). Therefore, measurements of free $T_4$, which represents about 0.02% of total $T_4$, are often viewed as being more reflective of thyroid activity and "biologically relevant." However, measuring free $T_4$ is in itself non-trivial and the RIA-based approach can give erroneous results if serum binding proteins are different [20]; therefore, the combination of serum-free and total $T_4$ and serum TSH is often used as a good index of thyroid function[21].

The thyroid system, as illustrated in Fig 13.2, is described below, with list numbering relating to the numbered parts within Fig. 13.2.

(1)  Nerve cells in the hypothalamus synthesize the neurohormone thyrotropin-releasing hormone (TRH) [22, 23]. Although TRH-containing neurons are widely distributed throughout the brain [24, 25], TRH neurons in the PVN project uniformly to the median eminence[26, 27], a neurohemal organ connected to the anterior pituitary gland by the hypothalamic–pituitary–portal vessels [28], and are the only TRH neurons to regulate the pituitary–thyroid axis [29, 30].

*Environmental Impacts on Reproductive Health and Fertility*, ed. T. J. Woodruff, S. J. Janssen, L. J. Guillette, and L. C. Giudice. Published by Cambridge University Press. ©Cambridge University Press 2010.

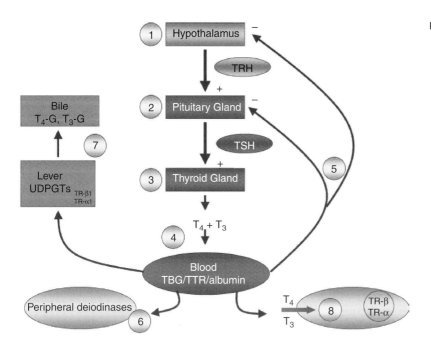

**Fig. 13.2.** The thyroid system.

(2) TRH stimulates the synthesis and release of thyroid stimulating hormone (TSH) or "thyrotropin" [31], which travels through the bloodstream to the thyroid gland where it stimulates thyroid function.

(3) Pituitary TSH binds to receptors on the surface of thyroid follicle cells stimulating adenylate cyclase [32, 33]. The effect of increased cAMP is to increase the uptake of iodide into thyroid cells, iodination of tyrosyl residues on thyroglobulin (TG) by thyroperoxidase, synthesis and oxidation of TG, TG uptake from thyroid colloid, and production of the iodothyronines $T_4$ and $T_3$. $T_4$ is by far the major product released from the thyroid gland [32].

(4) Thyroid hormones are carried in the blood by specific proteins. In humans, about 75% of $T_4$ is bound to thyroxine-binding globulin (TBG), 15% is bound to transthyretin (TTR) and the remainder is bound to albumin [18]. The presence and abundance of the different binding proteins varies among the vertebrates and may be developmentally regulated in a generalized manner. In the rat, high serum levels of TBG are found in the fetus and the early postnatal pup [34, 35]; adult levels of TBG are undetectable, but low serum $T_4$ appears to increase both serum TBG and liver biosynthesis in the rodent [35].

(5) Thyroid hormones exert a negative feedback effect on the release of pituitary TSH and on the activity of hypothalamic TRH neurons [22, 36, 37]. In addition, fasting suppresses the activity of TRH neurons by a neural mechanism that may involve leptin [38, 39]. Circulating levels of $T_4$ and of $T_3$ fluctuate considerably within an individual; therefore, TSH measurements are considered to be diagnostic of thyroid dysfunction [40–42]. However, individual $T_4$ levels in humans vary within far narrower limits than the population limits (i.e. the population reference range). In addition, variance in serum $T_4$ in pairs of monozygotic twins is far more correlated than that in pairs of dizygotic twins or the general population [43]. Thus, the set-point around which negative feedback appears to function has a very strong genetic component in humans and perhaps in other animals.

(6) Thyroid hormones are actively transported into target tissues [44–51]. $T_4$ can be converted to $T_3$ by the action of outer-ring deiodinases (ORD, Type I and Type II) [52]. Peripheral conversion of $T_4$ to $T_3$ by these ORDs accounts for nearly 80% of the $T_3$ found in the circulation [41].

(7) Thyroid hormones are cleared from the blood in the liver following sulfation or sulfonation by sulfotransferases, or following glucuronidation

by UDP-glucuronosyl transferase [53, 54]. These modified thyroid hormones are then eliminated through the bile.

(8) Thyroid hormones are actively concentrated in target cells about ten-fold over that of the circulation, although this is tissue dependent. The receptors for $T_4$ and $T_3$ (TRs) are nuclear proteins that bind to DNA and regulate transcription [55–59]. There are two genes that encode the TRs, c-erbA-alpha (TR-α) and c-erbA-beta (TR-β). Each of these genes is differentially spliced, forming three separate TRs, TR-α1, TR-β1, and TR-β2. The effects of thyroid hormone are quite tissue-, cell-, and developmental stage-specific and it is believed that the relative abundance of the different TRs in a specific cell may contribute to this selective action.

Recent studies also indicate that individual tissues can autonomously regulate thyroid hormone action employing mechanisms of TH uptake and $T_4$ metabolism, in the absence of overt changes in serum concentrations of thyroid hormone. This is becoming particularly well illustrated in the photoperiodic regulation of reproduction in seasonal animals [60–62], or of metabolism in brown fat [63]. The ability of tissues to individually regulate their sensitivity to TH also leads to the notion of "compensation" to low thyroid hormone. That is, tissues could up-regulate their ability to trap $T_4$ and $T_3$ and to up-regulate their ability to convert $T_4$ to $T_3$ so as to ameliorate the impacts of low $T_4$. Although provocative, there is little empirical evidence to support this concept in experimental systems, other than the recognition that low serum $T_4$ leads to an up-regulation of mechanisms that would appear to maintain tissue levels of $T_3$ [64–67]. Little has been done to show empirically that these adaptive responses can ameliorate the consequences of low $T_4$; this represents an important data gap in this field.

## Environmental impacts on thyroid hormone signaling

Much of the basic and applied research in this area has focused on the role of thyroid disruptors on brain development largely because of the critical importance of thyroid hormone to that process. It has long been recognized that there are environmental influences on thyroid function [68], but our ability to identify environmental factors that affect thyroid hormone

action during development is limited by the lack of information about thyroid hormone action in specific developing tissues [69]. Moreover, because all known "thyroid toxicants" have been identified solely by their ability to reduce circulating TH levels [5], the default approach to identify such chemicals is by their effects on hormone levels and on thyroid histology (e.g. size of the colloid, qualitative appearance of hypertrophic or hyperplastic effects) [70]. However, as reviewed above, tissue sensitivity to thyroid hormone action can change in the absence of changes in circulating levels of thyroid hormones, and chemicals that act directly on thyroid hormone receptors (TRs) could produce variable and perhaps unpredicted effects on hormone levels as well as to produce effects on development that do not completely mimic TH insufficiency (or action). Therefore, there is a critical weakness in our ability to identify compounds that interfere with thyroid hormone signaling directly, or to measure their effects in the human population.

A large number of man-made chemicals in the environment are known to influence thyroid hormone action [5, 6]. In general, these chemicals can be categorized as affecting serum thyroid hormone levels, or those that also directly interact with TRs [3, 9]. A number of chemicals can interfere with iodine uptake, including perchlorate, nitrates, chlorates, thiocyanates, and other ions. Other chemicals can block iodine organification, such as thiocyanates and isoflavones [71]. Several of the organochlorines, including PCBs, PBBs, PBDEs, and dioxin not only cause a reduction in serum thyroid hormones, but can also bind to the TR, although in some cases only after hydroxylation [9, 72].

## Implications for reproduction

A rich literature of thyroid hormone action in brain development, and the mechanisms by which TH signaling can be disrupted by environmental chemicals, provides important insight into the possible role of thyroid hormone in the development and function of tissues important for reproduction. A fundamental aspect of thyroid hormone action may well be that it is necessary but not sufficient for most, if not all, of its actions – including potentially those actions impacting reproduction. In other words, environmentally mediated thyroid disruption could interact with other events to impact reproductive measures. Recent studies indicate that thyroid hormone is important in pregnancy outcome. For example, Casey [73] found that pregnancies in women with subclinical hypothyroidism were

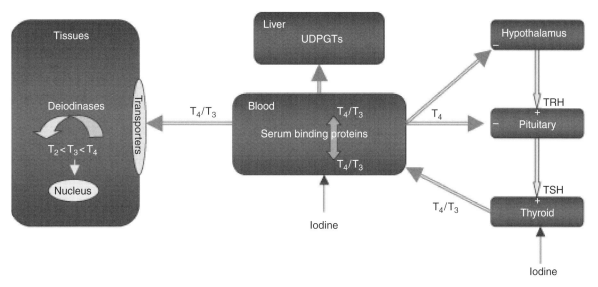

**Fig. 13.3.** Thyroid hormone regulation and action. The hypothalamic–pituitary–thyroid axis is "tuned" to control circulating levels of $T_4$ and $T_3$ within relatively narrow limits and environmental contaminants can interfere with this at many points of regulation. Changes in the rate of synthesis and release of $T_4$ into the bloodstream are controlled by pituitary TSH, and this system is normally kept in balance because serum $T_4$ exerts a negative feedback action on both hypothalamic TRH and pituitary TSH. However, changes in the rate of $T_4$ elimination (i.e. serum half-life) are controlled by complex physiological processes of $T_4$ clearance in the liver and uptake of $T_4$ into tissues, and these in turn are related to some degree to the serum-binding proteins. $T_4$ derived from serum is the main contributor to tissue $T_3$ after conversion of $T_4$ to $T_3$ by deiodinases. However, $T_3$ in some tissues is more directly controlled by serum $T_3$. Environmental contaminants can exert complex actions on the functioning of this system and there are specific chemicals known to interfere with each of the steps shown here [6].

three times more likely to be complicated by placental abruption and twice as likely to end in a preterm birth; the same did not apply to subclinical hyperthyroidism [74]. Overt hypothyroidism occurs in about 0.5–0.7% of women of reproductive age [75]. Hypothyroidism may alter estrogen metabolism and result in impaired ovulation [76].

Hypothyroidism is less common in men, and may have less predictable effects on reproduction [77]. Thyroid hormone receptors are selectively expressed in Sertoli cells [78] and may play an important role in Sertoli cell proliferation early in development, in part by regulating the expression of connexin 43 [79, 80]. Thyroid hormones are also likely important for Leydig cell differentiation and steroidogenesis in the postnatal testis [81], and for normal testicular physiology and antioxidant defense throughout development and maturation [82]. The role of thyroid hormone in adult male reproductive function has not been well studied, though there is evidence that it may stimulate testosterone and estradiol production and secretion by varying the pituitary's LH response to GnRH and/or Leydig cell steroidogenic response to LH [83, 84]. There is limited human data to suggest that subtle changes in thyroid hormone could be associated with sperm production

and quality, as a recent cross-sectional epidemiological study reported positive associations between serum-free $T_4$ and sperm concentration and motility [85] and inverse associations between free $T_4$ and measures of sperm DNA damage [86].

Thus, there is a growing body of research highlighting the importance of thyroid signaling on reproduction, but more work is clearly needed to improve our understanding of these relationships and whether thyroid-hormone deficits or surpluses considered subclinical may have important implications on reproductive development and function. Environmental chemicals that act solely on circulating levels of thyroid hormones may have predictable effects on reproductive outcome, based on our working knowledge of the effects of thyroid hormone insufficiency or excess on these measures. However, environmental chemicals that directly interfere with the TR could produce quite unpredicted effects on fertility or reproductive outcome, especially if they act in ways that are not fully explored.

## Conclusions

The human population is exposed to a large number of specific polyhalogenated aromatic hydrocarbons, and biomonitoring studies now detect these chemicals in adults, children, pregnant women, and in the fetal compartment [87]. Increasing numbers of reports are revealing that a broad array of compounds can bind to the TR and affect thyroid hormone-regulated gene expression, both in vivo and in vitro. However, considering the tremendously pleiotropic effects of thyroid hormone, it is predictable that these synthetic compounds may have very complex effects on the TR. In addition, these studies suggest that chemicals may interact with other important thyroid hormone-binding proteins. For example, deiodinase enzymes appear to control the sensitivity of different brain regions to thyroid hormone exposure during development [88]; thus, if exogenous chemicals alter the activity of these enzymes, it may influence the sequence of thyroid hormone-sensitive developmental events. Likewise, specific transporters appear to control the availability of $T_3$ to cells in the brain [89, 90]; thus, if environmental chemicals interfere with tissue uptake of thyroid hormone, adverse human health effects could result (Fig. 13.3). Our ability to identify chemical effects on TR function in vitro far exceeds our ability to identify chemical effects on TR function in vivo, in part because the mechanisms of thyroid hormone action in important developmental stages is less well understood. However, it will be important to define the role of thyroid hormone in brain and gonadal development, in addition to fully developed tissues and systems, and to identify the mechanisms by which thyroid hormone exerts these actions if we are to understand the potential human health effects of pervasive exposure to environmental compounds. Therefore, it is important to distinguish between changes in hormone levels in blood, changes in thyroid gland activity, changes in thyroid hormone metabolism, and changes in thyroid hormone action in tissues.

# References

1. Zoeller RT, Rovet J. Timing of thyroid hormone action in the developing brain: clinical observations and experimental findings. *J Neuroendocrinol* 2004; **16**: 809–18.

2. Bernal J. Thyroid hormone receptors in brain development and function. *Nat Clin Pract Endocrinol Metab* 2007; **3**: 249–59.

3. Darras VM. Endocrine disrupting polyhalogenated organic pollutants interfere with thyroid hormone signalling in the developing brain. *Cerebellum* 2007; 1–12.

4. Kahaly GJ, Dillmann WH. Thyroid hormone action in the heart. *Endocr Rev* 2005; **26**: 704–28.

5. Brucker-Davis F. Effects of environmental synthetic chemicals on thyroid function. *Thyroid* 1998; **8**: 827–56.

6. Howdeshell KL. A model of the development of the brain as a construct of the thyroid system. *Environ Health Perspect* 2002; **110** (Suppl. 3): 337–48.

7. Zoeller RT. Thyroid hormone and brain development: environmental influences. *Curr Opin Endocrinol Diabetes* 2005; **12**: 31–5.

8. Zoeller RT. Environmental chemicals as thyroid hormone analogues: new studies indicate that thyroid hormone receptors are targets of industrial chemicals? *Mol Cell Endocrinol* 2005; **242**: 10–15.

9. Zoeller RT. Environmental chemicals impacting the thyroid: targets and consequences. *Thyroid* 2007; **17**: 811–17.

10. Taurog A. Hormone synthesis: thyroid iodine metabolism. In Braverman LE, Utiger RD, eds. *The Thyroid: A Fundamental and Clinical Text*. 9th Edition. Philadelphia: Lippincott-Raven, 2004; 61–85.

11. Flamant F, Baxter JD, Forrest D. *et al.* International Union of Pharmacology. LIX. The pharmacology and classification of the nuclear receptor superfamily: thyroid hormone receptors. *Pharmacol Rev* 2006; **58**: 705–11.

12. Harvey CB, Williams GR. Mechanism of thyroid hormone action. *Thyroid* 2002; **12**: 441–6.

13. Bradley DJ, Towle HC, Young WS. Spatial and temporal expression of alpha- and beta-thyroid hormone receptor mRNAs, including the beta-2 subtype, in the developing mammalian nervous system. *J Neurosci* 1992; **12**: 2288–302.

14. Harvey CB, Bassett JH, Maruvada P, Yen PM, Williams GR. The rat thyroid hormone receptor (TR) Deltabeta3 displays cell-, TR isoform-, and thyroid hormone response element-specific actions. *Endocrinology* 2007; **148**: 1764–73.

15. Nunez J, Celi FS, Ng L, Forrest D. Multigenic control of thyroid hormone functions in the nervous system. *Mol Cell Endocrinol* 2008; **287**: 1–12.

16. Zoeller RT, Tan SW, Tyl RW. General background on the hypothalamic-pituitary-thyroid (HPT) axis. *Crit Rev Toxicol* 2007; **37**: 11–53.

17. McLanahan ED, Campbell JL Jr., Ferguson DC. *et al.* Low-dose effects of ammonium perchlorate on the hypothalamic-pituitary-thyroid axis of adult male rats pretreated with PCB126. *Toxicol Sci* 2007; **97**: 308–17.

18. Schussler GC. The thyroxine-binding proteins. *Thyroid* 2000; **10**: 141–9.

19. Brent GA. Maternal thyroid function: interpretation of thyroid function tests in pregnancy. *Clin Obstet Gynecol* 1992; **40**: 3–15.

20. Mandel SJ, Spencer CA, Hollowell JG. Are detection and treatment of thyroid insufficiency in pregnancy feasible? *Thyroid* 2005; **15**: 44–53.

21. Ladenson PW. Diagnosis of hypothyroidism. In Braverman LE, Utiger RD, eds. *The Thyroid: A Fundamental and Clinical Text*, 8th Edition. Philadelphia: Lippincott, Williams and Wilkins, 2000; 848–52.

22. Segersen TP, Kauer J, Wolfe HC. *et al.* Thyroid hormone regulates TRH biosynthesis in the paraventricular nucleus of the rat hypothalamus. *Science* 1987; **238**: 78–80.

23. Segersen TP, Hoefler H, Childers H. Localization of thyrotropin-releasing hormone prohormone messenger ribonucleic acid in rat brain by in situ hybridization. *Endocrinology* 1987; **121**: 98–107.

24. Jackson IMD, Wu P, Lechan RM. Immunohistochemical localization in the rat brain of the precursor for thyrotropin releasing hormone. *Science* 1985; **229**: 1097–9.

25. Lechan RM, Wu P, Jackson IMD. Immunolocalization of the thyrotropin-releasing hormone prohormone in the rat central nervous system. *Endocrinology* 1986; **119**: 1210–16.

26. Ishikawa K, Taniguchi Y, Inoue K, Kurosumi K, Suzuki M. Immunocytochemical delineation of the thyrotrophic area: origin of thyrotropin-releasing hormone in the median eminence. *Neuroendocrinology* 1988; **47**: 384–8.

27. Merchenthaler I, Liposits Z. Mapping of thyrotropin-releasing hormone (TRH) neuronal systems of rat forebrain projecting to the median eminence and the OVLT. Immunocytochemistry combined with retrograde labeling at the light and electron microscopic levels. *Acta Biol Hung* 1994; **45**: 361–74.

28. Martin JB, Reichlin S. *Clinical Neuroendocrinology*, 2nd Edition. F.A. Davis Company, 1987.

29. Aizawa T, Greer MA. Delineation of the hypothalamic area controlling thyrotropin secretion in the rat. *Endocrinology* 1981; **109**: 1731–8.

30. Taylor T, Wondisford FE, Blaine T, Weintraub BD. The paraventricular nucleus of the hypothalamus has a major role in thyroid hormone feedback regulation of thyrotropin synthesis and secretion. *Endocrinology* 1990; **126**: 317–24.

31. Haisenleder DJ, Ortolano GA, Dalkin AC, Yasin M, Marshall JC. Differential actions of thyrotropin (TSH)-releasing hormone pulses in the expression of prolactin and TSH subunit messenger ribonucleic acid in rat pituitary cells in vitro. *Endocrinology* 1992; **130**: 2917–23.

32. Taurog A, Dorris ML, Doerge DR. Minocycline and the thyroid: antithyroid effects of the drug, and the role of thyroid peroxidase in minocycline-induced black pigmentation of the gland. *Thyroid* 1996; **6**: 211–19.

33. Wondisford FE, Magner JA, Weintraub BD. Thyrotropin. In Braverman LE, Utiger RD, eds. *The Thyroid: A Fundamental and Clinical Text*, 7th Edition. Philadelphia: Lippincott-Raven, 1996; 190–206.

34. Vranckx R, Rouaze M, Savu L. *et al.* The hepatic biosynthesis of rat thyroxine binding globulin (TBG): demonstration, ontogenesis, and up-regulation in experimental hypothyroidism. *Biochem Biophys Res Commun* 1990; **167**: 317–22.

35. Vranckx R, Rouaze-Romet M, Savu L. *et al.* Regulation of rat thyroxine-binding globulin and transthyretin: studies in thyroidectomized and hypophysectomized rats given tri-iodothyronine or/and growth hormone. *J Endocrinol* 1994; **142**: 77–84.

36. Koller KJ, Wolff RS, Warden MK, Zoeller RT. Thyroid hormones regulate levels of thyrotropin-releasing hormone mRNA in the paraventricular nucleus. *Proc Natl Acad Sci USA* 1987; **84**: 7329–33.

37. Rondeel JMM, de Greef WJ, van der Vaart PDM, van der Schoot P, Visser TJ. In vivo hypothalamic release of thyrotropin-releasing hormone after electrical stimulation of the paraventricular area: comparison between push-pull perfusion technique and collection of hypophysial portal blood. *Endocrinology* 1989; **125**: 971–5.

38. Lagradi G, Emerson CH, Ahima RS, Flier JS, Lechan RM. Leptin prevents fasting-induced suppression of prothyrotropin-releasing hormone messenger ribonucleic acid in neurons of the hypothalamic paraventricular nucleus. *Endocrinology* 1997; **138**: 2569–76.

39. Fekete C, Mihaly E, Luo LG. *et al.* Association of cocaine- and amphetamine-regulated transcript-immunoreactive elements with thyrotropin-releasing hormone-synthesizing neurons in the hypothalamic paraventricular nucleus and its role in the regulation of the hypothalamic-pituitary-thyroid axis during fasting. *Journal of Neuroscience* 2000; **20**: 9224–34.

40. Roti E, Minelli R, Gardini E, Braverman LE. The use and misuse of thyroid hormone. *Endocrine Rev* 1993; **14**: 401–23.

41. Chopra IJ. Nature, source, and relative significance of circulating thyroid hormones. In Braverman LE, Utiger RD, eds. *The Thyroid: A Fundamental and Clinical Text*. 7th Edition. Philadelphia: Lippincott-Raven, 1996; 111–24.

42. Stockigt Jr. Serum thyrotropin and thyroid hormone measurements and assessment of thyroid hormone transport. In Braverman LE, Utiger RD, eds. *The Thyroid: A Fundamental and Clinical Text*. 8th Edition. Philadelphia: Lippincott-Raven, 2000; 376–92.

43. Hansen PS, Brix TH, Sorensen TI, Kyvik KO, Hegedus L. Major genetic influence on the regulation of the pituitary-thyroid axis: a study of healthy Danish twins. *J Clin Endocrinol Metab* 2004; **89**: 1181–7.

44. Oppenheimer JH. The nuclear receptor-triiodothyronine complex: relationship to thyroid hormone distribution, metabolism, and biological action. In Oppenheimer JH, Samuels HH, eds. *Molecular Basis of Thyroid Hormone Action*, New York: Academic Press, 1983; 1–35.

45. Everts ME, Docter R, Moerings EP. *et al.* Uptake of thyroxine in cultured anterior pituitary cells of euthyroid rats. *Endocrinology* 1994; **134**: 2490–7.

46. Everts ME, Visser TJ, Moerings EP. *et al.* Uptake of triiodothyroacetic acid and its effect on thyrotropin secretion in cultured anterior pituitary cells. *Endocrinology* 1994; **135**: 2700–7.

47. Everts ME, Visser TJ, Moerings EP. *et al.* Uptake of 3,5',5,5'-tetraiodothyroacetic acid and 3,3',5'-triiodothyronine in cultured rat anterior pituitary cells and their effects on thyrotropin secretion. *Endocrinology* 1995; **136**: 4454–61.

48. Kragie L. Membrane iodothyronine transporters, Part II: Review of protein biochemistry. *Endocr Res* 1996; **22**: 95–119.

49. Docter R, Friesema ECH, Van Stralen PGJ. *et al.* Expression of rat liver cell membrane transporters for thyroid hormone in *Xenopus laevis* oocytes. *Endocrinology* 1997; **138**: 1841–6.

50. Friesema ECH, Docter R, Moerings EP. *et al.* Identification of thyroid hormone transporters. *Biochem Biophys Res Commun* 1999; **254**: 497–501.

51. Moreau X, Lejeune PJ, Jeanningros R. Kinetics of red blood cell T3 uptake in hypothyroidism with or without hormonal replacement, in the rat. *J Endocrinol Invest* 1999; **22**: 257–61.

52. St Germain DL, Galton VA. The deiodinase family of selenoproteins. *Thyroid* 1997; **7**: 655–68.

53. Hood A, Klaassen CD. Differential effects of microsomal enzyme inducers on in vitro thyroxine (T(4)) and triiodothyronine (T(3)) glucuronidation. *Toxicol Sci* 2000; **55**: 78–84.

54. Hood A, Klaassen CD. Effects of microsomal enzyme inducers on outer-ring deiodinase activity toward thyroid hormones in various rat tissues. *Toxicol Appl Pharmacol* 2000; **163**: 240–8.

55. Lazar MA. Thyroid hormone receptors: multiple forms, multiple possibilities. *Endocr Rev* 1993; **14**: 184–93.

56. Lazar MA. Thyroid hormone receptors: Update 1994. *Endocr Rev Monogr* 1994; **3**: 280–3.

57. Oppenheimer JH, Schwartz HL, Strait KA. Thyroid hormone action 1994: the plot thickens. *Eur J Endocrinol* 1994; **130**: 15–24.

58. Mangelsdorf DJ, Evans RM. The RXR heterodimers and orphan receptors. *Cell* 1995; **83**: 841–50.

59. Oppenheimer JH, Schwartz HL. Molecular basis of thyroid hormone-dependent brain development. *Endocrine Rev* 1997; **18**: 462–75.

60. Watanabe T, Yamamura T, Watanabe M. *et al.* Hypothalamic expression of thyroid hormone-activating and -inactivating enzyme genes in relation to photorefractoriness in birds and mammals. *Am J Physiol Regul Integr Comp Physiol* 2007; **292**: R568–72.

61. Ebling FJ, Barrett P. The regulation of seasonal changes in food intake and body weight. *J Neuroendocrinol* 2008; **20**: 827–33.

62. Nakao N, Ono H, Yamamura T. *et al.* Thyrotrophin in the pars tuberalis triggers photoperiodic response. *Nature* 2008; **452**: 317–22.

63. Watanabe M, Houten SM, Mataki C. *et al.* Bile acids induce energy expenditure by promoting intracellular thyroid hormone activation. *Nature* 2006; **439**: 484–9.

64. Silva JE, Larsen PR. Peripheral metabolism of homologous thyrotropin in euthyroid and hypothyroid rats: acute effects of thyrotropin-releasing hormone, triiodothyronine, and thyroxine. *Endocrinology* 1978; **102**: 1783–96.

65. Leonard JL, Kaplan MM, Visser TJ, Silva JE, Larsen PR. Cerebral cortex responds rapidly to thyroid hormones. *Science* 1981; **214**: 571–3.

66. Silva JE, Larsen PR. Comparison of iodothyronine 5'-deiodinase and other thyroid-hormone-dependent enzyme activities in the cerebral cortex of hypothyroid neonatal rat. Evidence for adaptation to hypothyroidism. *J Clin Invest* 1982; **70**: 1110–23.

67. Burmeister LA, Pachucki J, St Germain DL. Thyroid hormones inhibit type 2 iodothyronine deiodinase in the rat cerebral cortex by both pre- and posttranslational mechanisms. *Endocrinology* 1997; **138**: 5231–7.

68. Gaitan E, ed. *Environmental Goitrogenesis.* Boca Raton: CRC Press, Inc., 1989.

69. Zoeller RT. Thyroid toxicology and brain development: should we think differently? *Environ Health Perspect* 2003; **111**: A628.

70. DeVito M, Biegel L, Brouwer A. *et al.* Screening methods for thyroid hormone disruptors. *Environ Health Perspect* 1999; **107**: 407–15.

71. Chen A, Rogan WJ. Isoflavones in soy infant formula: a review of evidence for endocrine and other activity in infants. *Annu Rev Nutr* 2004; **24**: 33–54.

72. You SH, Gauger KJ, Bansal R, Zoeller RT. 4-Hydroxy-PCB106 acts as a direct thyroid hormone receptor agonist in rat GH3 cells. *Mol Cell Endocrinol* 2006; **257–258**: 26–34.

73. Casey BM. Subclinical hypothyroidism and pregnancy. *Obstet Gynecol Surv* 2006; **61**: 415–20; quiz 423.

74. Casey BM, Dashe JS, Wells CE. *et al.* Subclinical hyperthyroidism and pregnancy outcomes. *Obstet Gynecol* 2006; **107**: 337–41.

75. Hollowell JG, Staehling NW, Flanders WD. *et al.* Serum TSH, T(4), and thyroid antibodies in the United States population (1988 to 1994): National Health and Nutrition Examination Survey (NHANES III). *J Clin Endocrinol Metab* 2002; **87**: 489–99.

76. Poppe K, Velkeniers B (2004) Female infertility and the thyroid. *Best Pract Res Clin Endocrinol Metab* 2004; **18**: 153–65.

77. Trokoudes KM, Skordis N, Picolos MK. Infertility and thyroid disorders. *Curr Opin Obstet Gynecol* 2006; **18**: 446–51.

78. Jannini EA, Crescenzi A, Rucci N.*et al.* (2000) Ontogenetic pattern of thyroid hormone receptor expression in the human testis. *J Clin Endocrinol Metab* 2000; **85**: 3453–7.

79. Hess RA, Cooke PS, Hofmann MC, Murphy KM. Mechanistic insights into the regulation of the spermatogonial stem cell niche. *Cell Cycle* 2006; **5**: 1164–70.

80. Sridharan S, Simon L, Meling DD. *et al.* Proliferation of adult sertoli cells following conditional knockout of the gap junctional protein GJA1 (Connexin 43). *Biol Reprod* 2007; **76**(5): 804–12.

81. Mendis-Handagama SM, Ariyaratane HB. Effects of thyroid hormones on Leydig cells in the postnatal testis. *Histol Histopathol* 2004; **19**: 985–97.

82. Sahoo DK, Roy A, Bhanja S, Chainy GB. Hypothyroidism impairs antioxidant defence system and testicular physiology during development and maturation. *Gen Comp Endocrinol* 2008; **156**: 63–70.

83. Velazquez EM, Bellabarba Arata G. Effects of thyroid status on pituitary gonadotropin and testicular reserve in men. *Arch Androl* 1997; **38**: 85–92.

84. Maran RR. Thyroid hormones: their role in testicular steroidogenesis. *Arch Androl* 2003; **49**: 375–88.

85. Meeker JD, Godfrey-Bailey L, Hauser R. Relationships between serum hormone levels and semen quality among men from an infertility clinic. *J Androl* 2007; **28**: 397–406.

86. Meeker JD, Singh NP, Hauser R. Serum concentrations of estradiol and free T4 are inversely correlated with sperm DNA damge in men from an infertility clinic. *J Androl* 2008; **29**: 379–88.

87. Takser L, Mergler D, Baldwin M. *et al.* Thyroid hormones in pregnancy in relation to environmental exposure to organochlorine compounds and mercury. *Environ Health Perspect* 2005; **113**: 1039–45.

88. Kester MHA, Martinez de Mena R, Obregon MJ. *et al.* Iodothyronine levels in the human developing brain: major regulatory roles of iodothyronine deiodinases in different areas. *J Clin Endocrinol Metab* 2004; **89**: 3117–28.

89. Friesema EC, Ganguly S, Abdalla A. *et al.* Identification of monocarboxylate transporter 8 as a specific thyroid hormone transporter. *J Biol Chem* 2003; **278**: 40 128–35.

90. Heuer H, Maier MK, Iden S. *et al.* The monocarboxylate transporter 8 linked to human psychomotor retardation is highly expressed in thyroid hormone-sensitive neuron populations. *Endocrinology* 2005; **146**(4): 1701–6.

# 13.3  The immune system

Robert W. Luebke and Dori R. Germolec

## Overview of the immune system

The immune system is a complex set of cellular, chemical, and soluble mediators that protects the body against foreign substances, including infectious agents and certain tumor cells. Immune cells are located throughout the body, either in discretely encapsulated organs, including the spleen, thymus, and lymph nodes or in diffuse accumulations of lymphoid and myeloid cells, as are found in association with the skin, lung, and the urogenital and GI tracts, which are primary locations for detection of entering pathogens and exogenous proteins.

Immune responses are classified as innate or adaptive. Innate responses occur within hours after the introduction of microbes, and provide the first line of defense against bacterial and viral infections. Innate responses are triggered by pattern recognition receptors that recognize components of microbes that are shared by broad classifications of potential pathogens. The interaction activates cells to release proteins that stimulate migration of additional cells to the site of infection, phagocytosis and destruction of microorganisms, and localized inflammation. Non-specific effector cells include macrophages and polymorphonuclear (PMN) leukocytes that phagocytize pathogens and produce proinflammatory molecules, natural killer (NK) cells that destroy some types of neoplastic and infected cells, and dendritic cells that are "professional" antigen-presenting cells. Cells and products of the innate immune system are critical to developing effective adaptive immunity. A summary of cellular origin, classification, function, and consequences of cell loss are presented in Table 13.1.

In contrast, adaptive immune responses are directed against specific proteins or carbohydrate antigens. These may be molecules such as bacterial cell wall proteins, virulence factors, proteolytic enzymes or peptides that initiate allergic responses. Foreign materials are broken down into peptide fragments by cells of the innate immune system and are presented to cells of the adaptive system, thus triggering a tightly controlled cascade of events that lead to cell division and maturation into effector cells. The process is relatively slow (a week or more to peak response) but very specific for the initiating antigen and results in long-lasting protection against future infections through the generation of long-lived antigen-specific memory cells.

Lymphocytes are the prime cellular effectors of adaptive responses. These cells are broadly classified by the organ in which they mature, and can be subdivided based on function (see Table 13.1). Lymphocyte progenitor cells arise from pluripotent hematopoietic stem cells in the bone marrow and mature in lymphoid organs, T cells in the thymus and B cells in the spleen and lymph nodes. Most (> 95%) immature T cells that initially migrate to the thymus are eliminated, either because of inefficient or overzealous recognition of host antigens. This process of T cell selection in the thymus is critical in establishing and maintaining tolerance to constitutively expressed "self" proteins (antigens) present on somatic cells and certain cell products. Subpopulations of T cells assist in and amplify other immune responses (T helper cells, Th), down-regulate other immune responses (T suppressor cells, TS) or destroy infected or neoplastic cells (cytotoxic T cells, TC). T helper cells produce cytokines that regulate immune function and can be further subdivided into subpopulations which stimulate other T cells (Th1) or stimulate and perpetuate antibody responses (Th2). T helper2 cytokine production predominates in newborns and is also associated with increased allergy and asthma. Soon after birth there is a switch to the Th1-dominated adult phenotype, which is important in eliminating certain bacteria and viruses. Modulation of these processes by xenobiotics can suppress the normally protective function of immune system cells and their products, increasing susceptibility to infection and some types of cancer, or may skew production of regulatory immune system proteins (cytokines) and inappropriately stimulate the immune system, increasing the risk of developing allergies, asthma, or autoimmune diseases.

Disclaimer: This report has been reviewed by the Environmental Protection Agency's Office of Research and Development, and approved for publication. Approval does not signify that the contents necessarily reflect the views and policies of the Agency nor does mention of trade names or commercial products constitute endorsement or recommendation for use. This work was supported by the Division of Intramural Research of the National Institute of Environmental Health Sciences, National Institutes of Health.

*Environmental Impacts on Reproductive Health and Fertility*, ed. T. J. Woodruff, S. J. Janssen, L. J. Guillette, and L. C. Giudice. Published by Cambridge University Press. ©Cambridge University Press 2010.

**Table 13.1.** Cells of the immune system, and consequences of compromised cell function.

| Cell type | Site of maturation | Cell function | Consequences of suppression |
|---|---|---|---|
| T cells | Thymus | | Reduced supply of naïve T cells |
| T helper cells | Thymus | Mediator production that stimulates the inflammatory response (Th1 cells) or antibody synthesis (Th2) | Reduced resistance to intracellular (Th1) or extracellular (Th2) pathogens |
| T regulatory cells | Thymus and peripheral lymphoid tissues | Homeostatic regulation of immune function, silencing of autoreactive T cells | Increased risk of immune mediated damage, including autoimmune disease |
| Cytotoxic T cells | Thymus | Destruction of infected or transformed cells | Reduced resistance to certain viruses, increased risk of certain tumors |
| B cells | Bone marrow, spleen, and lymph nodes | Antibody synthesis | Reduced resistance to extracellular bacteria and some viruses |
| Natural killer (NK) cells | Bone marrow, lymph nodes | Rapid destruction of certain tumors and virally infected cells, cytokine production | Severe or recurrent viral infections, tumors of hematological origin |
| Dendritic cells and macrophages | Bone marrow | Antigen processing and "presentation" to lymphocytes, phagocytosis and killing of pathogens. | Increased susceptibility to infections, suppressed or inappropriate immune responses |
| Polymorphonuclear granulocytes | Bone marrow | Phagocytosis and killing of pathogens | Recurrent infections with extracellular bacteria |

Generally, induction of immune responses follows a process where small lymphocytes divide and differentiate into cells responsible for effector function and immunologic memory. Naïve circulating B cells encounter antigen in lymph nodes, or tissue-associated lymphoid tissues and become activated. The B cells recognize antigen via membrane-bound immunoglobulin (Ig) molecules that act as antigen receptors. Cross-linking of the receptors initiates a signal transduction cascade, and, with the appropriate stimulus from Th2 cytokines, leads to activation, clonal expansion and differentiation into antibody-secreting plasma cells. Five classes of antibodies – IgM, IgG, IgE, IgA, and IgD – have been described and each has distinct expression patterns and functional properties during the immune response.

## Homeostatic control of the immune system

Immune responses that protect the host against infection and neoplasia have the potential to cause significant collateral damage to healthy tissue if the intensity and duration of the response are not controlled. Homeostasis is maintained in part by input from the neuroendocrine system, particularly products of the hypothalamic–pituitary–adrenal axis, which reduces inflammation and attenuates lymphocyte responses by altering cell circulation patterns and inducing apoptosis over the course of an individual response. Subpopulations of cells from the innate and adaptive arms of the immune systems also participate in regulating immune response via soluble mediators that suppress cell function, including inappropriate responses to self antigens. Inherited and acquired defects in regulatory cell performance are associated with inflammatory diseases and autoimmune diseases. The physical and chemical nature of the antigen, and the region of the body where the antigen is encountered, affect antigen processing and presentation, the pattern of cytokines produced by Th cells and, ultimately, the predominant type (humoral or cellular) of adaptive response. T helper1 cytokines favor inflammation and activation of cytotoxic cells whereas Th2 cytokines stimulate antibody responses, resistance to parasitic helminths and allergy. Key members of each cytokine type suppress production of the opposite group, typically to the benefit of the host, although environmental contaminants may skew the balance of Th cytokines, increasing the risk of allergy and, in theory, reducing resistance to certain types of bacterial infection.

## Gender, pregnancy, and the immune response

Modulation of immune function by endocrine hormones is complex in health and disease states, and a

189

comprehensive discussion of the interactions is beyond the scope of this chapter. Studies in laboratory animals have shown that gonadectomy or supraphysiological doses of opposite gender hormones will reverse gender differences in responsiveness. However, there is ample evidence that endocrine hormones modulate immune function, and that xenobiotics present in the environment may mimic, stimulate, or modulate the effects of endocrine hormones on the immune system, causing direct or indirect toxicity.

Innate and adaptive immune responses are influenced by endocrine hormones, particularly the balance between estrogen (17β-estradiol; E2) and testosterone [1, 2]. In general, cell-mediated immunity (e.g. cytotoxic T cell activity), antibody responses (e.g. total concentrations of immunoglobulins in the serum, antibody responses to vaccination) and resistance to infectious diseases are more robust in females, although greater immunoreactivity in females comes at the price of a significantly greater risk of autoimmune disease. Genetic and environmental factors that modulate sex hormone metabolism (e.g. peripheral estrogen hydroxylation, increased aromatase activity) may modify the development and pathogenesis of autoimmune and inflammatory diseases [3]. In addition, genetic differences in the rate of estrogen conversion to proinflammatory metabolites, such as 16-hydroxyestrone, or the relative abundance of naturally occurring antagonists (i.e. 2-hydroxyestrogens), may account for some of the hormonal effects on inflammatory processes. Immune function in females is further regulated by the relative concentration of hormones present during the menstrual cycle, pregnancy, and lactation.

Cells of the innate and adaptive immune systems express both androgen and estrogen receptors, and modulation of immune function is mediated by binding of sex steroids to their cognate receptor. Effects include stimulated differentiation and maturation of antigen-presenting cells (APCs) and B lymphocytes when levels of estrogen are increased, which translates to elevated antibody responses in pregnant versus virgin mice [4]. This observation has toxicological implications, as a possible mode of action responsible for enhanced antibody titers in animals exposed to endocrine-disrupting chemicals during gestation (e.g. propanil [5]; atrazine [6]) or as adults (e.g. malathion [7]; synthetic pyrethroids [8]; hexachlorobenzene [9]; and TCDD [10]). Some of the same compounds have been shown to exacerbate autoimmune disease in animal models of autoimmunity, although the

link between elevated antibody responses in immunotoxicity screening studies and increased risk of autoimmunity has not been thoroughly explored. Studies are currently underway to evaluate the role of physiological estrogen, EDC activity, elevated antibody responses and autoimmunity (Luebke et al., unpublished data).

Pregnancy is generally associated with reduced proinflammatory Th1 responses which are responsible for resistance to intracellular infections, and increased Th2 cytokine production, associated with increased humoral function. This evolutionary adaptation allows viviparous reproduction by preventing rejection of the fetus by the same mechanism that rejects organ grafts from non-identical twins. Paternal histocompatibility antigens are expressed by fetal cells and are readily accessible to and recognized by the maternal immune system. Elevated estrogen levels, in pregnancy or following exogenous administration, skews cytokine production away from the normal profile of Th1 dominance in adults. The shift to Th2 dominance has been described as the primary driver of pregnancy-associated immunosuppression and prevention of fetal rejection [11]. Reduction of Th1 responses also reduces the severity of autoimmune diseases that are primarily inflammatory (e.g. rheumatoid arthritis); however, symptoms of other autoimmune diseases that have a significant humoral component (e.g. systemic lupus erythematosus, SLE) typically worsen during pregnancy and improve after parturition [12]. Recent work suggests that other factors contribute to preventing the immune system from attacking the developing fetus. Early in pregnancy, E2 stimulates development of regulatory T cells that suppress immune responses to paternal antigens; E2 acts by binding to the estrogen receptors present on precursors to these cells [13]. In addition, *Fas-Fas*-ligand interaction mediates apoptosis of maternal T cells, and local production by macrophages of an enzyme that reduces synthesis of tryptophan, required for T cell division, occurs at the maternal–placental interface [14].

Prolactin, commonly recognized for its role in the promotion and support of lactation, also functions as a cytokine in immune tissues. It is structurally related to growth-promoting cytokines and prolactin receptors are members of the cytokine receptor superfamily. Elevated serum prolactin levels are associated with disease flares that occur during pregnancy and the postpartum period in individuals with SLE, rheumatoid arthritis, and multiple sclerosis. Thus, the endocrine system has a determinant role in protecting the fetus from the maternal immune system and also influences the severity, positively and negatively, of autoimmune diseases that affect overall maternal health.

While many of these shifts in the immune response stabilize after childbirth, some changes may be persistent and result in lingering disease. For example, Graves' disease is an autoimmune disease in which autoantibodies are formed to the TSH receptor; the autoantibodies act as a thyrotropic agonist, resulting in hyperthyroidism. The disease frequently becomes quiescent during pregnancy, with a corresponding decrease in antithyroid microsomal, antithyroglobulin, and thyroid-stimulating antibody levels [15]. It has been suggested that disease remission is a result of pregnancy-induced reductions in Th1 responses, and the concomitant increase in Th2 responses. Not surprisingly, the clinical manifestations of Graves' disease are exacerbated in the first several months following delivery as the maternal immune system returns to the "normal" Th1/Th2 balance. The estimated prevalence of postpartum autoimmune thyroiditis is 7.2% in women who were asymptomatic prior to pregnancy, and while the majority of women re-establish normal thyroid function within the first year, approximately 25% will develop permanent hypothyroidism [16].

Concern has been raised with regard to persistent immunologic effects in the children of women who received diethylstilbestrol (DES) during pregnancy to prevent pre-term delivery or pregnancy loss. Diethylstilbestrol, an estrogenic pharmaceutical, was prescribed between the 1940s and 1970s under the erroneous assumption that it would prevent miscarriage, but was discontinued because it increased risk of a rare vaginal cancer in the female offspring. Since that time prenatal exposure to DES has been linked to a number of adverse outcomes in the children and grandchildren. The overall frequency of autoimmune diseases has been reported to be elevated in DES-exposed daughters, when compared with a control group [17]. Other studies suggest that the offspring of DES-treated women exhibit a variety of immune system perturbations, including enhanced T cell proliferation and elevated NK cell activity that could contribute to altered immune function and an elevated risk for autoimmune disease.

## Endocrine-disrupting chemicals, reproductive outcomes, fetal origin of adult disease, and the immune system

Environmental toxicants that modify immune responses and inflammatory processes have the potential to affect reproductive outcomes and the development of adult-onset disease. This may be particularly important when exposures occur during gestation or early in life. Numerous reviews have described the greater sensitivity of the developing immune system to a variety of xenobiotics, and the potential risk assessment implications of conducting hazard identification studies in adults [18–21]. Greater sensitivity during development may be expressed as greater persistence of effects, effects produced at lower doses during immune system ontogeny, or adverse effects in offspring that are not observed in following adult exposure [19]. A variety of chemical classes that have endocrine or endocrine-disrupting activity, including heavy metals, polycyclic aromatic hydrocarbons, dioxins and related compounds, pesticides and drugs have been identified as developmental immunotoxicants (Table 13.2).

Gender-dependent effects on the immune system, manifested either as greater dose sensitivity or as the presence of immune system effects in only one gender, have been reported following exposure to EDCs. For example, Luster et al. [23] determined that humoral immunity was suppressed in female and enhanced in male offspring of dams exposed to DES, whereas Rooney et al. [24] determined that the herbicide atrazine affected only male offspring. These examples suggest that disruption of critical hormone-mediated events during ontogeny of both the immune and reproductive systems may have a profound impact on the observed immune deficits. However, gender-dependent effects on immune function following gestational exposure is not restricted to EDCs, as exposure to 250 ppm of lead in the drinking water during gestation suppressed cellular immunity only in female rats [25]. Although developmental exposure to lead has been reported to reduce body-weight gain and testosterone levels, the authors of the study concluded that effects were not due to "endocrine imprinting" [26].

Inflammation is an important component of many known causes of infertility, and exposure to EDCs may indirectly affect reproductive success through the altered secretion of inflammatory mediators, changes

**Table 13.2.** Examples of endocrine-disrupting developmental toxicants that affect immune function [22].

| Chemical Class | Example |
| --- | --- |
| Pesticides | Atrazine |
| | p,p′-DDE |
| | Heptachlor |
| | Hexachlorobenzene |
| | Methoxychlor |
| | Tributyltin dichloride |
| Industrial chemicals | PCBs |
| | TCDD |
| | Bisphenol-A |
| | Cadmium |
| Drugs/food | DES |
| | Genistein |

p,p′-DDE, 1,1-dichloro-2,2-bis(p-chlorophenyl)ethylene; PCBs, polychlorinated biphenyls; TCDD, 2,3,7,8-tetrachlorodibenzo-p-dioxin; DES, diethylstilbestrol.

in disease resistance, and dysregulation of tolerance. Several epidemiologic studies have linked body-burdens of TCDD or dioxin-like PCBs with increased incidence of endometriosis, an estrogen-dependent disease that affects approximately 10% of women in their reproductive years and has been associated with infertility [27]. The disease is characterized by adhesion of endometrial cells to the peritoneum, subsequent cell proliferation and an inflammatory response. While it has been suggested that defects in NK cell activity and immune surveillance may promote the growth of ectopic endometrial cells, the disease also presents a clinical picture common to a number of autoimmune disorders, including increased levels of autoantibodies specific for histones, endometrial, and ovarian proteins, and Th1-mediated macrophage activation [28]. TCDD has been shown to promote both chronic inflammation and the progression of autoimmune disease, and it has been suggested that TCDD may disrupt the function of both endometrial and immune cells leading to the development of endometriosis [29].

## Conclusions

Endogenous hormones, xenobiotics, and drugs that alter endocrine function have the potential to alter the immune system, and exposure to these entities during gestation may directly or indirectly affect women during pregnancy and subsequent health outcomes in the child. The primary adverse immune system effects include an increased risk of infection secondary to immunosuppression in adults and offspring and an increased risk of autoimmune or inflammatory disease in susceptible populations. Reduced resistance to infectious disease caused by EDC exposure may also contribute to infertility through increased incidence of infection-based pelvic inflammatory disease. There is a growing body of evidence that many aspects of both female and male infertility have at least some autoimmune component, and hormonally active compounds which promote self-reactivity are likely to contribute to these effects. While there is a significant gap in our understanding of the interplay between endocrine-disrupting xenobiotic exposure, reproductive success, and immune system health, multidisciplinary teams have demonstrated the practicality of investigating reproductive, immuno- and neurotoxicity in the same cohorts of offspring [30]. Additional studies of this type, with a focus on dose response and modes of action, will help to clarify the relationship between unintentional immune system modulation and reproductive success.

## References

1. Nalbandian G, Kovats S. 2005. Understanding sex biases in immunity. *Immunol Res* 2005; **31**; 91–106.
2. Verthelyi D. Sex hormones as immunomodulators in health and disease. *Int Immunopharmacol* 2001; **1**: 983–93.

3. Cutolo M, Sulli A, Capellino S. *et al*. Sex hormones influence on the immune system: basic and clinical aspects in autoimmunity. *Lupus* 2004; **13**: 635–8.

4. Dresser, DW. The potentiating effect of pregnancy on humoral immune responses of mice. *J Reprod Immunol* 1991; **20**: 253–66.

5. Salazar KD, Miller MR, Barnett JB. *et al*. Evidence for a novel endocrine disruptor: the pesticide propanil requires the ovaries and steroid synthesis to enhance humoral immunity. *Toxicol Sci* 2006; **93**: 62–74.

6. Rowe AM, Brundage KM, Schafer R. *et al*. Immunomodulatory effects of maternal atrazine exposure on male Balb/c mice. *Toxicol Appl Pharmacol* 2006; **214**: 69–77.

7. Johnson VJ, Rosenberg AM, Lee K. *et al*. Increased T-lymphocyte dependent antibody production in female SJL/J mice following exposure to commercial grade malathion. *Toxicology* 2002; **170**: 119–29.

8. Madsen C, Claesson MH, Röpke C. Immunotoxicity of the pyrethroid insecticides deltametrin and alpha-cypermetrin. *Toxicology* 1996; **107**: 219–27.

9. Michielsen CC, van Loveren H, Vos JG. The role of the immune system in hexachlorobenzene-induced toxicity. *Environ Health Perspect* 1999; **107** (Suppl 5): 783–92.

10. Smialowicz RJ, Riddle MM, Williams WC. *et al*. Effects of 2,3,7,8-tetrachlorodibenzo-p-dioxin (TCDD) on humoral immunity and lymphocyte subpopulations: differences between mice and rats. *Toxicol Appl Pharmacol* 1994; **124**: 248–56.

11. Wegmann TG, Lin H, Guilbert L. *et al*. Bidirectional cytokine interactions in the maternal-fetal relationship: is successful pregnancy a TH2 phenomenon? *Immunol Today* 1993; **14**: 353–6.

12. Verthelyi, D. 2001. Sex hormones as immunomodulators in health and disease. *Int. Immunopharmacol* 2001; **1**: 983–93.

13. Tai P, Wang J, Jin H. *et al*. Induction of regulatory T cells by physiological level estrogen. *J Cell Physiol* 2008; **214**: 456–64.

14. Aluvihare VR, Kallikourdis M, Betz, AG. Regulatory T cells mediate maternal tolerance to the fetus. *Nature Immunol* 2004; **5**: 266–71.

15. Amino N, Izumi Y, Hidaka Y. *et al*. No increase of blocking type anti-thyrotropin receptor antibodies during pregnancy in patients with Graves' disease. *J Clin Endocrinol Metab* 2003; **88**: 5871–4.

16. Stagnaro-Green A. Clinical Review 152: Postpartum thyroiditis. *Clin Endocrinol Metab* 2002; **87**: 4042–7.

17. Noller KL, Blair PB, O'Brien PC. *et al*. Increased occurrence of autoimmune disease among women exposed in utero to diethylstilbestrol. *Fertil Steril* 1988; **49**: 1080–2.

18. Dietert RR, Piepenbrink MS. Perinatal immunotoxicity: why adult exposure assessment fails to predict risk. *Environ Health Perspect* 2006; **114**: 477–83.

19. Luebke RW, Chen DH, Dietert RR. *et al*. The comparative immunotoxicity of 5 selected compounds following developmental or adult exposure. *J Toxicol Environ Health B* 2006; **9**: 1–26.

20. van Loveren H, Piersma A. Immunotoxicological consequences of perinatal chemical exposures. *Toxicol Lett* 2004; **149**: 141–5.

21. Holsapple MP, West LJ, Landreth, KH. Species comparison of anatomical and functional immune system development. *Birth Defects Res* B 2003; **68**: 321–34.

22. World Health Organization. Environmental Health Criteria Documents 180, 236 and 237, Geneva. http://www.inchem.org/pages/ehc.html.

23. Luster MI, Faith RE, McLachlan JA. Alterations of the antibody response following in utero exposure to diethylstilbestrol. *Bull Environ Contam Toxicol* 1978; **20**: 433–7.

24. Rooney AA, Matulka RA, Luebke RW. Developmental atrazine exposure suppresses immune function in male, but not female Sprague–Dawley rats. *Toxicol Sci* 2003; **76**: 366–75.

25. Bunn TL, Parsons PJ, Kao E. *et al*. Gender-based profiles of developmental immunotoxicity to lead in the rat: assessment in juveniles and adults. *J Toxicol Environ Health A* 2001; **64**: 223–40.

26. Ronis MJ, Badger TM, Shema SJ. *et al*. Effects on pubertal growth and reproduction in rats exposed to lead perinatally or continuously throughout development. *J Toxicol Environ Health A* 1998; **53**: 327–41.

27. Foster WG. Endocrine toxicants including 2,3,7,8-terachlorodibenzo-*p*-dioxin (TCDD) and dioxin-like chemicals and endometriosis: is there a link? *J Toxicol Environ Health B Crit Rev* 2008; **11**: 177–87.

28. Minici F, Tiberi F, Tropea A. *et al*. Paracrine regulation of endometriotic tissue. *Gynecol Endocrinol* 2007; **23**: 574–80.

29. Bruner-Tran KL, Yeaman GR, Crispens MA. *et al*. Dioxin may promote inflammation-related development of endometriosis. *Fertil Steril* 2008; **89**: 1287–98.

30. Chapin RE, Harris MW, Davis BJ. *et al*. The effects of perinatal/juvenile methoxychlor exposure on adult rat nervous, immune, and reproductive system function. *Fundam Appl Toxicol* 1997; **40**: 138–57.

# Environmental contaminants and cancers of the reproductive tract

Gail S. Prins and Esther L. Calderon

## Introduction

Many environmental contaminants have been shown to directly or indirectly contribute to carcinogenesis and/or cancer progression of reproductive tract organs. These include endocrine-disrupting chemicals (EDCs), industrial compounds, cigarette smoke, air pollution, radiation, electromagnetic fields, processed foods, alcohol, and pharmaceuticals. This review will focus on EDCs as they relate to reproductive tract cancers due to their unique capacity to contribute to carcinogenesis through hormonal signaling pathways that normally control growth of these end-organs. The readers are referred to other recent review articles for information regarding other environmental contaminants and cancer risk [1–3].

The US Environmental Protection Agency (EPA) defines an EDC as an exogenous agent that interferes with the synthesis, secretion, transport, binding, action, or elimination of natural hormones in the body that are responsible for the maintenance of homeostasis, reproduction, development, and/or behavior [4]. Descriptions of the various types of EDCs that impact reproductive structures and their mechanisms of action are provided in other chapters of this book and the readers are referred to them for detailed information. The present discussion is organized around the major reproductive tract cancers that occur in the human population. In males, evidence for risks of testicular and prostate cancer as a function of exposure to endocrine-disrupting agents will be examined while in females, cancers of the breast, ovaries, and endometrium will be evaluated. As a cross-reference, Table 14.1 summarizes the evidence and provides references for the individual chemicals with regards to reproductive tract tumors. This chapter will primarily review evidence for cancer risks in humans and highlight research conducted on animal models as supportive, or when human data are minimal or lacking altogether, as predictive of potential human risks. In addition to exposures during adult life that may contribute to cancer initiation and growth, we also will emphasize EDC exposures during the critical developmental periods. It has long been appreciated that reproductive tract structures are particularly sensitive to hormones, especially estrogens, during early-life developmental periods. Consequently, it is becoming increasing clear that early-life exposures to EDCs may contribute to adult reproductive tract disorders including hormone-driven cancers, thus providing a developmental basis for these diseases.

## Testicular cancer

Testicular cancer is the most commonly diagnosed malignancy in men between 15–44 years of age in developed countries worldwide. Since incidence for this cancer peaks during early adulthood, its presence at an early life stage is suggested. Likewise, carcinoma *in situ*, the precursor of virtually all germ-cell tumors, is believed to be generated in utero. The vast majority of testicular cancers are germ-cell malignancies which are classified histologically as seminomas and non-seminomas. Interestingly, there is a ten-fold variation in incidence rates of testicular cancers across different populations with the highest rates in Nordic countries (Denmark being the highest) and lowest rates in African countries followed by Asian populations [5]. In the USA, there is also considerable variability among racial groups with Whites having the highest and Blacks and Latinos having the lowest incidence rates.

Testis cancer rates have increased worldwide over the past 35 years with the greatest increase observed in populations of European ancestry. While the causes for this increase remain unresolved, it has been suggested that environmental factors including endocrine-disrupting agents may be contributory [6, 7]. This is

*Environmental Impacts on Reproductive Health and Fertility*, ed. T. J. Woodruff, S. J. Janssen, L. J. Guillette, and L. C. Giudice. Published by Cambridge University Press. © Cambridge University Press 2010.

**Table 14.1.** Summary of evidence for reproductive tract cancer risks in humans and animal model systems as a result of exposure to endocrine-disrupting chemicals.

| Endocrine- disrupting chemicals | Evidence for cancer risk in humans | References | Evidence for cancer risk in experimental models | References |
|---|---|---|---|---|
| Diethylstilbestrol | Elevated testicular cancer risk | [9, 13] | | |
| | | | Elevated prostate cancer risk | [47–50] |
| | Elevated breast cancer risk | [94, 95] | Elevated breast cancer risk | [96] |
| | Elevated ovarian cancer risk | [97, 131] | Elevated ovarian cancer risk | [133] |
| | No correlation to ovarian cancer risk | [132] | | |
| | | | Elevated endometrial cancer risk | [143–145] |
| Chlorinated compounds | | | | |
| PCBs | Elevated testicular cancer risk | [14, 15] | | |
| | Elevated prostate cancer risk | [62–65] | Elevated prostate cancer risk | [66] |
| | No correlation to breast cancer risk | [105] | | |
| Chlordanes | Elevated testicular cancer risk | [14, 15] | | |
| Hepatochlor epoxide | Elevated breast cancer risk | [104] | | |
| DDT/DDE | Elevated testicular cancer risk | [14, 15] | | |
| | Elevated breast cancer risk | [98–100, 102] | | |
| | No correlation to breast cancer risk | [101, 103–105] | | |
| | Elevated ovarian cancer risk | [136] | Elevated ovarian cancer risk | [137] |
| | Elevated endometrial cancer risk | [146] | | |
| | Decreased endometrial cancer risk | [147] | | |
| | No correlation to endometrial cancer risk | [148, 149] | | |
| PBDE | Elevated testicular cancer risk | [14, 15] | | |
| Atrazine | Elevated testicular cancer risk | [20] | | |
| | Elevated prostate cancer risk | [68, 69] | Elevated prostate cancer risk | [67] |
| | Decreased prostate cancer risk | [70, 71] | | |

**195**

*(Continued)*

**Table 14.1.** (cont.).

| Endocrine- disrupting chemicals | Evidence for cancer risk in humans | References | Evidence for cancer risk in experimental models | References |
|---|---|---|---|---|
| | | | Elevated breast cancer risk | [106, 107] |
| | No correlation to breast cancer risk | [108–110] | | |
| | Elevated ovarian cancer risk | [134] | | |
| | Decreased ovarian cancer risk | [108] | Decreased ovarian cancer risk | [153] |
| | No correlation to ovarian cancer risk | [135] | | |
| Vinclozolin | | | Decreased prostate cancer risk | [85] |
| | | | Elevated prostate cancer risk | [86–88] |
| Dieldrin | Elevated breast cancer risk | [98, 99] | | |
| | No correlation to breast cancer risk | [105] | | |
| Aldrin | Elevated breast cancer risk | [103] | | |
| Lindane | Elevated breast cancer risk | [103] | | |
| Phthalates | | | | |
| DBP | | | Elevated testicular cancer risk | [25] |
| PVC | Elevated testicular cancer risk | [26] | | |
| Phenols | | | | |
| BPA | Elevated prostate cancer risk | [60] | Elevated prostate cancer risk | [57–59] |
| | | | Elevated breast cancer risk | [111, 112] |
| Heavy metals | | | | |
| Arsenic | Elevated prostate cancer risk | [79, 83] | Elevated prostate cancer risk | [80–82] |
| | | | Decreased ovarian cancer risk | [138–142] |
| | | | Elevated endometrial cancer risk | [152] |
| Cadmium | Elevated and decreased prostate cancer risk | [75] | Elevated prostate cancer risk | [76, 77] |
| | Elevated breast cancer risk | [113–115] | Elevated breast cancer risk | [116] |
| | Elevated endometrial cancer risk | [150, 151] | Elevated endometrial cancer risk | [116] |

**Table 14.1.** (*cont.*).

| Endocrine- disrupting chemicals | Evidence for cancer risk in humans | References | Evidence for cancer risk in experimental models | References |
|---|---|---|---|---|
| Pesticides | | | | |
| Methyl bromide | Elevated prostate cancer risk | [32] | | |
| Chlorpyrifos | Elevated prostate cancer risk | [32, 34] | | |
| Fonofos | Elevated prostate cancer risk | [32, 34] | | |
| Coumaphos | Elevated prostate cancer risk | [32, 34] | | |
| Phorate | Elevated prostate cancer risk | [32, 34] | | |
| Permethrin | Elevated prostate cancer risk | [32, 34] | | |
| Butylate | Elevated prostate cancer risk | [32, 34] | | |
| UV filters | | | | |
| 4-methyl-benzylidene camphor (4-MBC) | | | Elevated prostate cancer risk | [72, 74] |
| 3-benzylidene camphor (3-BC) | | | Elevated prostate cancer risk | [72, 74] |
| Dioxin | | | | |
| TCDD | Elevated breast cancer risk | [118–120] | | |

See text for chemical names in full.

based, in part, on the recently described testicular dysgenesis syndrome (TDS), a collection of disorders of the male reproductive tract – hypospadias, cryptorchidism, low sperm counts, testicular cancer – that have a common link to abnormal testicular development during fetal/neonatal life. Although multiple disturbances can contribute to this syndrome such as premature birth, intrauterine growth restriction, maternal stress, or genetic abnormalities, there is emerging evidence that inadvertent exposures to EDCs may disrupt in utero testicular development and drive some or all of these disorders which have increased in incidence during the past 10–30 years [8]. Although direct evidence for increased testicular cancer due to EDC exposures is very limited [9], it is noteworthy that men with cryptorchidism and infertility are at increased risk for testicular cancer [10]. Since cryptorchidism and male infertility have been directly linked to EDC exposures, a potential link to testicular cancer is implied.

# Environmental estrogens

Environmental estrogens or xenoestrogens are man-made, non-steroidal chemicals with identified estrogenic activity (estrogen mimics), mostly through activation of nuclear or membrane-associated estrogen receptors. Humans are typically exposed to these chemicals through ingestion, adsorption, or transplacental transfer. Xenoestrogens with possible carcinogenic potential include chlorinated compounds in pesticides and herbicides (methoxychlor, kepone, DDT/DDE, chlordane, dieldrin, aldrin) and industrial products (polychlorinated biphenols or PCBs, tetrachloro-p-dioxin), phenolic derivatives (bisphenol-A, butylated hydroxyanisole), phthalates (di-(2-ethylhexyl) phthalate or DEHP, 1,4-dioxane), atrazine, and heavy metals (arsenic, uranium, cadmium).

### Diethylstilbestrol

Diethylstilbestrol exposure is considered an important model of endocrine disruption and provides proof-of-principle for exogenous estrogenic agents as disruptors of multiple end-organs. A synthetic and potent estrogenic compound, DES was prescribed to pregnant women from the 1950s to1970s to prevent spontaneous abortions with an estimated usage of 2–10 million women worldwide. Its utilization during pregnancy was discontinued in the USA in 1972 and worldwide by 1980 when it was discovered that maternal DES treatment was linked to an increased incidence of vaginal clear-cell adenocarcinoma in DES-exposed daughters [11]. Importantly, DES-exposed sons were identified early as having an increased incidence of reproductive tract abnormalities including hypospadias, cryptorchidism, and reduced sperm counts [12]. More recent assessments reveal an increase in testicular cancer cases in DES sons as compared with controls [9, 13]. The DES outcomes thus raise the possibility that other EDCs may also increase testicular cancer risk.

### Persistent organic pollutants

Persistent organic pollutants are fat-soluble chemicals that bioaccumulate in the human body. Many have estrogenic or antiandrogenic activity and, as such, may perturb male reproductive activity. A link between chlorinated chemicals and testicular cancer has been suggested by studies that found higher levels of PCBs, chlordanes, p,p'-dichlorodiphenyldichloroethylene (DDE) and polybrominated diphenyl ethers (PBDEs) in the serum of mothers of men with testicular cancers as compared with controls [14, 15]. These findings are particularly interesting since serum measurements of organochlorine levels in the men themselves were not associated with cancer risk. Rather, the findings implicate that fetal exposure to these environmental estrogens may predispose to testicular cancer later in life [16]. Recently, a large case-controlled study of military personnel participating in the Servicemen's Testicular Tumor Environmental and Endocrine Determinants (STEED) registry found a significant association between testicular germ cell tumors and higher levels of DDE and chlordanes in prediagnostic serum samples [17]. While both DDE and chlordanes were associated with increased seminomas risk, only DDE levels were associated with elevated risk of non-seminomas. Since these organochlorine pesticides are persistent and bioaccumulate in the body, the authors suggest that early-life exposures may have contributed to the development of testicular cancer in these young men.

### Atrazine

Atrazine, a triazine herbicide, is a high-volume contaminant in agricultural communities and ~60% of individuals in the USA are exposed to it on a daily basis. It acts as an EDC through multiple effects and is considered a xenoestrogen due to its ability to increase aromatase activity and thus increase synthesis of estradiol in cells [18]. Atrazine has been classified as a possible human carcinogen by the International Agency for Research on Cancer [19]. While studies have shown associations with atrazine and cancers of the prostate and ovary (see below), assessment of testicular cancer data is limited. In one epidemiologic assessment of cancer rates in Californian agricultural workers exposed to pesticides, an association was observed between increased testicular cancer and atrazine exposure in Hispanic males but not in other ethnic groups [20]. This now requires further analysis in other exposed populations.

## Phthalates

Phthalates are high-production compounds used as plasticizers in polyvinyl chloride (PVC) products, as constituents in various personal-care products such as cosmetics, perfumes, and baby lotions as well as in medical tubing and catheters. Humans are exposed to ~ 2 mg/day in the general population but occupational and medical exposures can reach much higher levels. Due to lack of metabolic clearance, infants and children are exposed to higher levels of these compounds. Phthalates are a large family of compounds and some have been shown to negatively impact reproductive structures in rodents [21]. These phthalates are believed to act through estrogenic and antiandrogenic mechanisms including alterations in testosterone synthesis and liver steroid metabolism [22]. There is compelling evidence for the involvement of phthalate exposures in TDS in animal models [16, 23]. Further, specific phthalates are associated with reduced ano-genital distance in male infants suggesting a connection to TDS in humans [24]. Unfortunately, rodent models used for TDS studies are not useful for testicular cancer research due to resistance of these species to develop germ-cell cancers. However, testicular carcinoma *in situ* was recently reported in rabbits treated in utero with di-*n*-butyl phthalate (DBP) [25] suggesting that rabbits may be a better model for testicular cancers as a function of EDCs. Importantly, this report suggests a potential for the involvement of early-life phthalate exposure and testicular cancer in humans which will require future investigation. It is noteworthy that a case-controlled study determined a six-fold increased risk for seminomas in plastic workers exposed to PVC suggesting a link to testicular cancer and phthalates in adulthood [26]. Clearly, further studies with robust animal models as well as exposed populations are required to determine whether phthalate exposures can lead to testicular cancers in humans.

## Prostate cancer

The prostate is an androgen-dependent male accessory sex gland. Androgens play a critical role in the initiation and progression of prostate cancer which is the basis for current hormonal treatment strategies. In addition to androgens, estrogen involvement in the etiology of prostatic cancer has been demonstrated and the use of antiestrogens has been recently recognized to have a therapeutic role in prostate cancer management. In the human population, direct connections between EDCs and prostate cancer risk have not been established. Nonetheless, due to the hormonal basis of this disease and the evidence that dietary compounds high in isoflavones (e.g. red clover, genistein) can control prostate cancer growth in humans [27, 28] and animal models [29], there is reasonable cause to evaluate and understand any potential relationship between EDCs and prostate cancer risk. In addition to epidemiologic studies, there are in vitro studies with human prostate cells and in vivo studies in animal models that indicate associations between EDCs and prostate cancer, carcinogenesis, and/or susceptibility.

### Farming and pesticides

Regarding links between prostate cancer and environmental factors in humans (outside of diet), the most compelling data come from the established occupational hazard of farming and increased prostate cancer rates [30–32]. While several variables may contribute to higher prostate cancer rates in farmers, chronic or intermittent exposures to pesticides is the most likely explanation [32, 33]. This is supported by a large epidemiology study (Agricultural Health Study) in a collaborative effort between the NCI, NIEHS, and EPA in the USA that has examined agricultural lifestyles and health in ~90 000 participants in North Carolina

and Iowa since 1993 (www.aghealth.org). Evaluation of > 55 000 pesticide applicators revealed a direct link between methyl bromide exposure, a fungicide with unknown mode of action, and increased prostate cancer rates [32]. Further, 6 out of 45 common agricultural pesticides showed correlation with exposure and increased prostate cancer in men with a familial history, suggesting gene–environment interactions. These six agents were chlorpyrifos, fonofos, coumaphos, phorate, permethrin, and butylate [32, 34]. The first four of these compounds are thiophosphates and share a common chemical structure. While these agents are regarded as acetylcholine esterase inhibitors and have not been shown to have direct estrogenic or antiandrogenic activities, a literature search revealed that these compounds have significant capacity as p450 enzyme inhibitors. In particular, chlorpyrifos, fonofos, and phorate strongly inhibit CYP1A2 and CYP3A4 which are the major p450s that metabolize estradiol, estrone, and testosterone in the liver [35, 36]. Furthermore, the human prostate constitutively expresses CYP1A2 and CYP3A4 enzymes that are involved in intraprostatic metabolism of steroids, drugs, and dietary compounds [37–39]. This raises the possibility that exposure to these compounds may interfere with steroid hormone metabolism by the liver as well as the prostate and, in so doing, alter steroid balance and availability which in turn may contribute to increased prostate cancer risk. A similar mechanism of endocrine disruption in vivo has been identified for PCBs and polyhalogenated aromatic hydrocarbons (including dioxins, BPA, and dibenzo-furans) through potent inhibition of estrogen sulfotransferase which effectively elevates bioavailable estrogens in various target organs [40, 41].

## Environmental estrogens

In men, chronically elevated estrogens have been associated with increased risk of prostate cancer [42]. In rodents, estrogens in combination with androgens induce prostate cancer [43]. There is some evidence that environmental estrogens may be involved in prostate cancers at some level.

### Diethylstilbestrol

Maternal exposure to DES during pregnancy was found to result in more extensive prostatic squamous metaplasia in human male offspring than observed with maternal estradiol alone [44]. While prostatic metaplasia eventually resolved following DES withdrawal, ectasia and persistent distortion of ductal architecture

199

remained [45]. This has lead to the postulation that men exposed prenatally to DES may be at increased risk for prostatic disease later in life although this has not been borne out in the limited population studies conducted to date [46]. However, extensive studies with DES in rodent models predict marked abnormalities in the adult prostate including increased susceptibility to adult-onset carcinogenesis following early DES exposures [47–50].

## Bisphenol-A

Bisphenol-A (BPA) is a synthetic polymer used in the production of polycarbonate plastics and epoxy resins, and significant levels have been found in the urine of 93% of the US population in a recent screen by the CDC [51]. While the affinity of BPA for nuclear estrogen receptors (ER-α and ER-β) is ~10 000 lower than estradiol or DES [52, 53], BPA induces membrane ER through non-genomic pathways with an $EC_{50}$ equivalent to 17β-estradiol suggesting that in vivo estrogenic activity of BPA may be due to non-genomic activation of ER [54, 55].

Effects of BPA with regards to carcinogenic potential, including the prostate gland, have recently been reviewed by an expert panel [56]. In short, there is evidence from rodent models and human prostate cell lines that BPA can influence carcinogenesis, modulate prostate cancer cell proliferation and for some tumors, stimulate progression. Recent reports have provided evidence that early life exposure to BPA may increase susceptibility to hormonal carcinogenesis in the prostate gland, possibly by developmentally reprogramming carcinogenic risk [57, 58]. Studies using a rat model showed that brief neonatal exposure to a low dose of BPA (10 μg/kg bw/day) significantly increased the incidence and grade of prostatic intraepithelial neoplasia (PIN) following adult estrogen exposure. This model of sensitivity to hormonal carcinogenesis is relevant to humans in that relative estradiol levels increase in the aging male and may contribute to prostate disease risk [59]. The above studies further identified alterations in DNA methylation patterns in multiple cell signaling genes in BPA-exposed prostates which suggests that environmentally relevant doses of BPA "imprint" the developing prostate through epigenetic alterations [57, 58].

Knudsen and colleagues examined the influence of BPA on human prostate cancer cells that contained an AR point mutation (AR-T877A) frequently found in advanced prostate cancers of patients who relapsed after androgen-deprivation therapy [60]. They first observed that 1nM BPA activates

AR-T877A in transcriptional assays and leads to unscheduled cell cycle progression and cellular proliferation in vitro in the absence of androgen. Since BPA had no impact on wild-type AR, these data indicate that this gain-of-function AR mutant attained the ability to utilize BPA as an agonist. Subsequent in vivo analyses of the impact of BPA on human prostate tumor growth and recurrence was performed utilizing a mouse xenograft of human cells containing the AR-T877A mutation [61]. At low doses that fall within the reported ranges of human exposure, prostate tumor size increased in response to BPA administration as compared with placebo control and mice in the BPA cohort demonstrated an earlier rise in PSA (biochemical failure). These findings indicate that BPA significantly shortened the time to therapeutic relapse. These outcomes underscore the need for further study of the effects of BPA on tumor progression and therapeutic efficacy.

## Polychlorinated biphenols

Polychlorinated biphenols or PCBs are persistent organic pollutants that bioaccumulate in body fat deposits. A recent analysis of adipose tissue concentrations of PCBs in Swedish men with and without prostate cancer revealed a significant association between PCB levels in the higher quadrants and prostate cancer odds-ratio with the most marked associations for PCB 153 and trans-chlordane [62]. A more extensive epidemiologic study of capacitor–manufacturing plant workers highly exposed to PCBs revealed a strong exposure–response relationship for prostate cancer mortality [63]. This supports previous findings of correlations between PCB 153 and 180 and prostate cancer risk in electric-utility workers [64, 65]. While estrogenic activity of these compounds is a suspected mode of action, there is also evidence that PCBs inhibit estrogen sulfotransferase activity in the liver and effectively increase bioavailable estrogen in the body [40]. Recently, Aroclor-1254, a mixture of 60 PCB pollutants, was tested on rat prostate cells in vitro and shown to disrupt gap junctions, expression of connexin 32 and 43, and increase double-stranded DNA breaks, suggesting that PCBs may be able to transform prostate cells leading to carcinogenesis [66]. Further investigation using animal models is warranted for PCBs and prostate cancer risk.

## Atrazine

Atrazine at environmentally relevant levels has been shown to result in chronic prostatitis in rats [67] which is believed to be a predisposing factor to prostate cancer. Atrazine exposure was associated with a four-to six-fold increase in prostate cancer in men working in an atrazine production facility [68, 69], however, this was refuted in a subsequent case-controlled analysis of these workers [70]. Furthermore, a large epidemiologic study of Californian agriculture workers exposed to atrazine found no increased risk for prostate cancer [71]. The effects of atrazine on the prostate are believed to be a result of its ability to increase aromatase and thus estradiol levels, but they may also be related to its capacity to elevate circulating prolactin levels which have been correlated to prostate cancer risk.

### Ultra violet light filters

There are a few recent reports that ultra violet light filters used in creams to protect against the sun have estrogenic activity [72]. Specifically, 4-methylbenzylidene camphor (4-MBC) and 3-benzyidene camphor (3-BC) are ER-β ligands [73]. While little if any work has been done with regards to these UV filters and human prostate cancer, a few recent reports indicate that developmental exposure to the compounds can alter prostate gland development and estrogen target gene expression in the rat [72, 74]. This raises the possibility that the fetal prostate may be affected following maternal use of these compounds.

### Cadmium

Cadmium has been classified as a known human carcinogen by the International Agency for Research on Cancer and the National Toxicology Program based on epidemiologic studies showing a causal association with lung cancer. Cadmium is known to ligand to ERs and function as an estrogenic mimic. While some large epidemiologic reports have indicated a relationship between cadmium exposure and prostate cancer rates, others have refuted these findings [75]. Nonetheless, there are intriguing reports in the literature which show that cadmium has proliferative action with human prostate cells in vitro through an ER-dependent mechanism and that this exposure is associated with acquisition of androgen-independence [76]. Furthermore, prostatic tumors have been shown to be experimentally induced by oral exposure to cadmium [77]. Since cadmium bioaccumulates in the body, further epidemiologic analysis of cadmium and prostate cancer risk is warranted, particularly in men with occupational exposures.

### Arsenic

Exposure to arsenic has long been associated with a number of diseases including cancers [78, 79]. A recent review of the epidemiologic data has shown an

association between inorganic arsenic exposure from the environment and prostate cancer incidence and mortality in the human population [80]. Importantly, it has been documented that arsenic may mediate some of these effects through endocrine disruption, specifically through interaction with ERs and activation of estrogen-regulated genes [81]. In this context, there is a recent report that arsenic can induce malignant transformation of prostate epithelial cells in vitro and drive them towards an androgen-independent state [82]. Interestingly, this was shown to be mediated through Ras-MAPK pathways and it is possible that membrane ERs may be involved in this process. Epidemiologic studies have shown an association between arsenic exposure and prostate cancer mortality in Taiwan [79], a finding that was substantiated by a later study in the USA [83]. Thus it is possible that endocrine disruption by arsenic can contribute to prostate cancer risk.

## Antiandrogens

While there are no known environmental androgens, endocrine disruptors can also function through antiandrogenic pathways. Since prostate cancer is an androgen-dependent disease, we will briefly examine the known effects of some of these agents on the prostate gland.

### Vinclozolin

Vinclozolin is a fungicide that is used as a pesticide on crops. It has known antiandrogenic properties by interfering with androgen receptor (AR) activity [84]. Since vinclozolin effects are driven through AR antagonism, it is not surprising that there are no reported associations between this compound and prostate cancer, an androgen-dependent disease. Exposure of rats to vinclozolin during development results in reduced prostate gland growth and size, which would be expected for an antiandrogen [85]. Of interest, however, are recent studies with maternal (i.e. in utero) exposure to vinclozolin in rats which produce transgenerational effects on offspring through epigenetic alterations [86]. These permanent perturbations include adverse consequences on the prostate gland such as premature acinar atrophy and aging-associated prostatitis for four generations [87]. This may be particularly significant in light of recent evidence that chronic inflammation may play a role in prostate cancer initiation [88].

### DDT/DDE

Dichlorodiphenyltrichloroethane (DDT) and its metabolic derivative dichlorodiphenyldichloroethylene

201

(DDE) were widely used as pesticides in the USA and their use is still in effect in other countries worldwide. In addition to AR antagonistic effects [89], DDE at high concentrations has been shown to function as an inhibitor of 5α-reductase, the intraprostatic enzyme responsible for converting testosterone to the more potent androgen, dihydrotestosterone [90]. While many reproductive abnormalities have been found with DDT/DDE exposure, including reduced prostate growth, there is no known association between exposure to DDT/DDE and prostate cancer risk.

# Breast cancer

Breast cancer is the most common invasive malignancy in women in the USA and is the second leading cause of cancer-related deaths in the female population [91]. Similar to the prostate, breast cancer is a hormonally driven cancer and one major identified risk factor for breast cancer is an increased lifetime exposure to estrogens [92]. A comprehensive analysis of published reports on chemicals causing mammary gland tumors in animal models has been recently published and is an excellent resource for many agents including EDCs [2]. Population-based studies have also examined human EDC exposures as they relate to breast-cancer risks and a searchable database for epidemiologic studies on environmental pollutants and breast cancer is available at www.komen.org/environment [93]. There is compelling evidence for a role of several EDCs, primarily acting through estrogenic pathways, on breast-cancer risk and progression. Beginning with DES as a model EDC during the developmental period, population-based evidence is presented below for several of these compounds.

## Environmental estrogens

### Diethylstilbestrol

Continued follow-up of mothers who used DES during pregnancy has shown a moderate increased risk for the development of breast cancer in the mothers with aging [94]. As mentioned previously, the DES-exposed daughters exhibited an increased incidence of vaginal clear-cell adenocarcinoma at a young age which led to discontinuation of its utilization during pregnancy [11]. Since animal models predicted an increased risk for the development of other female reproductive tract tumors in DES-exposed offspring, follow-up analysis of case-controlled cohorts of exposed populations has continued. A recent report of a large cohort of women

prenatally exposed to DES and followed since the 1970s revealed an increased risk for the development of breast cancer after 40 years of age [95]. The incidence rate ratio of breast cancer occurring after 40 years of age was 1.91 compared with case controls and increased to 3.00 for breast cancers occurring after 50 years, suggesting a heightened risk with aging. The highest relative risk was observed for cohorts receiving the highest cumulative dose of DES exposure, further suggesting a dose–response effect for breast cancer development. Studies using animal models for fetal DES exposure now suggest that adverse effects may be transmitted to the third generation male and female offspring [96]. Since the human population of DES-exposed granddaughters and grandsons is limited in size at this time and relatively young, studies have not yet observed a significant increase in breast-cancer rates in the third generation and this possibility will require continued monitoring for decades to come [97].

### Persistent organochlorine pesticides

Many organochlorine pesticides used at high volumes worldwide, such as dieldrin, aldrin, chlordanes, and DDT/DDE, are classified as EDCs since they either possess estrogenic or antiandrogenic activity or they modulate estrogen action through changes in metabolism or excretion of steroids. These persistent chemicals accumulate in fatty tissues such as the breast with half-lives lasting many years and thus have the potential to contribute to the development of breast cancer. In 1998, a cohort-nested case–control study was undertaken on Danish women who had blood specimens collected and stored for 17 years as participants in a Copenhagen City Heart Study [98]. Several organochlorines were measured in these stored serum samples and breast cancer incidence, stage, and survival were determined by record linking to the Denmark national registry. Serum dieldrin levels were associated with a significantly increased dose-related risk of breast cancer and in a follow-up study, had a significant adverse effect on breast cancer survival [99]. These studies suggest that exposures to dieldrin in the distant past affect not only breast-cancer risk but also survival from the disease decades later. It is noteworthy that these studies did not find a correlation of breast-cancer risk with DDE levels although a linear trend was noted for higher DDE concentrations and breast cancer survival. In a recent prospective, nested case–control study in California, serum samples from young women collected between 1959–1967, when DDT was widely used as a pesticide, were measured for DDT and DDE, and breast-cancer cases were analyzed from the state cancer registry in 1998 [100]. High serum levels of DDT correlated with a significant five-fold increased risk of breast cancer before the age of 50 years, again suggesting that early-life DDT exposures may increase cancer risk during adulthood. However, a recent nested case–control Japanese study found no relationship between serum DDT or DDE levels and breast cancer incidence after 10 years of follow-up [101]. The differences in these studies may be in the age that serum was collected for organochlorine measurements since the positive associations were noted in samples collected in young adulthood.

Other population-based studies have examined the relationship of breast cancer to serum or tissue organo-chlorine levels at the time of cancer diagnosis. A case–control study of women living in Mexico City evaluated serum DDE levels and compared them against levels in matched control women without cancer [102]. Women in the top quartile of DDE levels were twice as likely to have a breast-cancer diagnosis and this association increased in postmenopausal women suggesting that current DDE exposures may increase breast-cancer risk. Adipose tissue levels of 16 organochlorine pesticides including DDE were measured in Spanish women at the time of breast cancer diagnosis in another case-controlled study [103]. While DDE levels were higher in cases than controls, the difference was not significant. Significant increases in breast-cancer risk were noted for all women with detectable aldrin levels and for postmenopausal women with measurable aldrin and lindane. Interestingly, risk was greatest in lean women with the highest quartile of total organochlorines as compared with those with higher body mass. While a small Texas study did not find a link between adipose DDE or chlordane levels and breast-cancer risk, heptachlor epoxide, another cyclodiene pesticide was positively associated with breast cancer prevalence [104]. In contrast, the Long Island Breast Cancer Study Project found no association of breast-cancer risk for any measured organochlorines including DDE, chlordane, dieldrin, or PCB congeners [105]. It is possible that racial and regional differences exist with regards to cancer susceptibility as a function of these specific environmental exposures.

## Atrazine

Atrazine has been linked to increased mammary tumors in rodent models, however, this was shown to be a function of neuroendocrine alterations that shift puberty and cause premature reproductive senescence rather than actions as a direct carcinogen [106, 107]. Although it has been shown to increase aromatase activity in human cancer-cell lines [18], population-based studies have not found a positive association between atrazine exposures or serum levels and increased risk of breast cancers in women [108–110].

## Bisphenol-A

The relationship between BPA exposures and breast-cancer risk has not been evaluated in the human population. Similar to the prostate gland, animal models for breast cancer predict that the fetal/neonatal developmental period may be the most sensitive for BPA exposures as they relate to reprogramming of the breast and increasing cancer susceptibility in later life. Rats perinatally exposed to low-dose BPA (2.5 µg/kg/bw per day) showed a three- to four-fold increase in the number of hyperplastic ducts in adulthood as compared with vehicle-treated animals and these lesions appeared to progress to carcinoma *in situ* [111]. In another study, rats treated with 25 µg BPA/kg/bw per day were evaluated for tumorigenic susceptibility of the mammary gland to subcarcinogenic doses of the known mammary carcinogen, N-nitroso-N-methylurea (NMU). At 4 and 7 months, histological tumors were observed in 20% of rats treated with BPA followed with NMU, whereas rats exposed only to NMU failed to form any tumors [112]. Together, these reports indicate that perinatal exposure to BPA results in the formation of an adult mammary gland that has an increased susceptibility to tumorigenic insults that may either be spontaneous in nature or the result of a later carcinogenic challenge. These findings provide concern for human exposures to this ubiquitous chemical and future population-based studies are considered necessary.

## Cadmium

In addition to occupational exposure, tobacco smoke and food are the largest intake sources for this heavy metal. As with prostate cancer, recent studies have indicated a link between cadmium exposure and human breast cancer. A prospective case–control study measured urinary cadmium levels in 500 women with or without breast cancer and found that women in the highest quartile of cadmium levels had greater than two-fold breast-cancer risk [113]. Further, there was a significant increase in risk with increasing cadmium levels suggesting a positive dose–response relationship. Studies in Europe found that tissue breast-cancer concentrations of cadmium were significantly higher in neoplastic regions compared with benign tissue suggesting a potential relationship between cadmium and carcinogenic effects within the affected cells [114, 115]. That these effects may be through endocrine disruption is supported by animal studies that show potent in vivo estrogen-like activity of cadmium in the mammary gland and uterus [116].

## Dioxins and industrial PCBs

Dioxins are polyhalogenated aromatic hydrocarbons that are known environmental toxicants and carcinogens for a variety of end-organs in all vertebrates. These persistent EDCs bioaccumulate and mediate responses via high-affinity binding to the aryl hydrocarbon receptor (AhR) [117]. The most common is 2,3,7,8-tetra-chlorodibenzo-*p*-dioxin (TCDD). The major sources for dioxins in the environment come from paper and pulp manufacturing, waste incineration and production of certain herbicides and they enter the food chain through accumulation in dietary fats in milk, fish, and meat. The manufacturing plant accident in Seveso, Italy in 1976 led to dioxin exposure at high levels to nearly 1000 women living in the area. Analysis of breast cancer in exposed women found a two-fold increased incidence between 1976–1998 associated with a ten-fold increase in serum TCDD levels [118] and follow-up of this population continues. Other studies of women living near a production facility [119] or occupationally exposed to dioxins [120] have also observed significant elevations in breast-cancer rates. Thus evidence is increasing for a direct relationship between PCB exposures and breast-cancer risk in the human population and this demands continued and increased monitoring as well as detailed research to explain the cellular and molecular pathways involved.

## Ovarian cancer

Ovarian cancer is the eighth most common cancer in women in the USA and has the highest mortality rate of any female reproductive tract cancer. While ovarian cancer can arise from granulosa cells, germ cells, and stromal cells, the vast majority of epithelial ovarian cancer (EOC) arises from the ovarian surface epithelium which itself comprises a tiny component of the normal ovary [121, 122]. Interestingly, in EOC, epithelial cells become more differentiated as they undergo neoplasia and it has been shown that they express multiple müllerian duct characteristics [123, 124]. The National Cancer Institute (NCI) classifies EOC as serous, endometrioid, mucinous, or clear-cell, in

which serous adenocarcinomas have a fallopian tube histology, endometrioid have an endometrium histology, mucinous carcinomas have an endocervix histology, and clear-cell tumors resemble urogenital tract histology [123, 125]. Among these types, the serous EOC remains the most common with approximately 80% incidence.

The high mortality rate of ovarian cancer is mainly due to its asymptomatic nature; hence diagnosis is usually assessed at later stages, when the disease has metastasized to other organs [126]. It has been noted that ovarian cancer develops mainly in postmenopausal women around 55 years of age or older. Although the etiology of ovarian cancer remains unclear, some suspected contributors are cyclic ovulation with continual rupture/repair of the surface epithelium [127], late age at menopause, infertility, and obesity. On the other hand, pregnancy, oral contraceptive use, and hysterectomy are protective of EOC [128] which is believed to be a function of anovulation. Other suggested potential causes of ovarian cancer are exposure to environmental agents such as talc, pesticides, and herbicides, and life-style factors.

## Environmental estrogens

In women, estradiol is produced by the action of aromatase on androgens in both granulosa and surface epithelial cells [128, 129]. Although the etiology of EOC remains unclear, estradiol has been long suspected to play a role in the development of the disease. A study looking at the effects of estradiol exposure on ovarian surface epithelial morphology in rabbits found that estradiol stimulates ovarian surface epithelial-cell proliferation and formation of a papillary ovarian surface morphology as seen on serous EOC [128, 130].

### Diethylstilbestrol

Early examination of women given DES during pregnancy reported a 2.83-fold increased relative risk of ovarian cancer in these mothers as compared with non-exposed mothers, although this was not statistically significant [131]. Continued observation of DES-exposed daughters exposed to DES in utero has not seen an increased incidence of ovarian cancer in that population [132]. However, in preliminary studies of DES-exposed granddaughters – those whose mothers were exposed to DES in utero (also referred to as the DES third generation) – a higher frequency was noted for ovarian cancer than predicted [97]. While the numbers are low and could be a chance occurrence, it is interesting to note that mouse models have also shown increased rates of ovarian cancer in the third generation following in utero DES [133]. In summary, there is provocative evidence for the involvement of early-life estrogen exposures and ovarian cancer risk, and this warrants examination of other EDCs for similar risks.

## Atrazine

Since atrazine has been shown to increase aromatase expression, there has been concern regarding its carcinogenic potential for the ovary, a tissue high in aromatase. A population-based, case–control study of Italian women exposed to herbicidal triazines as farmers reported a 2.7 relative risk for ovarian epithelial neoplasms with trends observed for both duration and probability of exposure [134]. Another epidemiologic study, conducted on 22 counties in central California for a period of 2 years, examined whether women with EOC had an increased occupational exposure to triazine herbicides. Analysis of ever versus never occupational exposure to triazines showed slight but not significant likelihood of exposure to the herbicides in EOC patients compared with controls [135]. In an ecological study using secondary data with atrazine concentrations in Kentucky's drinking water, increased atrazine exposure was associated with a decreased incidence in ovarian cancer over a 5-year period [108]. Furthermore, an experimental study in which ovarian cancer was induced in Sprague–Dawley rats also showed a reduced incidence of ovarian cancer after dietary intake of atrazine for a period of 50 weeks at concentrations of 5, 50, and 500 ppm. In summary, although the more recent findings do not support a relationship between atrazine exposure and increased ovarian cancer risk and provide evidence that it may decrease risk, the studies are limited in number as well as lacking in actual atrazine measurements in the exposed populations. This area will require more detailed work to determine if a risk exists.

## Persistent organic pollutants

An epidemiologic study examined the effects of organochlorine compounds (OCC) on ovarian hormones of 50 Laotian-born immigrant women of reproductive ages 18–40 residing in the San Francisco Bay area who consumed fish on a regular basis [136]. Since this area has been shown to have high levels of several organochlorine pesticides, PCBs, and mercury, serum samples were analyzed for these compounds. The investigators found that serum samples contained organochlorine compounds including DTT, its metabolite DDE, and 10 polychlorinated biphenyl (PCB) congeners, all of which had mean levels higher than typical US populations. The urine samples collected from these women were tested for metabolites of estrogen and progesterone as well as women's menstrual cycle parameters. The investigators found that the progesterone metabolite levels during the luteal phase were decreased with higher concentrations of DDE. Mean cycle length was approximately 4 days shorter and the adjusted mean luteal phase length was 1.5 days shorter in the highest quartile concentration of DDT and DDE as compared with the lowest quartile. This study indicates a potential effect of DDE on ovarian function which may in turn influence fertility, pregnancy, and reproductive cancers. Williams and colleagues examined the effects of TCDD on the protein kinase C pathway in the ID8 ovarian surface epithelial cancer-cell line. They found that TCDD increased protein expression, kinase activity and induces the subcellular redistribution of PCK-$\delta$ which suggests a potential role for this kinase as an effecter molecule for TCDD-mediated events in EOC cells [137]. While these studies are provocative, they have not been substantiated with in vivo studies due to a paucity of available animal models for spontaneous ovarian cancer. Currently, there is a lack of epidemiologic evidence for a role of persistent organic pollutants in ovarian cancer risks in humans and this is an area of study that requires investigation.

## Arsenic

In contrast to studies that have linked estrogen-mimic heavy metals with cancer induction, several studies with arsenic have found that arsenic has potential use as a therapeutic agent for ovarian cancer. An in vitro study using prostate cancer-cell lines DU145 and PC-3 and the ovarian cancer-cell line MDAH2774 found that arsenic at different concentrations had a cytotoxic effect through induction of apoptosis [138]. This was replicated in a study using cisplatin-sensitive 3AO ovarian cancer cells and cisplatin-resistant 3AO/CDDP cells where arsenic induced apoptosis and inhibited cell proliferation in both cell lines [139]. A separate study used MDAH2774 cells to determine the effect of arsenic on topoisomerase II levels. This enzyme changes the topology of DNA by separating and recombining the DNA helix during cell replication and studies have shown that topoisomerase II expression is elevated in ovarian cancer. Increasing concentrations of arsenic decreased topoisomerase II levels in MDAH2774 cells suggesting a protective effect of arsenic in ovarian cancer [140]. Another interesting study demonstrated antiproliferative and cytotoxic effects of arsenic loaded into MDAH2774 cells via microemulsion [141]. Additionally, the investigators observed that by delivering higher dilution microemulsion, there was a 1.5-fold increase in apoptosis. A recent study examined the potential for arsenic in regulating peritoneal invasive activity in ovarian cells in vitro and in vivo. The results demonstrated a protective effect of arsenic in vitro and in vivo against peritoneal invasiveness in a dose-dependent manner [142]. In conclusion, studies with arsenic suggest that it may be protective against ovarian cancer and may hold therapeutic promise. It is important to note, however, that there is a lack of animal studies to support this at present as well as epidemiologic evidence to suggest a protective effect. Since arsenic is an estrogen mimic, future therapeutic studies using arsenic for ovarian cancer must proceed with caution.

# Endometrial cancer

Endometrial cancer is the most common cancer found in the reproductive tract of American women. This uterine cancer arises from the uterine lining in contrast to uterine sarcoma, which develops in the myometrium, and cervical cancer, which begins in the cervix. In addition, the uterus can also present with common benign conditions such as myometrial fibroids, endometriosis in which endometrial tissue grows outside the uterus, and endometrial hyperplasia in which cells of the lining of the uterus increase in number. Unlike ovarian cancer, endometrial cancer presents with symptoms such as unusual vaginal bleeding, abnormal discharge, and pelvic pain. Endometrial cancer risks proposed by the American Cancer Society include aging, late onset of menopause, nulliparity, infertility, obesity, diabetes, and the use of estrogen treatments. Since a major risk factor for this cancer is estrogen action unopposed by progesterone, exposure to estrogens or estrogen agonists from pesticides, herbicides, and other environmental contaminants have the potential to play a role in endometrial cancer initiation or promotion. A few studies have been conducted to evaluate this possibility and they are discussed below.

## Environmental estrogens

### Diethylstilbestrol

Animal studies have shown that developmental exposure to DES results in a high incidence of uterine adenocarcinoma with aging in a murine model [143, 144]. Although increased rates of uterine cancers have not been observed in DES-exposed daughters in the human population, the rodent data could be predictive of cancers yet to arise. It is of particular interest that onset of uterine adenocarcinoma in neonatal DES-exposed mice required a secondary hormonal "push" by pubertal steroids since prepubertally ovariectomized mice did not develop cancers [143]. A new study has shown that this is a direct function of specific DNA methylation changes induced by the secondary pubertal hormones that occur only in mice that were first exposed neonatally to DES or genistein [145]. This serves to emphasize the subtle influences of adult life experiences on disease manifestation from early-life exposures.

### Persistent organic pollutants

There is conflicting evidence on the association of persistent organic pollutants with endometrial cancer risk in humans. A case-controlled study in Sweden examined the adipose tissue concentration of DDE, PCBs, hexachlorobenzene, chlordanes and polybrominated biphenyls (PBBs) in women with benign endometrial hyperplasia and findings suggested an interaction between DDE and abnormal endometrial growth (odds-ratio of 1.9) which further increased to 2.3 if women also used estrogen-replacement therapy [146]. However, in another case-controlled study, serum concentrations of organochlorine compounds, DDT, DDE, and PCBs showed no link between organochlorine compounds and the risk of endometrial cancer [147]. Further, a separate epidemiologic study in Sweden looking at serum concentrations of 10 chlorinated pesticides and 10 PCB congeners in females with endometrial cancer found no significant association between high levels of organochlorine compound exposure with the incidence of the cancer [148]. In summary, while epidemiologic data on endometrial cancer are limited, the ecological and occupational studies performed thus far have not provided a clear association between organochlorine exposure and increased risk of endometrial cancer [149].

### Cadmium

An in vivo study using female Sprague–Dawley rats examined whether cadmium could act as an estrogen agonist in the uterus [116]. Rats were ovariectomized at 4 weeks, exposed to an environmentally relevant level of cadmium or estradiol 3 weeks later and their uteri were examined 4 days after exposure. Similar to estradiol, there was a 1.9-fold increase in uterine weight following cadmium exposure which could be blocked by the estrogen receptor antagonist ICI 182,780. Histologic studies revealed that the increased weight was due to a mitogenic response of endometrial cells which resulted in uterine hyperplasia and hypertrophy. Rats treated with cadmium in utero exhibited an early onset of puberty. Taken together, these provide clear evidence that cadmium functions as an estrogen mimic in endometrial tissue. In humans, cadmium levels were found to be markedly decreased in uterine tissue of women with myomas but only modestly suppressed in uterine samples obtained from women with endometrial cancer as compared with age-matched women with a lesion-free uterus [150]. While this does not support a role for cadmium acting as an estrogen mimic to drive uterine pathology, the authors note that altered cadmium was associated with changes in levels of other trace elements with which cadmium interacts, suggesting a potential indirect effect. In a recent long-term population cohort study (Swedish Mammography Cohort), the incidence of postmenopausal endometrial cancer was examined in association to dietary intake of cadmium. The results found a significant association between cadmium dietary intake and increased risk of endometrial cancer over 16 years of follow-up, with an overall relative risk of 1.39 when comparing women in the highest and lowest cadmium tertile [151]. Among never-smoking women with normal body mass index, the relative risk for endometrial cancer increased to 1.86. Further, there was a 2.9-fold increased risk associated with long-term cadmium intake above the median for over 10 years. The authors propose that these findings support the hypothesis that cadmium may increase the risk of this hormone-related cancer through its estrogenic effects. In total, the scanty amount of literature thus far suggests that cadmium may increase the risk of endometrial cancer; however, further evidence in vivo and in vitro, as well as cellular and molecular mechanisms of action, are needed to fully understand the effects and risks of this metal on endometrial cancer.

### Arsenic

Evidence for a relationship between arsenic and endometrial cancer is limited to a single interesting study with CD1 mice that investigated fetal arsenic exposure at environmentally relevant doses without or with subsequent neonatal exposure to DES [152]. Over a 90-week period, in utero arsenic alone produced a 6%

incidence of uterine adenocarcinoma, neonatal DES alone produced no uterine malignancies while combined in utero arsenic with neonatal DES resulted in a uterine cancer incidence of 21%. Prenatal arsenic increased uterine estrogen receptor-α expression and with subsequent neonatal DES treatment, there was marked overexpression of pS2 (also known as trefoil factor 1), an estrogen-regulated gene. When combined with vaginal and ovarian tumors, mice treated prenatally with arsenic and postnatally with DES showed a 48% incidence of malignant tumors. These findings are similar to those of DES cited above where in utero exposures can be influenced by subsequent lifetime estrogenic exposures to alter uterine cancer risks. Clearly, early-life arsenic exposure requires further examination for its potential risk in predisposing or inducing endometrial cancer in combination with lifetime estrogenic exposures.

## Summary

There is accumulating and consistent evidence across the hormone-dependent reproductive tract organs that exposures to endocrine-disrupting chemicals over a lifetime are associated with an increased risk of cancers. Published findings for the individual chemicals are summarized in Table 14.1 as they pertain to risks for reproductive tract cancers. While the findings for individual compounds, classes of compounds, and individual organs in humans may be somewhat limited and at times contradictory, the evidence must be considered as a whole. Overall, there are clear trends that support a link between early-life EDC exposures as well as accumulation of persistent EDCs throughout life and an increased risk of testicular, prostate, breast, ovarian, and endometrial cancers. This is supported with a wealth of research using animal models as well as in vitro systems that has allowed researchers to dissect potential mechanisms of action. It appears that specific chemicals or classes of compounds may show an association and role in some but not necessarily all of the reproductive organ cancers. In fact, this is to be expected since the separate organs express different levels and types of steroid receptors as well as many other genes in differential amounts which will render a unique response to each chemical. At the same time, there are also common responses to some agents (e.g. DES) across all five organs with regards to carcinogenic potential which likely reflects a response by receptors common to all of these organs (e.g. estrogen receptor-α). Clearly, continued animal and epidemiologic studies are required over the next several years to accurately determine risks of cancers as a function of accumulating EDCs in the environment. These evaluations will be critical for the establishment of proper guidelines and federal regulations regarding use, exposure, and dispersal of these compounds. The development of biomarkers for EDC exposures would also be of great future benefit to the medical and regulatory community as we try to link exposures with disease outcomes. In summary, while there has been significant progress in determining human cancer risks from environmental factors, there is much that remains to be done in the decades to come.

# References

1. Belpomme D, Irigaray P, Hardell L. *et al.* The multitude and diversity of environmental carcinogens. *Environ Res* 2007; **105**: 414–29.

2. Rudel RA, Attfield KR, Schifano JN, Brody JG. Chemicals causing mammary gland tumors in animals signal new directions for epidemiology, chemical testing and risk assessment for breast cancer prevention. *Cancer Suppl* 2007; **109**: 2635–66.

3. National Cancer Institute, Cancer and the Environment, U. S. Department of Health and Human Services 2003; http://www.cancer.gov/images/Documents/5d17e03e-b39f-4b40-a214-e9e9099c4220/

4. U. S. Environmental Protection Agency, Office of Prevention, Pesticides and Toxic Substances, 2002; http://www.epa.gov/scipoly/oscpendo/history/glossary.html

5. Purdue MP, Devesa SS, Sigurdson AJ, McGlynn KA. International patterns and trends in testis cancer incidence. *Int J Cancer* 2005; **115**: 822–7.

6. Skakkebaek NE, Rajpert-De Meyts E, Jørgensen N. *et al.* Germ cell cancer and disorders of spermatogenesis: an environmental connection? *Acta Pathologica, Microbiologica, Immunologica Scand* 1998; **106**:3–11.

7. Safe S. Environmental estrogens:roles in male reproductive tract problems and in breast cancer. *Rev Environ Health* 2002; **17**: 253–62.

8. Vidaeff AC, Sever LE. In utero exposure to environmental estrogens and male reproductive health: a systematic review of biological and epidemiologic evidence. *Reprod Toxicol* 2005; **20**: 5–20.

9. Martin OV, Shialis T, Lester JN. *et al.* Testicular dysgenesis syndrome and the estrogen hypothesis: a quantitative meta-analysis. *Environ Health Perspect* 2008; **116**: 149–57.

10. Garner MJ, Turner MC, Ghadirian P, Krewski D. Epidemiology of testicular cancer: an overview. *Int J Cancer* 2005; **116**: 331–9.

11. Herbst AL, Ulfelder H, Poskanzer DC. Adenocarcinoma of the vagina: association of maternal stilbestrol therapy with tumor appearance in young women. *New Engl J Med* 1971; **284**: 878–81.

12. Gill WB, Schumacher GF, Bibbo M, Straus FH, Schoenberg HW. Association of diethylstilbestrol exposure in utero with cryptorchidism, testicular hypoplasia and semen abnormalities. *J Urology* 1979; **122**: 36–9.

13. Strohsnitter W, Noller KL, Hoover RN. *et al.* Cancer risk in men exposed in utero to diethylstilbestrol. *J Nat Cancer Inst* 2001; **93**: 545–51.

14. Hardell L, van Bavel B, Lindstrom G. *et al.* Increased concentrations of polychlorinated biphenyls, hexachlorobenzene, and chlordanes in mothers of men with testicular cancer. *Environ Med* 2003; **111**: 930–4.

15. Hardell L, Bavel B, Lindström GA. In utero exposure to persistent organic pollutants in relation to testicular cancer risk. *Int J Andrology* 2006; **29**: 228–34.

16. Sonne SB, Kristensen DM, Novotny GW. *et al.* Testicular dysgenesis syndrome and the origin of carcinoma in situ testis. *Int J Androl* 2008; **31**: 275–87.

17. McGlynn KA, Quaraishi SM, Graubard B. *et al.* Persistent organochlorine pesticides and risk of testicular germ cell tumors. *J Natl Cancer Inst* 2008; **100**: 663–71.

18. Fan W, Yanase T, Morinaga H. *et al.* Atrazine-induced aromatase expression is SF-1 dependent: implications for endocrine disruption in wildlife and reproductive cancers in humans. *Environ Health Perspect* 2007; **115**: 720 – 7.

19. IARC. *Evaluating Carcinogenic Risks in Humans: Some Chemicals that Cause Tumors of the Kidney or Urinary Bladder in Rodents and Some Other Substances*. Lyon, France: World Health Organization, 1999.

20. Mills PK. Correlation analysis of pesticide use data and cancer incidence rates in California counties. *Arch Environ Health* 1998; **53**: 410–13.

21. Fischer JS. Environmental anti-androgens and male reproductive health: focus on phthalates and testicular dysgenesis syndrome. *Reproduction* 2004; **127**: 305–15.

22. Ge RS, Chen GR, Tanrikut C, Hardy MP. Phthalate ester toxicity in Leydig cells: developmental timing and dosage considerations. *Reprod Toxicol* 2007; **23**: 366–73.

23. Gray LE, Ostby J, Furr J. *et al.* Perinatal exposure to the phthalates DEHP, BBP, and DINP, but not DEP, DMP, or DOTP, alters sexual differentiation of the male rat. *Toxicol Sci* 2000; **58**: 350–65.

24. Swan SH, Main KM, Liu F. *et al.* Decrease in anogenital distance among male infants with prenatal phthalate exposure. *Environ Health Perspect* 2005; **113**: 1056–61.

25. Veeramachaneni DN. Impact of environmental pollutants on the male: effects on germ cell differentiation. *Animal Reprod Sci* 2008; **105**: 144–57.

26. Ohlson CG, Hardell L. Testicular cancer and occupational exposures with a focus on xenoestrogens in polyvinyl chloride plastics. 2000; *Chemosphere* **40**: 1277–82.

27. Jarred RA, Keikha M, Dowling C. et al. Induction of apoptosis in low to moderate-grade human prostate carcinoma by red clover-derived dietary isoflavones. *Cancer Epidemiol Biomarkers Prev* 2002; **11**: 1689–96.

28. Lakshman M, Xu L, Ananthanarayanan V. et al. Dietary genistein inhibits metastasis of human prostate cancer in mice. *Cancer Res* 2008; **68**: 2024–32.

29. McCormick DL, Johnson WD, Bosland MC, Lubet RA, Steele VE. Chemoprevention of rat prostate carcinogenesis by soy isoflavones and by Bowman–Birk inhibitor. *Nutr Cancer* 2007; **57**: 184–93.

30. Morrison H, Savitz D, Semenciw R. et al. Farming and prostate cancer mortality. *Am J Epidemiol* 1993; **137**: 270–80.

31. Meyer TE, Coker AL, Sanderson M., Symanski E. A case-control study of farming and prostate cancer in African-American and Caucasian men. *Occup Environ Med* 2007; **64**: 155–60.

32. Alavanja MC, Samanic C, Dosemeci M. et al. Use of agricultural pesticides and prostate cancer risk in the Agricultural Health Study cohort. *Am J Epidemiol* 2003; **157**: 800–14.

33. Van Maele-Fabry G, Libotte V, Willems J, Lison D. Review and meta-analysis of risk estimates for prostate cancer in pesticide manufacturing workers. *Cancer Causes Control* 2006; **17**: 353–73.

34. Mahajan R, Bonner MR, Hoppin JA, Alavanja MC. Phorate exposure and incidence of cancer in the agricultural health study. *Environ Health Perspect* 2006; **114**(8): 1205–9.

35. Usmani KA, Rose RL, Hodgson E. Inhibition and activation of the human liver microsomal and human cytochrome P450 and 3A4 metabolism of testosterone by deployment-related chemicals. *Drug Metab Dispos* 2003; **31**: 384–91.

36. Usmani KA, Cho TM, Rose RL, Hodgson E. Inhibition of the human liver microsomal and human cytochrome P450 1A2 and 3A4 metabolism of estradiol by deployment-related and other chemicals. *Drug Metab Dispos* 2006; **34**: 1606–14.

37. Lawson T, Kolar C. Human prostate epithelial cells metabolize chemicals of dietary origin to mutagens. *Cancer Lett* 2002; **175**: 141–6.

38. Finnström N, Bjelfman C, Söderström T. G, et al. Detection of cytochrome P450 mRNA transcripts in prostate samples by RT-PCR. *Eur J Clin Invest* 2001; **31**: 880–6.

39. Sterling KM, Cutroneo UR. Constitutive and inducible expression of cytochromes P4501A (CYP1A1 and CYP1A2) in normal prostate and prostate cancer cells. *J Cell Biochem* 2004; **91**: 423–9.

40. Kester MH, Bulduk S, Tibboel D. et al. Potent inhibition of estrogen sulfotransferase by hydroxylated PCB metabolites: a novel pathway explaining the estrogenic activity of PCBs. *Endocrinology* 2000; **141**: 1897–900.

41. Kester MH, Bulduk S, van Toor H. et al. Potent inhibition of estrogen sulfotransferase by hydroxylated metabolites of polyhalogenated aromatic hydrocarbons reveals alternative mechanism for estrogenic activity of endocrine disrupters. *J Clin Endocrinol Metab* 2002; **87**: 1142–50.

42. Modugno F, Weissfeld JL, Trump DL, et al. Allelic variants of aromatase and androgen and estrogen receptors: toward a multigenic model of prostate cancer risk. *Clin Cancer Res* 2001; 7: 3092–6.

43. Leav I, Ho S, Ofner P. et al. Biochemical alterations in sex hormone-induced hyperplasia and dysplasia of the dorsolateral prostates of Noble rats. *J Natl Cancer Inst* 1988; **80**: 1045–53.

44. Driscoll SG, Taylor SH. Effects of prenatal maternal estrogen on the male urogenital system. *Obstet Gynecol* 1980; **56**: 537–42.

45. Yonemura CY, Cunha GR, Sugimura Y, Mee SL. Temporal and spatial factors in diethylstilbestrol-induced squamous metaplasia in the developing human prostate. II. Persistent changes after removal of diethylstilbestrol. *Acta Anat* 1995; **153**: 1–11.

46. Giusti RM, Iwamoto K, Hatch EE. Diethylstilbestrol revisited: a review of the long-term health effects. *Ann Int Med* 1995; **122**: 778–88.

47. Arai Y, Mori T, Suzuki Y, Bern HA. Long-term effects of perinatal exposure to sex steroids and diethylstilbestrol on the reproductive system of male mammals. In: Bourne GHaD, J. F.,eds. *International Review of Cytology*. New York: Academic Press, 1983; 235–68.

48. Rajfer J, Coffey DS. Sex steroid imprinting of the immature prostate. *Invest Urol* 1978; **16**: 186–90.

49. Prins GS, Birch L, Habermann H. et al. Influence of neonatal estrogens on rat prostate development. *Reprod Fertil Dev* 2001; **13**: 241–52.

50. Huang L, Pu Y, Alam S, Birch L, Prins GS. Estrogenic regulation of signaling pathways and homeobox genes during rat prostate development. *J Andrology* 2004; **25**: 330–7.

51. Calafat AM, Ye X, Wong LY, Reidy JA, Needham LL. Exposure of the U.S. population to bisphenol A and 4-tertiary-octylphenol: 2003–2004. *Environ Health Perspect* 2008; **116**: 39–44.

52. Kuiper GG, Lemmen JG, Carlsson B. et al. Interaction of estrogenic chemicals and phytoestrogens with estrogen receptor beta. *Endocrinology* 1998; **139**: 4252–63.

53. Lemmen JG, Arends RJ, van der Saag PT, van der Burg B. In vivo imaging of activated estrogen receptors in

utero by estrogens and bisphenol A. *Environ Health Perspect* 2004; **112**: 1544–9.

54. Song KH, Lee K, Choi HS. Endocrine disruptor bisphenol A induces orphan nuclear receptor Nur77 gene expression and steroidogenesis in mouse testicular Leydig cells. *Endocrinology* 2002; **143**: 2208–15.

55. Walsh DE, Dockery P, Doolan CM. Estrogen receptor independent rapid non-genomic effects of environmental estrogens on [Ca2+]i in human breast cancer cells. *Mol Cell Endocrinol* 2005; **230**: 23–30.

56. Keri R, Ho SM, Hunt PA. *et al.* An evaluation of evidence for the carcinogenic activity of bisphenol A: report of NIEHS Expert Panel on BPA. *Reprod Toxicol* 2007; **24**: 240–52.

57. Ho SM, Tang WY, Belmonte J, Prins GS. Developmental exposure estradiol and bisphenol A (BPA) increases susceptibility to prostate carcinogenesis and epigenetically regulates phosphodiesterase type 4 variant (PDE4D4) in the rat prostate. *Cancer Res* 2006; **66**: 5624–32.

58. Prins GS, Tang WY, Belmonte J, Ho SM. Perinatal exposure to oestradiol and bisphenol A alters the prostate epigenome and increases susceptibility to carcinogenesis. *Basic Clin Pharmacol Toxicol* 2008; **102**: 134–8.

59. Kaufman JM, Vermeulen A. The decline of androgen levels in elderly men and its clinical and therapeutic implications. *Endocrine Rev* 2005; **26**: 833–76.

60. Wetherill YB, Fisher NL, Staubach A. *et al.* Xenoestrogen action in prostate cancer: pleiotropic effects dependent on androgen receptor status. *Cancer Res* 2005; **65**: 54–65.

61. Wetherill YB, Hess-Wilson JK, Comstock CE. *et al.* Bisphenol A facilitates bypass of androgen ablation therapy in prostate cancer. *Mol Cancer Therapy* 2006; **5**: 3181–90.

62. Hardell L, Andersson SO, Carlberg M. *et al.* Adipose tissue concentrations of persistent organic pollutants and the risk of prostate cancer. *J Occup Environ Med* 2006; **48**: 700–7.

63. Prince MM, Ruder AM, Hein MJ. *et al.* Mortality and exposure response among 14,458 electrical capacitor manufacturing workers exposed to polychlorinated biphenyls (PCBs). *Environ Health Perspect* 2006; **114**: 1508–14.

64. Ritchie JM, Vial SL, Fuortes LJ. *et al.* Organochlorines and risk of prostate cancer. *J Occup Environ Med* 2003;**45**: 692–702.

65. Charles LE, Loomis D, Shy CM. *et al.* Electromagnetic fields, polychlorinated biphenyls, and prostate cancer mortality in electric utility workers. *Am J Epidemiol* 2003; **157**: 683–91.

66. Cillo F, de Eguileor M, Gandolfi F, Brevini T. Aroclor-1254 affects mRNA polyadenylation, translational activation, cell morphology, and DNA integrity of rat primary prostate cells. *Endocrin Relat Cancer* 2007; **14**: 257–66.

67. Stoker TE, Robinette C, Cooper RL. Maternal exposure to atrazine during lactation suppresses suckling-induced prolactin release and results in prostatitis in the adult offspring. *Toxicol Sci* 1999; **52**: 68–79.

68. MacLennan PA, Delzell E, Sathiakumar N. *et al.* Cancer incidence among triazine herbicide manufacturing workers. *J Occup Environ Med* 2002; **44**: 1048–58.

69. Sass J. Cancer incidence among triazine herbicide manufacturing workers: reply. *J Occup Environ Med* 2004; **45**: 343–4.

70. Hessel PA, Kalmes R, Smith TJ. *et al.* A nested case-control study of prostate cancer and atrazine exposure. *J Occup Environ Med* 2004; **46**: 379–85.

71. Rusiecki JA, De Roos A, Lee WJ. *et al.* Cancer incidence among pesticide applicators exposed to atrazine in the Agricultural Health Study. *J Natl Cancer Inst* 2004; **96**: 1375–82.

72. Schlumpf M, Schmid P, Durrer S. *et al.* Endocrine activity and developmental toxicity of cosmetic UV filters – an update. *Toxicology* 2004; **205**: 113–22.

73. Schlumpf M, Jarry H, Wuttke W, Ma R, Lichtensteiger W. Estrogenic activity and estrogen receptor beta binding of the UV filter 3-benzylidene camphor. Comparison with 4-methylbenzylidene camphor. *Toxicology* 2004; **199**: 109–20.

74. Hofkamp L, Bradley S, J. T, Lichtensteiger W, Schumpf M, Timms B. Region-specific growth effects in the developing rat prostate following developmental exposure to estrogenic UV filters. *Environ Health Perspect* 2008; **116**: 867–72.

75. Parent ME, Siemiatycki J. Occupation and prostate cancer. *Epidemiol Rev* 2001; **23**: 138–43.

76. Benbrahim-Tallaa L, Liu J, Webber MM, Waalkes MP. Estrogen signaling and disruption of androgen metabolism in acquired androgen-independence during cadmium carcinogenesis in human prostate epithelial cells. *Prostate* 2007; **67**: 135–45.

77. Waalkes MP. Cadmium carcinogenesis in review. *J Inorg Biochem* 2000; **79**: 241–4.

78. Watson WH, Yager JD. Arsenic: extension of its endocrine disruption potential to interference with estrogen receptor-mediated signaling. *Toxicol Sci* 2007; **98**: 1–2.

79. Chen CJ, Kuo T, Wu M. Arsenic and cancers. *Lancet* 1988; **1**: 414–5.

80. Benbrahim-Tallaa L, Waalkes MP. Inorganic arsenic and human prostate cancer. *Environ Health Perspect* 2008; **116**: 158–64.

81. Davey JC, Bodwell JE, Gosse JA, Hamilton J. Arsenic as an endocrine disruptor: effects of arsenic on estrogen receptor-mediated gene expression in vivo and in cell culture. *Toxicol Sci* 2007; **98**: 75–86.

82. Benbrahim-Tallaa L, Webber MM, Waalkes MP. Mechanisms of acquired androgen independence during arsenic-induced malignant transformation of human prostate epithelial cells. *Environ Health Perspect* 2007; **115**: 2.

83. Lewis DR, Southwick JW, Ouellet-Hellstrom R, Rench J, Calderon R. Drinking water aresenic in Utah: A cohort mortality study. *Environ Health Prospect* 1999; **107**: 359–65.

84. Kavlok R, Cummings A. Mode of action: inhibition of androgen receptor function – vinclozolin-induced malformations in reproductive development. *Crit Rev Toxicol* 2005; **35**: 721–6.

85. Yu W, Lee B, Nam S. *et al.* Reproductive disorders in pubertal and adult phase of the male rats exposed to vinclozolin during puberty. *J Vet Med Sci* 2004; **66**: 847–53.

86. Anway MD, Cupp AS, Uzumcu M, Skinner MK. Epigenetic transgenerational actions of endocrine disuptors and male fertility. *Science* 2005; **308**: 1466–9.

87. Anway M, Skinner M. Transgenerational effects of the endocrine disruptor vinclozolin on the prostate transcriptome and adult onset disease. *Prostate* 2008; **68**: 515–29.

88. Nelson WG, DeWeese TL, DeMarzo AM. The diet, prostate inflammation, and the development of prostate cancer. *Cancer Metast Rev* 2002; **21**: 3–16.

89. Gray LE, Wolf C, Lambright C. *et al.* Administration of potentially antiandrogenic pesticides (procymidone, linuron, iprodione, chlozolinate, p,p'-DDE, and ketoconazole) and toxic substances (dibutyl- and diethylhexyl phthalate, PCB 169, and ethane dimethane sulphonate) during sexual differentiation produces diverse profiles of reproductive malformations in the male rat. *Toxicol Ind Health* 1999; **15**: 94–118.

90. Lo S, King I, Alléra A, Klingmüller D. Effects of various pesticides on human 5alpha-reductase activity in prostate and LNCaP cells. *Toxicol in Vitro* 2007; **21**: 502–8.

91. Jemal A, Siegel R, Ward E. *et al.* Cancer Statistics, 2008. *CA Cancer J Clin* 2008; **58**: 71–96.

92. Laden F, Hunter DJ. Environmental risk factors and female breast cancer. *Annu Rev Public Health* 1998; **19**: 101–23.

93. Brody JG, Moysich KB, Humblet O. *et al.* Environmental pollutants and breast cancer: epidemiologic studies. *Cancer* 2007; **109**: Suppl. 12.

94. Veurink M, Koster M, Berg LT. The history of DES, lessons to be learned. *Pharm World Sci* 2005; **27**: 139–43.

95. Palmer JR, Wise LA, Hatch EE. *et al.* Prenatal diethylstilbesterol exposure and risk of breast cancer. *Cancer Epidemiol Biomarkers Prev* 2006; **15**: 1509–14.

96. Newbold RR, Padilla-Banks E, Jefferson WN. Adverse effects of the model environmental estrogen diethylstilbestrol are transmitted to subsequent generations. *Endocrinology* 2006; **147**: S11–17.

97. Titus-Ernstoff L, Troisi R, Hatch EE. *et al.* Offspring of women exposed in utero to diethylstilbestrol (DES): a preliminary report of benign and malignant pathology in the third generation. *Epidemiology* 2008; **19**: 251–7.

98. Hoyer AP, Grandjean P, Jorgenson T, Brock JW, Hartving HB. Organochlorine exposure and risk of breast cancer. *Lancet* 1998; **352**: 1816–20.

99. Hoyer AP, Jorgenson T, Brock JW, Grandjean P. Organochlorine exposure and breast cancer survival. *J Clinical Epidemiology* 2000; **53**: 323–30.

100. Cohn BA, Wolff MS, Cirillo PM, Sholtz RI. DDT and breast cancer in young women: new data on the significance of age at exposure. *Environ Health Perspect* 2007; **115**: 1406–14.

101. Iwasaki M, Inoue M, Sasazuki S. *et al.* Plasma organochlorine levels and subsequent risk of breast cancer among Japanese women: a nested case-control study. *Sci Total Environ* 2008; **402**: 176–83.

102. Romieu I, Hernandez-Avila M, Lazcano-Ponce E, Weber JP, Dewailly E. Breast cancer, lactation history, and serum organochlorines. *Am J Epidemiol* 2000; **152**: 363–70.

103. Ibarluzea JJ, Fernández MF, Santa-Marina L. *et al.* Breast cancer risk and the combined effect of environmental estrogens. *Cancer Causes Control* 2004; **15**: 591–600.

104. Cassidy RA, Natarajan S, Vaughan GM. The link between the insecticide heptachlor epoxide, estradiol, and breast cancer. *Breast Cancer Res Treat* 2006; **90**: 55–64.

105. Gammon MD, Wolff MS, Neugut AI. *et al.* Environmental toxins and breast cancer on Long Island. II. Organochlorine compound levels in blood. *Cancer Epidemiol Biomarkers Prev* 2002; **11**: 686–97.

106. Eldridge JC, Wetzel LT, Stevens JT, Simpkins JW. The mammary tumor response in triazine-treated female rats: a threshold-mediated interaction with strain and species-specific reproductive senescence. *Steroids* 1999; **64**: 672–8.

107. Cooper RL, Laws SC, Das PC. *et al.* Atrazine and reproductive function: mode and mechanism of action studies. *Birth Defects Res B Dev Reprod Toxicol* 2007; **80**: 98–112.

108. Hopenhayn-Rich C, Stump ML, Browning SR. Regional assesment of atrazine exposure and incidence of breast and ovarian cancers in Kentucky. *Arch Environ Contam Toxicol* 2002; **42**: 127–36.

109. Gammon DW, Aldous CN, Carr WC, Sanborn JR, Pfeifer KF. A risk assessment of atrazine use in

California: human health and ecological aspects. *Pest Manag Sci* 2005; **61**: 331–55.

110. McElroy JA, Gangnon RE, Newcomb PA. *et al.* Risk of breast cancer for women living in rural areas from adult exposure to atrazine from well water in Wisconsin. *J Expo Sci Environ Epidemiol* 2007; **17**: 207–14.

111. Murray TJ, Maffini MV, Ucci AA, Sonnenschein C, Soto AM. Induction of mammary gland ductal hyperplasias and carcinoma in situ following fetal bisphenol A exposure. *Reprod Toxicol* 2007; **23**: 383–90.

112. Durando M, Kass L, Piva J. *et al.* Prenatal bisphenol A exposure induces preneoplastic lesions in the mammary gland in Wistar rats. *Environ Health Perspect* 2007; **115**: 80–6.

113. McElroy JA, Shafer MM, Trentham-Dietz A, Hampton JM, Newcomb PA. Cadmium exposure and breast cancer risk. *J Natl Cancer Inst* 2006; **98**: 869–73.

114. Rydzewska A, Król I, Lipin'ski L. Concentration of cadmium in breast cancer tissue of women living in the Wielkopoiska region. *Przeql Lek* 2004; **61**: 786–8.

115. Strumylaite L, Bogusevicius A, Ryselis S. *et al.* Association between cadmium and breast cancer. *Medicina* 2008; **44**: 415–20.

116. Johnson MD, Kenney N, Stoica A. *et al.* Cadmium mimics the in vivo effects of estrogen in the uterus and mammary gland. *Nature Med* 2003; **9**: 1081–4.

117. Van den Berg M, Birnbaum L, Bosveld AT. *et al.* Toxic equivalency factors (TEFs) for PCBs, PCDDs, PCDFs for humans and wildlife. *Environ Health Perspect* 1998; **106**: 775–92.

118. Warner M, Eskenazi B, Mocarelli P. *et al.* Serum dioxin concentrations and breast cancer risk in the Seveso Women's Health Study. *Environ Health Perspect* 2002; **110**: 625–8.

119. Revich B, Aksel E, Ushakova T. *et al.* Dioxin exposure and public health in Chapaevsk, Russia. *Chemosphere* 2001; **43**: 951–66.

120. Flesch-Janys D, Becher H, Manz A. *et al.* Epidemiologic investigation of breast cancer incidence in a cohort of female workers with high exposure to PCDD/F and HCH. *Organohalogen Compounds* 1999; **44**: 379–82.

121. Leung PC, Choi JH. Endocrine signaling in ovarian surface epithelium and cancer. *Human Reprod Update* 2007; **13**: 143–62.

122. Wang G, Shang HL, Xie Y. *et al.* Effects of mifepristone on the proliferation, apoptosis and cis-diaminedichloroplatinum sensitivity of cultured chemoresistant human ovarian cancer cells. *Chin Med J (Engl)* 2005; **118**: 333–6.

123. Auersperg N, Wong AS, Choi KC, Kang SK, Leung PC. Ovarian surface epithelium: biology, endocrinology, and pathology. *Endocrin Rev* 2001; **22**: 255–88.

124. Auersperg N, Ota T, Mitchell GW. Early events in ovarian epithelial carcinogenesis: progress and problems in experimental approaches. *Int J Gynecol Cancer* 2002; **12**: 691–703.

125. National Cancer Institute. *National Institutes of Health* 2008; http://www.cancer.gov/cancertopics/types/ovarian

126. McGuire WP, Markman M. Primary ovarian cancer chemotherapy: current standards of care. *Br J Cancer* 2003; **89**: S3–8.

127. Fathalla M. Incessant ovulation – a factor in ovarian neoplasia? *Lancet* 1971; **2**(7716): 163.

128. Salehi F, Dunfield L, Phillips KP, Krewski D, Vanderhyden BC. Risk factors for ovarian cancer: an overview with emphasis on hormonal factors. *J Toxicol Environ Health B Crit Rev* 2008; **11**: 301–21.

129. Cunat S, Rabenoelina F, Daurès JP. *et al.* Aromatase expression in ovarian epithelial cancers. *J Steroid Biochem Mol Biol* 2005; **93**: 15–24.

130. Bai W, Oliveros-Saunders B, Wang Q, Acevedo-Duncan ME, Nicosia SV. Estrogen stimulation of ovarian surface epithelial cell proliferation. *In Vitro Cell Dev Biol Anim* 2000; **36**: 657–66.

131. Hadjimichael OC, Meigs JW, Falcier FW, Thompson WD, Flannery JT. Cancer risk among women exposed to exogenous estrogens during pregnancy. *J Natl Cancer Inst* 1984; **73**: 831–4.

132. Troisi R, Hatch EE, Titus-Ernstoff L. *et al.* Cancer risk in women prenatally exposed to diethylstilbestrol. *Int J Cancer* 2007; **121**: 356–60.

133. Walker BE. Tumors of female offspring of mice exposed prenatally to diethylstilbestrol. *J Natl Cancer Inst* 1984; **73**: 1133–40.

134. Donna A, Crosignani P, Robutti F. *et al.* Triazine herbicides and ovarian epithelial neoplasms. *Scand J Work Environ Health* 1989; **15**: 47–53.

135. Young HA, Mills PK, Riordan DG, Cress RD. Triazine herbicides and epithelial ovarian cancer risk in Central California. *J Occup Environ Med* 2005; **47**: 1148–56.

136. Windham GC, Lee D, Mitchell P. *et al.* Exposure to organochlorine compounds and effects on ovarian function. *Epidemiology* 2005; **16**: 182–90.

137. Williams SR, Son DS, Terranova PF. Protein kinase C delta is activated in mouse ovarian surface epithelial cancer cells by 2,3,7,8-tetrachlorodibenzo-p-dioxin (TCDD). *Toxicology* 2004; **195**: 1–17.

138. Uslu R, Sanli UA, Sezgin C. *et al.* Arsenic trioxide-mediated cytotoxicity and apoptosis in prostate and ovarian carcinoma cell lines. *Clin Cancer Res* 2000; **6**: 4957–64.

139. Kong B, Huang S, Wang W. *et al.* Arsenic trioxide induces apoptosis in cisplatin-sensitive and -resistant

ovarian cancer cell lines. *Int J Gynecol Cancer* 2005; **15**: 872–7.

140. Askar N, Cirpan T, Toprak E. *et al.* Arsenic trioxide exposure to ovarian carcinoma cells leads to decreased level of topoisomerase II and cytotoxicity. *Int J Gynecol Cancer* 2006; **16**: 1552–6.

141. Terek MC, Karabulut B, Selvi N. *et al.* Arsenic trioxide-loaded, microemulsion-enhanced cytotoxicity on MDAH 2774 ovarian carcinoma cell line. *Int J Gynecol Cancer* 2006; **16**: 532–7.

142. Zhang J, Wang B. Arsenic trioxide (As(2)O(3)) inhibits peritoneal invasion of ovarian carcinoma cells in vitro and in vivo. *Gynecol Oncol* 2006; **103**: 199–206.

143. Newbold RR, Bullock BC, McLachlan JA. Uterine adenocarcinoma in mice following developmental treatment with estrogens: a model for hormonal carcinogenesis. *Cancer Research* 1990; **50**: 7677–81.

144. Caserta D, Maranghi L, Mantovani A. *et al.* Impact of endocrine disruptor chemicals in gynaecology. *Hum Reprod Update* 2008; **14**: 59–72.

145. Tang WY, Newbold RR, Mardilovich K. *et al.* Persistent hypomethylation in the promoter of nucleosomal binding protein 1 (Nsbp1) correlates with overexpression of Nsbp1 in mouse uteri neonatally exposed to diethylstilbestrol or genistein. *Endocrinology* 2008; **149**: 5919–21.

146. Hardell L, van Bavel B, Lindström G. *et al.* Adipose tissue concentrations of p,p'-DDE and the risk for endometrial cancer. *Gynecol Oncol* 2004; **95**: 706–11.

147. Sturgeon SR, Brock JW, Potischman N. *et al.* Serum concentrations of organochlorine compounds and endometrial cancer risk (United States). *Cancer Causes Control* 1998; **9**: 417–24.

148. Weiderpass E, Adami HO, Baron JA. *et al.* Organochlorines and endometrial cancer risk. *Cancer Epidemiol Biomarkers Prev* 2000; **9**: 487–93.

149. Adami HO, L. L, Titus-Ernstoff L, Hsieh CC, *et al.* Organochlorine compounds and estrogen-related cancers in women. *Cancer Causes Control* 1995; **6**: 551–66.

150. Nasiadek M, Krawczyk T, Sapota A. Tissue levels of cadmium and trace elements in patients with myoma and uterine cancer. *Hum Exp Toxicol* 2005; **24**: 623–30.

151. Akesson A, Julin B, Wolk A. Long-term dietary cadmium intake and postmenopausal endometrial cancer incidence: a population-based prospective cohort study. *Cancer Res* 2008; **68**: 6435–41.

152. Waalkes MP, Liu J, Ward JM, Powell DA, Diwan BA. Urogenital carcinogenesis in female CD1 mice induced by in utero arsenic exposure is exacerbated by postnatal diethylstilbestrol treatment. *Cancer Res* 2006; **66**: 1337–45.

153. Terasaka S, Aita Y, Inoue A. *et al.* Using a customized DNA microarray for expression profiling of the estrogen-responsive genes to evaluate estrogen activity among natural estrogens and industrial chemicals. *Environ Health Perspect* 2004; **112**: 773–81.

# Communicating with patients and the public about environmental exposures and reproductive risk

Gina M. Solomon and Sarah J. Janssen

## Communication of environmental health risks

There is widespread concern among the general public about environmental health risks, especially risks to infants and children [1]. Patients frequently come in to their health-care provider's office with questions about environmental hazards but health-care providers often do not feel prepared to address these concerns. A survey to assess provider knowledge and behavior on reproductive environmental health in members of the Association for Reproductive Health Professionals (ARHP) found nearly 60% of those surveyed reported their knowledge of environmental health was less than adequate [2].

Discussions about reproductive risk and the environment can occur in an office setting with an individual patient, in a group at a workplace or community meeting, or in a public policy context. These contexts will be discussed separately in this chapter because there are different scientific issues, different needs from the listener, and different roles for the clinician.

## Communication about individual risk

In the patient-care setting, environmental health concerns tend to focus on questions about individual risk. People bring worries about specific exposures or illnesses to their personal physician. Because the science on environmental health does not pertain to individual risk but rather to population risk, the challenge to the health-care professional is substantial.

Even assuming that the health-care provider is familiar with the scientific data relevant to the issue in question, there remains a challenge in translating a combination of complex and sometimes conflicting results from a variety of sources such as in vitro assays, laboratory rodent studies, and limited human epidemiological research to practical advice for a patient's individual situation. This problem is further complicated by difficulties in exposure assessment, the fact that individuals are exposed to mixtures and not single chemicals, and differing effects of chemicals when exposure occurs during vulnerable periods of the lifespan. The resulting conversation must therefore move away from a focus on trying to "answer the question" toward a more open discussion of scientific uncertainty, risk, and prevention.

## Risk communication contexts

Individuals may come to their health-care provider either after an adverse event (such as a miscarriage or a birth defect) has occurred, or they may have concerns of potential future harm while they are pregnant or planning a pregnancy. They may have had exposure to an occupational or environmental hazard, or there may be no obvious exposures. These possibilities allow patient risk-communication encounters to be categorized in four ways (Table 15.1).

Patients who have suffered from an *adverse event* are generally focused on exploring causation. They may be trying to understand what happened, to assign blame, or to recover compensation for the event. Individuals who have suffered a *known hazardous exposure*, irrespective of dose or of whether an adverse event has occurred, may require counseling about their future risk and may have questions about biological monitoring for their body burden of the chemical, and potential treatment options to reduce their risk. In all cases of a known exposure to an environmental hazard, it is wise to involve specialists in occupational and environmental medicine or environmental health. In addition, these are situations where public health agency

*Environmental Impacts on Reproductive Health and Fertility*, ed. T. J. Woodruff, S. J. Janssen, L. J. Guillette, and L. C. Giudice. Published by Cambridge University Press. © Cambridge University Press 2010.

**Table 15.1.** Categories of patient presentations requiring risk communication.

| | Adverse event | No adverse event |
|---|---|---|
| Known exposure | Causality questions<br>Worker's compensation<br>Medico-legal<br>Need for public health intervention | Counseling about future risk<br>Reduction of other risk factors<br>Treatment questions<br>Need for public health intervention |
| Unknown or no known exposure | Occupational/environmental history<br>Biomonitoring questions | Occupational/environmental history<br>Anticipatory guidance |

intervention may be needed to identify other exposed individuals and to reduce or eliminate future risk.

The most common patient-care situations involve individuals with no known unusual environmental exposures, who are seeking routine preconception or prenatal care. The health-care provider should take a screening occupational and environmental health history in all patients to assess for potential reproductive hazards. Anticipatory guidance is a cornerstone of prenatal care and should include occupational and environmental health hazards. In addition, the provider should be prepared to respond to common questions from patients.

## Tools for communicating with patients

### Explaining the problem of scientific uncertainty

Many patients believe that science "proves" or "disproves" links between potential environmental hazards and health effects. The many shades of uncertainty, data gaps, and data quality problems are not issues most people have grappled with in their personal or professional lives. Yet communicating about reproductive risk requires the clinician to convey these uncertainties as a way of explaining why there are no clear answers to most questions.

Most people believe that all chemicals in commerce have been scientifically tested for toxicity, and would not be allowed for use if they had not been proven safe. Unfortunately, only approximately 23% of chemicals produced in excess of a million pounds or more have been tested for reproductive toxicity [3]. The statistics are even grimmer for smaller volume chemicals. Of the 80 000 plus chemicals that have been registered for use over the past 65 years, only a handful have reproductive toxicity data and usually this information comes to light because of academic, not industry or government, research. When people are told that there is no information related to the reproductive risk of a chemical, they often respond with disbelief and anxiety.

Many scientific links between exposure and adverse effects are based on animal toxicology studies. People respond to rodent data based on their preconceptions about risk, with some people dismissing such results as irrelevant to humans, and others finding any such results alarming, irrespective of data quality. The clinician can point out the animal toxicology findings and add cautions appropriate to the situation, either to encourage precautionary action to reduce exposure, or to indicate the difficulty of establishing causation based on limited animal toxicology data.

Even when the hazard associated with an environmental agent is known, the dose a patient may have received is often unknown. Route of exposure, dose, and timing of exposure are important determinants of risk. Some people may be falsely reassured, for example, learning that an exposure to a known reproductive toxicant was below the OSHA Permissible Exposure Limit (PEL), even though these limits are not designed to protect against reproductive toxicity. Other people may be extremely anxious about a single low-dose, short-term exposure and require extensive counseling and reassurance.

Even with known developmental toxicants such as lead, and known blood lead levels, it remains difficult to communicate risk, since epidemiological studies allow prediction of neurodevelopmental deficits on a population level, but are not predictive for an individual. For example, if a mother has a blood lead level of 10 micrograms per deciliter ($\mu$g/dL), it is not possible to predict that her child will lose 3 IQ points and will be more hyperactive, inattentive, and prone to violent behavior, even though many epidemiologic studies have shown these associations on a population level. Due to the multifactorial determinants of health, the child of such a mother could grow up to be a genius or could be profoundly developmentally delayed. Predicting or attributing risk on an individual basis is a tricky business and must be done with great caution.

It is often helpful for the clinician to describe his or her own frustration with the lack of sufficient data and the inability to use the existing data to predict individual risk. Most patients can understand the scientific uncertainty once it is explained to them. It is helpful for the clinician to empower the patient by offering some actions that they can take to help protect themselves and their family (see anticipatory guidance below).

### Taking an occupational and environmental history

All patients should undergo a screening occupational and environmental history. This history can identify potential risks at an early enough stage to prevent adverse outcomes, and can allow for intervention and prevention. The key components of a history are the following:

- Occupational information, including job duties, chemical and physical hazards at work, and occupation of others living in the household (because of the risk of "take-home" exposures).
- Hobbies, including arts, crafts, recreational fishing, "do it yourself" home repairs, and gardening.
- Household information, including the age of the home, water source, heating, pets, household pesticide use, and neighborhood environmental hazards.
- Personal habits, including dietary choices, cultural and magic-religious practices, herbal remedies, cosmetic use, plastics for food and water-contact, smoking and alcohol use.

A more detailed occupational and environmental history is outlined in Table 15.2.

Table 15.3 lists sources of common occupational and environmental reproductive toxicants.

### The emerging role of biomonitoring

It is increasingly common for patients to seek out tests for residues of chemicals or heavy metals in their bodies. Patients may request such testing from their health-care provider, or they may come to their health-care provider with results obtained elsewhere and with questions about health risk. There is fairly extensive information to allow interpretation of biomonitoring for a few environmental agents, such as lead, mercury, cadmium, and PCBs, in blood and urine. Several hundred other environmental agents have some age-, sex- and race-specific normative data from the National Health and Nutrition Examination Survey (NHANES) conducted by the Centers for Disease Control and Prevention (CDC) [4]. However these data simply allow comparison with the general US population and provide no information on whether the levels are safe or unsafe.

Hair testing for contaminants has become quite popular among some practitioners due to the convenience of collecting a sample and the low expense of analysis. Hair testing also is marketed directly to consumers over the Internet. Although it can be of some utility in screening for a few metals (lead, mercury, arsenic), studies have shown that correlations between hair and blood concentrations of metals is generally poor, indicating that hair may not be a good biomarker of absorbed dose for many metals [5].

A Californian survey of commercial laboratories providing hair analysis found very poor reliability, including a greater than ten-fold variation for 12 minerals in identical hair samples, and statistically significant extreme values for 14 of the 31 minerals that were analyzed by three or more laboratories [6]. If a hair test indicates elevated levels of any toxic metals, the results should be confirmed with a blood test prior to taking any action. There are very few laboratories that can reliably conduct biomonitoring for chemicals other than heavy metals in blood and urine, and most of these laboratories only do research, or survey studies, and are not available for testing individual patients. It is likely that biomonitoring will become more widespread and reliable in the next few years. Until biomonitoring becomes more reliable, it is important for the clinician to repeat the test using blood or urine (as appropriate) at an accredited laboratory, to take a careful exposure history for the chemical or metal in question, and seek an expert opinion when necessary.

### Treatment of occupational/environmental reproductive toxicity

When individuals learn that they may have been exposed to a hazardous substance, or when a biomonitoring test reveals an elevated concentration of a toxicant, people often seek ways to eliminate the substance from their body. Some practitioners advocate chelation to remove metals from the body, and various herbal remedies or detoxifying strategies to remove other contaminants. For the most part, there are no data on the efficacy of these treatments, and some of them have been shown to have harmful side-effects [7]. Detoxifying treatments and chelation have not been shown to be safe during pregnancy, and their use is generally not recommended [8].

If a specific contaminant has been identified, it is important first to determine if the patient truly has an elevated or hazardous level in their body, and second to consider the natural elimination time of the chemical.

**Table 15.2.** Occupational and environmental exposure history.

| **Work/hobbies** |
|---|
| What is your occupation? What are your hobbies? |
| What are the occupations and hobbies of other members of your household? |
| Are you exposed to any of the following substances at work, home or school? |
|    Fumes, vapors, dusts, pesticides, painting materials, lead, mercury or other metals. |
| Have you ever felt sick after contact with a chemical? |
| Do you wear personal protective equipment at work or while doing hobbies? |
| Do your symptoms get better away from work/hobbies? |
| **Residence** |
| Was your home built before 1978? If so, has it been tested for lead paint? |
| If your home has lead paint, is it flaking? Have you done any recent remodeling? |
| Where does your drinking water come from? |
| Have you had your water tested for lead? |
| If you have a private well, has the water been tested? |
| Do you know of any industrial emissions near your house (hazardous waste sites, dry cleaners, auto repair shops)? |
| Do you live in an agricultural area? |
| Do you use pesticides? In your home? Garden? On pets? |
| Do you use any traditional medications or remedies? * |
| Do you ever smell chemical odors while you are at home? |
| Do your symptoms get better away from home? |
| **Diet** |
| What kind of fish do you eat? How often do you eat fish? |
| Do you or anyone in your home fish in local waters? |
| Do you eat a lot of foods high in animal fat (fast food, ice cream, cheese, whole milk, fatty meats)? |
| Do you grow your own vegetables? Has the soil been tested? |
| Do you take any dietary supplements? * |

* May involve exposure to heavy metals such as mercury or lead.

For example, most organic solvents have a half-life in the body of only 2–3 days, and many metals have a half-life of a couple of months. Since virtual elimination occurs naturally over approximately five half-lives, watchful waiting is generally a reasonable option as the body clears the contaminant.

### Reporting sentinel events

Patients with known exposures or adverse outcomes can be sentinels for potential public health problems. An adverse event or a toxic exposure in an individual can signal a workplace or community hazard requiring attention. In the USA, physicians are legally required to report work-related illnesses or injuries, and some states have additional requirements. For example, the State of California requires that health-care providers report pesticide-related illnesses. Likewise other developed countries require reporting of occupational illnesses and injury, and some have occupational disease registries designed for capturing sentinel events [9].

Many important reproductive hazards were initially identified because of clusters of adverse events. For example, the potent testicular toxicant and pesticide, dibromochloropropane (DBCP), was first identified when a group of workers at a chemical plant discovered that they all had been unable to father children. The teratogenic and neurotoxic effects of methylmercury were first discovered when numerous severely developmentally disabled children were born in the community of Minamata, Japan. The reproductive toxicity of several glycol ethers was first identified due to reports of spontaneous abortions among women working in "clean rooms" at semiconductor manufacturing facilities [10]. The link between a common

**Table 15.3.** Common occupational and environmental exposures.

| Chemical exposure | Occupational source | Environmental source |
|---|---|---|
| Lead | Battery manufacture or recycling, smelting, car repair, painting, welding, soldering, firearm cleaning or shooting, stained glass ornament making, jewelry making | Paint, water pipes, imported ceramics or pottery, herbal remedies, traditional cosmetics, hair dyes, contaminated soil, toys, costume jewelry |
| Cadmium | Smelting, battery manufacture or recycling, painting, welding, electroplating | Toys, cigarette smoke, intake of contaminated food, paints and pigments |
| Mercury | Medical devices and electronics, jewelry making, taxidermy, tanning, dentistry, laboratory uses. | Herbal remedies, skin-lightening creams, thermometers, thermostats, barometers, antique clocks, dental amalgams, fish |
| Arsenic | Semiconductor and electronics manufacturing, mining, agriculture, smelting, glass manufacturing | Water or soil contamination, pressure-treated wood decks or playground equipment |
| Solvents | Degreasing, automotive, laboratory work, pesticide use, industrial cleaning, dry cleaning, painting, furniture refinishing, embalming | Automotive products, degreasers, thinners, varnish removers, spot removers, pesticides, nail polish |
| Pesticides | Manufacturing, exterminators, agricultural work, landscapers, lawn care, janitorial work | Gardening, pets, home extermination, agricultural drift, food and water contamination |

solvent used in many consumer products and stillbirth was first described in a case report [11]. Unfortunately, although the toxicity for many of these chemicals became apparent in the workplace, many of them were not banned for several decades and continued to cause harm (see Box 15.1).

Health-care providers should remain alert to sentinel events such as these. The decision to report a problem and to intervene may prevent many future adverse reproductive outcomes in the population.

<br>

**Box 15.1.   The case of DBCP.**

1,2-dibromo-3-chloropropane (DBCP) is a pesticide that was used as a soil fumigant against nematodes that attack the roots of banana trees, pineapple plants, and other fruit crops. DBCP was widely and heavily used from 1959–1979 in the USA and 14 other countries. In 1974 alone, 9.8 million pounds of this chemical were used on crops in the USA [12]. At the time of use, its persistence in soil, with a half-life of decades, was considered an attribute. Now over 40 years later, DBCP continues to contaminate water near agricultural fields.

In the 1970s, several workers in a DBCP production unit at an Occidental Chemical plant in Southern California reported to their labor union representative that they had been unable to father children. They were seen as a group by a local physician and were found to all have testicular failure and infertility. Subsequent investigations revealed that in a cohort of over 26 000 workers exposed to DBCP from 12 different countries, over 60% had low sperm counts or no sperm and these effects were permanent [13]. DBCP is also recognized as a carcinogen.

This whole tragedy could have been avoided, however, if animal research done during development by the chemical manufacturers had not been kept secret. Laboratory studies conducted by DBCP manufacturers, Shell and Dow Chemical Companies, found DBCP exposure led to testicular failure in at least three different animal species. This information was not submitted to government agencies and the final label and material safety data sheets (MSDS) did not provide complete information about DBCP's toxicity.

After the human health effects became known, the State of California banned DBCP in 1977, but it took 2 more years for the US EPA to restrict use and DBCP continued to be allowed for use on pineapples until 1985. However, the ban in the USA did not prevent continued exposure in workers outside of the US. The USA manufacturers continued to sell DBCP to Latin America for use in banana plantations.

As a result, thousands of plantation workers now are infertile or have reduced fertility that could have been predicted and prevented.

## The importance of knowing your community

Although some exposures to reproductive toxicants are nearly universal at low levels (e.g. through consumer products), and others are difficult to predict, some exposures are predictable and localized. Clinicians should learn about potential environmental hazards in the communities they serve so that they are better prepared to prevent and respond to potential problems.

(1) Water source – Which major public water systems serve the community? In the USA, every water utility is required to distribute an annual "Consumer Confidence Report" (CCR) detailing measured levels of regulated contaminants in local water systems. The CCRs are available to anyone, and can usually be obtained with a simple phone call or on-line search. CCRs should be studied for any contaminants that exceed the Maximum Contaminant Level Goal (MCLG), which is the health-based exposure limit and is generally lower than the legal limit (the Maximum Contaminant Level (MCL)).

What fraction of the community is supplied by private wells? If that fraction is significant, it will be important to identify whether there are any local or state agencies that offer free or subsidized testing of well water. If not, it is worthwhile to seek private water testing laboratories that are state certified and learn how much it costs to test well water for a variety of common contaminants such as total coliform, metals, nitrates, and perhaps pesticides or other contaminants depending on the region.

In other regions in the world, there is not a universal standard for regulating drinking water contaminants or for reporting requirements. The World Health Organization has recommended drinking water standards [14] and the United Nations Environment Programme has a database on international water quality[15].

(2) Major industry – What are the major local employers and the health hazards associated with those industries? In the USA, facilities that emit federally listed toxic chemicals are required to report these emissions. Check a website such as the Scorecard (www.scorecard.org) to learn what industrial sources of toxic chemicals exist in the community. In the EU, the European Pollutant Emission Register reports on the emissions of industrial facilities into air and water and maintains an on-line database [16]. The report covers 50 pollutants and is produced triennially.

(3) Hazardous waste sites – Are there any toxic waste sites in the community? Where are they located, what contaminants do they contain, and how have they been ranked according to health threat? A list of Superfund sites in the US can be found at: http://www.epa.gov/superfund/sites/npl/npl.htm.

(4) Air quality – Are there problems with ambient air quality in the community? If so, which pollutants are the biggest problem? Some air pollutants have been associated with adverse reproductive effects. In the USA, sign up for email alerts from EPA or your local air district to know when there are unhealthy levels of air pollution. The EPA website www.airnow.gov is the best resource for this information. In the EU, daily air quality information can be obtained from http://www.airqualitynow.eu/index.php.

(5) Pesticide use – In the USA, most states do not collect information on patterns of pesticide use. California is the only state with a comprehensive pesticide use reporting system. US data and international information on pesticide resources are compiled at www.pesticideinfo.org.

(6) Lead hazards – Lead paint was banned in most western European countries by the early 1930s. However it was not banned in the USA until 1978 and as a consequence, in the USA, houses built prior to 1978 may contain lead paint, and those built prior to the 1960s are almost always significantly contaminated with lead. If the paint on these homes is peeling or is disturbed during renovations, they can generate a serious lead hazard. In addition, communities criss-crossed with major roadways or freeways are likely to have significant soil contamination from historical use of leaded gasoline. Many industrial sources of lead exist in the USA. These can be identified at: http://www.nrdc.org/health/effects/lead/lead_Emitters_maps.asp.

## Precautionary anticipatory guidance that clinicians can offer

People are routinely exposed to a wide variety of chemicals, including reproductive toxicants, in the food they eat, the water they drink, the air they breathe, and in consumer products used on a daily basis.

Patients may not be aware of their ongoing exposures and a visit to their health-care provider can be an opportunity for patient education on topics they were not previously aware of. Instead of focusing the conversation on past exposures and unpredictable health outcomes, health-care providers can use this opportunity to educate patients about prevention. The provider does not need to be an expert in environmental health to discuss environmental exposures. Simple, common-sense guidance for reducing exposure to known or suspected reproductive hazards can prevent unnecessary risks.

Provided here are a few topics that health providers can discuss with their patients during the course of a routine office visit. Not all topics can be covered in one visit, nor is there one best way to avoid all exposures. By starting the conversation, providers empower a patient with information and a course of action.

### Dietary advice

Eat more fruits, vegetables, grains, and reduce consumption of fatty animal products (beef, pork, and full-fat dairy). Eat a variety of fish and avoid those known to be high in contaminants such as mercury (e.g. swordfish, shark, tuna, and fish caught from contaminated waterways). Many reproductive toxicants, such as PCBs and dioxins, are lipophilic and accumulate in fat. Eating fatty foods can increase the body burden and fat accumulation of these chemicals in humans over years and even decades. When a woman breastfeeds, these contaminants are mobilized from fat and end up in breast milk. Therefore, animal fat intake should be reduced beginning in childhood.

### Reducing pesticide exposure

Many pesticides are known or suspected reproductive toxicants. Pesticides are commonly used around the home and garden and on pets. To reduce pesticide exposure, choose non-chemical alternatives for home, garden, and pet use. If the use of a pesticide is necessary, use the least toxic alternative. For examples of some alternatives see: www.pesticide.org/factsheets.html–alternatives. For insect and rodent control, baits and traps are the best approach in conjunction with sealing cracks and cleanliness. Avoid insecticide sprays or "bombs". Pregnant women and children should not mix or apply pesticides and should not be present in a home when treatments are applied.

### Reduce exposure to heavy metals – such as lead and mercury

Lead is still commonly found in the paint and pipes of older housing and can be found in the consumer marketplace in some imported pottery with lead glaze, some candies imported from Mexico, and personal-care products such as hair dyes. People can reduce their exposure to lead by having their drinking water tested for lead, by having a professional remove any peeling lead paint in their home, and avoiding use of products containing lead. Lead may be present in garden soil and can end up in vegetables or be tracked into the home on shoes. If soil is suspected to be contaminated, it can be tested at a low cost.

In addition to dietary exposure, mercury exposure can occur through occupations, hobbies, magic-religious practices, and consumer products. The most common occupational exposures occur in dentistry. Some Caribbean religious practices involve sprinkling metallic mercury inside the home or car as a purification ceremony. The resulting exposures to mercury vapor can be very high. Imported skin-lightening creams and acne remedies may contain inorganic mercury. Finally, thermometers, fluorescent bulbs, thermostats, and some types of switches may all contain mercury. People should recycle fluorescent bulbs and batteries, and exchange their mercury thermometer for a digital one. Many communities sponsor collections of these products.

### Smoking

Both active and second-hand tobacco smoke exposure have been associated with a number of adverse reproductive outcomes, including infertility, low sperm counts, spontaneous abortion, low birthweight, preterm labor, and premature menopause. All couples should be advised to stop smoking and to avoid second-hand smoke exposure when attempting to become pregnant, while pregnant, and when there is an infant or child in the home.

### Reducing solvent exposure

Solvents are used to dilute or dissolve other substances into a solution and are also used in some cleaning agents, degreasers, oil-based paints, and paint removers. Solvents can be inhaled from fumes or vapors or can be absorbed across the skin. Once in the body, solvents dissolve quickly in the bloodstream. Solvent exposure has been linked to cancer, infertility, and miscarriage. Patients can reduce their solvent exposures by substituting use with less toxic chemicals and if this is not possible by working in a well-ventilated area with suitable proper personal protection including impermeable gloves and eye protection.

### Reducing exposure to the plastic chemical, bisphenol-A

Bisphenol-A (BPA) is a hormone-disrupting chemical that has been associated with reproductive harm, cancer, and neurological damage. BPA exposure is particularly a concern for babies, young children, and pregnant women. This chemical is commonly used to make polycarbonate plastic (baby bottles, sippy cups, and reusable water containers). BPA is also used in the resin lining of metal food and soda cans. BPA leaches out of the can liner into the food or drink, especially when the food is acidic such as tomato-based products or sodas. Pregnant women may want to cut back on canned food and canned soda, and parents should avoid using liquid infant formula packaged in metal cans. More adults are exposed to BPA by eating canned food or drinking canned soda than by drinking out of a polycarbonate bottle. Nevertheless, there are a number of alternatives to polycarbonate plastic and people should avoid using these containers for food or beverages.

## Communicating with groups

Although health-care providers tend to focus on communication about environmental health issues with individual patients, health professionals are also often called upon to communicate with groups of people in a variety of settings, such as workplaces, schools, and communities. These types of communications are different from the discussions that occur with individuals.

## The workplace setting

Occupational exposures to industrial chemicals or pesticides are often significantly higher than are usually encountered in the general environment. In addition, some chemicals used in workplaces are not found in the community, and the toxicity may be distinct. Occupational Safety and Health Administration (OSHA) standards generally focus on preventing undue acute toxicity, but rarely are set on the basis of chronic effects. In fact, for only four chemicals are the OSHA standards designed specifically to protect against adverse reproductive outcomes [17]. This is concerning given that the working population in the USA now includes a large percentage of women, and it is not unusual for women to work during their reproductively active years.

Communicating with workers about workplace exposures requires a careful job history, some understanding of the workplace setting, collection of material safety data sheets (MSDS) for the products or chemicals handled, and an effort to gather as much information as possible about exposure pathways, duration, and magnitude. It is important to be aware that OSHA compliance does not necessarily imply that a workplace is safe,

especially for pregnant women, and that MSDS information is frequently incomplete, especially for reproductive and developmental toxicity. In fact, one review of MSDSs for lead and ethylene glycol ethers (both known reproductive toxicants) found that 60% of the 700 MSDSs surveyed failed to even mention reproductive effects [18]. Before communicating with a group of workers, it is helpful to tour the workplace and review the scientific literature on the chemicals used.

Although it can be very difficult to answer questions about causation of specific adverse events, it is possible to use these communication opportunities to offer precautionary guidance to the employer and workers about reducing exposures within the workplace. In this context, the hierarchy of controls for management of risk in the workplace specifies elimination of the hazard, such as substitution with less toxic chemicals and/or processes whenever possible. When elimination of the hazard is not possible, engineering controls that prevent worker exposure are far preferable to administrative changes (e.g. rotating workers through the most dangerous jobs) or to personal protective equipment (PPE) such as respirators (which can fail or may not be worn properly). If workers do need to wear PPE, it is important that they are properly trained. Because the workplace is a more controlled environment than the community, if an employer is willing to make the effort, it is often possible to substantially reduce or eliminate exposures. If exposure is truly prevented, then there is little need to worry about health risk.

Health-care providers should also be aware of the potential for take-home exposures, which occur when the worker brings home hazardous materials either on their clothing, shoes, tools, or other items. If there are young children, pregnant women, or preconception women in the home, these exposures could potentially cause serious harm. Contaminants that are commonly brought home include lead, arsenic, mercury, cadmium, asbestos, pesticides, and infectious agents. These exposures can be avoided by changing and leaving soiled clothes and boots at work, washing work clothing separately from other household clothing, showering before leaving work, and leaving tools and other equipment at work (see Box 15.2).

Unfortunately, in the USA even when a reproductive hazard is identified and recognized in the workplace, the exposed worker has very few opportunities for avoiding the exposure without having to leave their job. Often the worker is faced with taking the risk of continued exposure or risk losing their job. For pregnant women, family leave is limited and if the worker does not belong to a union, there is no job protection. Finally, a 1990 Supreme Court decision (UAW v. Johnson Controls) established a legal precedent that prevented discrimination against women of reproductive age in the workplace but fell short of protecting pregnant women. The US policies are in sharp contrast to the EU where pregnant workers have guaranteed rights, extended maternity leave, and job protection [19].

---

**Box 15.2.** A case of take-home lead exposure.

A 5-year-old boy was found to have an elevated blood lead level of 18 µg/dL at his well-child check (a level over 10 µg/dL is considered to be lead poisoning in children). A home investigation revealed markedly elevated levels of lead dust in the garage, in the carpeting, and on furniture. However, soil samples taken outside of the home revealed only background levels of lead contamination and water samples taken from the tap were also at very low levels. An interview with the large extended family who lived in the house and further blood testing of family members revealed that two adult male members and another child also had elevated blood lead levels. Both men had blood lead levels above 40 µg/dL and the 3-year-old child who was only in the home part time had a blood lead level of 10 µg/dL. Although the men were asymptomatic, the younger man reported that he and his wife had difficulty conceiving another child. The two adult men worked at a shooting range where lead bullets were used. At the end of each day, they came home in their work clothes, wearing their work boots and sometimes bringing home bullets for refilling in their garage. A thorough decontamination of the home, the family car and removal of the carpets reduced levels of contamination in the home. The men changed their clothes and shoes at work and hired a laundry service to wash their work clothes. Within 2 months, everyone's blood lead levels had started to decline.

---

## The school and community setting

Conversations about environmental health risks in a community setting require that the health-care provider consider and address the exposures or illnesses that have already occurred, the future risks to people in the local community, and the need for public health action to protect the health of the people in the community. Physicians are one of the most trusted and credible sources of information about environmental health risks [20]. It is important that health-care providers listen to community concerns and respond with honesty. Blanket reassurances are rarely appropriate and rarely believed.

Understanding different perceptions of risk is important to help understand how to communicate about risk in a community setting. If the person who is attempting to explain a risk does not realize that the community may perceive risks differently, the discussion is not likely to be productive or effective. One important issue related to discussing risks in the community setting is the reality of environmental injustice. Low-income communities of color have become increasingly concerned about a disproportionate and unfair burden of environmental risk in their communities. Even a relatively small risk may be seen in the context of a history of racial and socioeconomic discrimination in the distribution of environmental risks, and is perceived as adding to an already unacceptable background of risk.

In the USA, three-fifths of Blacks and Hispanics live in communities with uncontrolled toxic waste sites, and the most significant predictor for the location of hazardous waste facilities nationwide is the race of the local community [21]. Low-income communities and communities of color are also more likely to contain multiple environmental pollution sources. Reviews of research have shown that children of color suffer disproportionate burdens of disease with potential environmental aspects, including asthma, neurodevelopmental disorders, and childhood cancer [22]. In part as a result of these disparities, people living in these communities may see a single incident such as a ruptured chemical tank near a day-care center, as part of a bigger picture of environmental hazards and a history of environmental injustice. If the health-care provider ignores the history and context behind an individual incident, the conversation can feel frustrating and confusing to all parties involved.

In many cases, the actual risk to people in the community is essentially unquantifiable. As a result, it may not be possible to assign a risk of an adverse outcome, even at a community level. Therefore, support and precautionary guidance may be the most useful information a health-care provider can offer to a community. Whenever possible, vulnerable populations such as pregnant women and children should be removed from situations of potential exposure to reproductive or environmental toxicants. Likewise, environmental pollution should be cleaned up and minimized whenever possible.

## The role of the clinician in public policy

Health-care providers can and should communicate to the press and the general public about the implications of population-level shifts in reproductive outcomes, such as birthweight, preterm labor, or age of onset of puberty. Contexts in which such discussions might occur include comments to the media, policy discussions at medical and nursing societies, and health policy discussions at the local, regional, and international level.

Although many health-care providers are reluctant to make public statements about population risk, there are at least three reasons why they should consider doing so. First, the scientific basis for extrapolating the results of environmental reproductive outcomes research is far stronger when the extrapolation is at the population level rather than at the level of the individual patient; second, health-care providers are a trusted and important voice that is rarely heard in public discussions about environmental health policy; and third, the foundation of medicine is prevention, and the most useful prevention activities around reproductive hazards can occur at the population, rather than individual, level.

Communicating with the media or with policy-makers requires a different set of considerations than communicating with individual patients or small groups of people. Prior to speaking with a reporter or a policymaker, it is important to review the policy proposal at issue and to determine whether it seems like a reasonable, precautionary, science-based step toward protecting public health. If the science and the policy seem reasonable, the next step is to either write out a statement of support or to develop key talking points. Communications experts suggest identifying three or four major "messages" that summarize the main points that need to be conveyed.

The conversation with the reporter or policymaker should remain "big-picture" and clear to the non-scientific listener and should stick to the talking points to avoid making mistakes or going astray into issues that are either irrelevant or outside the speaker's area of expertise. It is generally possible to answer almost any question by restating a talking point, even if it means saying something such as: "I don't know the answer to your question, but the real issue here is …" By pre-identifying a set of talking points within a scientific and policy comfort zone and staying within those points, the health-care provider can assure both that the major issues will come through clearly in any news story or policy hearing, and also that his or her credibility will remain intact.

## Examples of responses to common questions about environmental exposures

It is difficult to predict what environmental health concerns or questions a health-care provider may encounter. Some questions can be anticipated due to their ongoing prevalence in the news media, popular press, or on the Internet. Others may be based on specific community concerns. The questions from an individual patient may be very similar to those asked in a public meeting and likewise, whether speaking to an individual or group, the clinician's response may be similar. The overall approach involves having some knowledge of the toxicity of the contaminant of concern, assessing the route and likelihood of exposure, and being able to communicate a science-based approach to reducing unnecessary exposures. Furthermore, health-care providers also can offer advice to groups or individuals about reducing exposure to other contaminants.

### Common questions

*A young pregnant woman comes in for a prenatal appointment. She has been reading a lot of information on the Internet and is worried about contaminants in her drinking water causing harm to her baby. She lives on a limited budget and wonders if investing in an expensive water filtration unit is worth the expense.*

Before investing in a water filter, check the local water utility company's annual water quality report. (For help in interpreting water quality reports, this website can help: www.safe-drinking-water.org/rtk.html). In most cities, healthy adults can drink tap water without concern. Pregnant women and young children may be more vulnerable to some contaminants in water, such as lead or trihalomethanes. People who have private wells should get their water tested for common contaminants. If any pollutants are identified in drinking water, a filter that is appropriate for removal of the specific contaminants can be chosen. Different types of filters take out different contaminants, so there is no "one size fits all" solution (see Box 15.3 for information about water filtration systems).

Bottled water is not necessarily a better alternative to filtered water. Up to 40% of bottled water is ordinary tap water that has been filtered and packaged. Bottled water quality is actually subject to less stringent regulatory standards than tap water and can contain residues of the plastic it is bottled in.

---

**Box 15.3.** Types of water filtration.

In general there are two types of water filters, point of entry and point of use. All filtration systems require regular maintenance for proper functioning.

- *Point of entry units* are more expensive, are installed in the pipes outside the home and treat all the water before it enters the house.

- *Point of use filters* such as countertop filters (e.g. filter pitchers), faucet filters, and under-the-sink units generally use activated charcoal to remove bad tastes, and odors and chemical contaminants. Charcoal water filters are simple to install, relatively economical and effectively remove many toxins found in the environment and comprise the majority of filters in use.

- For many people, an *activated carbon filter bearing NSF Standard 53 certification* will filter out most pollutants of concern, including endocrine disruptors such as heavy metals and pesticides. However, some contaminants that are suspected endocrine disruptors, such as arsenic or perchlorate, may not be removed by charcoal filters.

- In *reverse osmosis filtration*, water is forced through a membrane and then filtered through charcoal; a method that removes most contaminants, including arsenic and perchlorate. However, this filtration system wastes a lot of water and is much more expensive.

---

*A farmer has been unable to conceive any children with his wife and was recently told his sperm count is low. His job involves mixing and applying pesticides and he does not always wear protective equipment. He wonders if the pesticides could have caused his infertility problems.*

Patients may approach their health provider with concerns that a past exposure is related to a specific condition, such as infertility or a pregnancy loss. In some cases the patient is simply struggling to understand a bad health outcome; in other situations a legal case may be pending. This is often a challenging case for a physician as most health outcomes have multifactorial causes, including, in some cases, chemical exposures.

Although health providers may not be able to give an immediate answer, they can take a thorough history to determine if the exposure was substantial (Table 15.2); give education about the health condition and the associated etiologies; discuss the uncertainty and challenges in determining individual risk; and provide guidance on how to avoid future exposure. Referral to an appropriate consulting specialist may be necessary for complex exposures and determination of causality.

## Special concerns and issues around breastfeeding and infant formula

*A pregnant woman who is near her due date is in for a check-up. She has been preparing for her new baby and has many questions about breastfeeding. She is concerned because she recently read that many chemicals have been found in breast milk. She worries about the effects of passing these contaminants onto her new baby and wonders if it would be better to use formula.*

Breast milk has been found to potentially contain many contaminants including endocrine disruptors such as PCBs, dioxins and furans, pesticide residues, flame retardants (PBBs and PBDEs), and plasticizers [23]. Providers should reassure their patients that despite this problem, the benefits of breastfeeding still outweigh the risks from pollution. Breastfeeding may even protect a baby against the adverse effects of exposures that occurred in utero [24].

Because of the benefits to baby and mother, the American Academy of Pediatrics recommends breastfeeding for at least the first 6 months of life and the World Health Organization recommends breastfeeding up until 2 years of age. Breast milk provides vital nutrients and antibodies that are passed from the mother to infant. These help prevent infections and promote growth of the brain and nervous system. Breastfeeding also is beneficial to the mother as it promotes bone strength, weight loss, and reduces the chances of pre-menopausal breast and ovarian cancer [25].

Baby formula is not an equivalent substitute for breast milk. Formula is lacking in many of the vital trace nutrients and antibodies found in breast milk. Studies have demonstrated that formula-fed babies get sick more often than breast-fed babies [25]. Although formula may not contain many of the contaminants found in breast milk, such as PCBs and dioxins, infant formula may contain other toxicants such as melamine, manganese, lead, or cadmium [26–29]. In addition, exposure to toxicants can occur if infant powder formula is diluted with water contaminated with pesticides, heavy metals, or micro organisms. Soy formulas are a particular concern due to very high levels of plant-derived estrogens (phytoestrogens) in soy products. The amounts of phytoestrogens are 2200–4500 times greater in soy milk than in breast milk and the long-term health effects are not well studied [29].

## Resources

Providers who are faced with questions of environmental or occupational exposures in their patients need quick, reliable sources of information. Provided here are scientifically based resources that health-care providers can use to help in the care of their patients with exposures to contaminants, including endocrine disruptors.

### Clinical referrals

*The Association of Occupational and Environmental Clinics* has a clinical directory for finding specialists in occupational and environmental medicine in the USA, Canada and Germany (www.aoec.org/directory)

*Pediatric Environmental Health Specialty Units (PEHSU)* (www.aoec.org/pehsu.htm) provides education and consultation for health professionals and others about the topic of children's environmental health in the USA, Mexico and Canada.

### Information on chemical toxicity

US Centers for Disease Control and Prevention (CDC):

*Agency for Toxic Substances Disease Registry (ATSDR)* produces "toxicological profiles" for hazardous substances. (www.atsdr.cdc.gov/toxpro2.html)

*The National Institute for Occupational Safety and Health (NIOSH)*(www.cdc.gov/niosh/homepage.html) provides information on chemical safety, workplace health hazard evaluations, and reproductive health and occupational exposures.

*The US National Library of Medicine* (www.nlm.nih.gov/) has links to databases including:

*PubMed* (www.pubmed.gov) references abstracts from thousands of biomedical journals

*ToxNet* (toxnet.nlm.nih.gov) is a network of databases on toxicology, hazardous chemicals, and environmental health.

*US Household Hazardous Substance Database* (householdproducts.nlm.nih.gov/products.htm) links over 6000 consumer brands to health effects from material safety data sheets (MSDS) and allows scientists and consumers to research products based on chemical ingredients.

The United Nations Environment Programme, Chemical Information Exchange Network / Réseau d'Echange d'Information sur les produits Chimiques (CIEN/REIC). High production volume chemicals are summarized in the Screening Information Data Set (SIDS).

International Chemical Safety Cards summarize information on chemicals for their use at the "shop floor" level by workers and employers in factories, agriculture, construction, and other workplaces. The ICSCs are available on the Internet in many languages: (www.ilo.org/public/english/protection/safework/cis/products/icsc/)

### Other useful websites

*Our Stolen Future* (www.OurStolenFuture.org.) provides regular updates about the cutting edge of science related to endocrine disruption and information about ongoing policy debates, as well as new suggestions about what people can do to minimize risks related to hormonally disruptive contaminants.

The National Pesticide Information Center (npic.orst.edu/) is a cooperative effort of Oregon State University and the US Environmental Protection Agency (EPA), providing on-line information about pesticide safety and toxicity. The organization also runs a toll-free hotline for pesticide questions (1–800–858–7378).

### References

1. Princeton Survey Research Associates. *National Survey of Public Perceptions of Environmental Health Risks.* April 2000. http://healthyamericans.org/docs/index.php?DocID=18

2. Gottlieb M, Miller M, Nelson J, Palmigiano M. *Tools for a Healthy Beginning: Prenatal Environmental Health Toolkit.* Web Survey completed September 2006 and presented as a poster presentation at UCSF-CHE Summit on Environmental Challenges to Reproductive Health and Fertility.

3. US EPA. *Chemical Hazard Data Availability Study. What do We Really Know about the Safety of High Production Volume Chemicals?* EPA's 1998 Baseline of Hazard Information that is Readily Available to the Public. Prepared by EPA's Office of Pollution Prevention and Toxics (April 1998). Available at: http://www.epa.gov/HPV/pubs/general/hazchem.pdf

4. Centers for Disease Control and Prevention. *Third National Report on Human Exposure to Environmental Chemicals.* Atlanta (GA): CDC, 2005. Available at: http://www.cdc.gov/ExposureReport/report.htm

5. Rodrigues JL, Batista BL, Nunes JA, Passos CJ, Barbosa F. Evaluation of the use of human hair for biomonitoring the deficiency of essential and exposure to toxic elements. *Sci Total Environ.* 2008. **405**(1–3): 370–6.

6. Seidel S, Kreutzer R, Smith D, McNeel S, Gilliss D. Assessment of commercial laboratories performing hair mineral analysis. *J Am Med Assoc* 2001; **285**(1): 67–72.

7. Risher JF, Amler SN. Mercury exposure: evaluation and intervention the inappropriate use of chelating agents in the diagnosis and treatment of putative mercury poisoning. *NeuroToxicology.* 2005; **26**(4): 691–9.

8. Weizsaecker K. Lead toxicity during pregnancy. *Primary Care Update Ob/Gyns* 2003; **10**(6): 304–9.

9. Driscoll T, Takala J, Steenland K, Corvalan C, Fingerhut M. Review of estimates of the global burden of injury and illness due to occupational exposures. *Am J Ind Med.* 2005; **48**(6): 491–502.

10. Schenker MB, Gold EB, Beaumont JJ. *et al.* Association of spontaneous abortion and other reproductive effects with work in the semiconductor industry. *Am J Ind Med.* 1995; **28**(6): 639–59.

11. Solomon GM, Morse EP, Garbo MJ, Milton DK. Stillbirth after occupational exposure to N-methyl-2-pyrrolidone. A case report and review of the literature. *J Occup Environ Med.* 1996; **38**(7): 705–13

12. Teitelbaum DT. The toxicology of 1,2-dibromo-3-chloropropane (DBCP): a brief review. *Int J Occup Environ Health* 1999; **5**(2): 122–6.

13. Slutsky M, Levin JL, Levy BS. Azoospermia and oligospermia among a large cohort of DBCP applicators in 12 countries. *Int J Occup Environ Health* 1999; **5**(2): 116–22.

14. World Health Organization *Guidelines for Drinking-water Quality.* http://www.who.int/water_sanitation_health/dwq/guidelines/en/index.html

15. United Nations Environment Programme Global Environment Monitoring System (GEMS). Water Programme. http://www.gemstat.org/

16. The European Pollutant Emission Register. http://eper.ec.europa.eu/eper/introduction.asp?i=

17. Occupational Safety and Health Administration. OSHA Standards: Reproductive Hazards. www.osha.gov/SLTC/reproductivehazards/standards.html

18. Paul M, Kurtz S. Analysis of reproductive health hazard information on material safety data sheets for lead and the ethylene glycol ethers. *Am J Ind Med* 1994; **25**(3): 403–15.

19. Council Directive 92/85/EEC of 19 October 1992. Protection of pregnant workers and workers who have recently given birth or are breastfeeding. http://europa.eu/scadplus/leg/en/cha/c10914.htm

20. Covello, V. Risk communication and occupational medicine. *J Occup Med* 1993; **35**(1): 18–19.

21. Commission for Racial Justice. *Toxic Wastes and Race in the United States: a National Report of the Racial and Socioeconomic Characteristics of Communities with Hazardous Waste Sites.* New York: United Church of Christ, 1987.

22. Mott L. The disproportionate impact of environmental health threats on children of color. *Environ Health Perspect* 1995; **103** (Suppl. 6): 33–5.

23. Solomon GM, Weiss PM. Chemical contaminants in breast milk: time trends and regional variability. *Environ Health Perspect.* 2002; **110**(6): A339–47.

24. Jacobson JL, Jacobson SW. Breast-feeding and gender as moderators of teratogenic effects on cognitive development. *Neurotoxicol Teratol.* 2002; **24**(3): 349–58.

25. Schack-Nielsen L, Larnkjaer A, Michaelsen KF. Long term effects of breastfeeding on the infant and mother. *Adv Exp Med Biol.* 2005; **569**: 16–23.

26. Hozyasz KK, Ruszczynska A. High manganese levels in milk-based infant formulas. *Neurotoxicology.* 2004 Jun; **25**(4): 733.

27. Eklund G, Oskarsson A. Exposure of cadmium from infant formulas and weaning foods. *Food Addit Contamin* 1999; **16**(12): 509–19.

28. Navarro-Blasco I, Alvarez-Galindo JI. Lead levels in retail samples of Spanish infant formulae and their contribution to dietary intake of infants. *Food Addit Contam.* 2005; **22**(8): 726–34.

29. Setchell KD, Zimmer-Nechemias L, Cai J, Heubi JE. Isoflavone content of infant formulas and the metabolic fate of these phytoestrogens in early life. *Am J Clin Nutr.* 1998; **68** (Suppl 6): 1453S–61S.

# Interpreting science in the policy context

Tracey J. Woodruff and Sarah J. Janssen

## Introduction

Over 40 years have passed since the publication of Rachel Carson's *Silent Spring* foretold the harmful effects of chemical pollution in wildlife [1] and the subsequent tragedies of Love Canal and Bhopal that brought critical attention to the human harm caused by environmental contamination. The overwhelming evidence catapulted public concern about environmental contaminants and led to a number of legislative and policy changes at the federal and state levels to address concerns about harm from environmental exposures. Focused effort in certain areas has brought about significant improvements, such as decreased blood lead level in children, improved air quality, and declines in several persistent pollutants, such as DDT, in the environment. Yet, there is remaining concern about existing chemicals that have not yet been addressed and newer ones that have since emerged.

Observed, unexplained increases in certain chronic conditions, such as childhood cancer, diabetes, impaired fecundity, and reproductive cancers, and a continuously growing base of science linking environmental contaminant exposure to increased risk of both reproductive and other health effects signifies further attention is needed. Preventing and reducing illness depends on public policies that focus on removing or limiting exposure to harmful chemicals. Public policies provide a structured, more universal approach that can address the broad, often non-specific sources of environmental exposures. Yet this relatively straightforward approach requires scientific knowledge and an understanding of exposure sources, what contributes to these sources, and knowledge about the potential health consequences of exposure to particular environmental contaminants (Fig. 16.1).

Environmental contaminants can come from a variety of sources. Traditionally "environmental contaminants" have been described as chemicals originating from outdoor sources either as direct emissions or by-products of industrial activity, applications, transportation, or waste generation. These chemicals contaminate outdoor media such as air, water bodies, or food crops, and then come into contact with people who breathe contaminated air, drink contaminated water or eat contaminated food. More recently, there has been increased attention on chemical contaminants found in indoor environments, where they often occur because of their use in various consumer products. Exposure to indoor environmental contaminants occurs either through use of the product or by leaching from the product and contamination of indoor air, surfaces, or dust (see Chapter 2).

Many chemicals are found in both outdoor and indoor environments, resulting in multiple sources of exposure. These exposures can increase the risk of subsequent illness; a risk that can be modified by extrinsic and intrinsic factors such as social and economic status, disease status, age, gender, and exposure to other environmental contaminants [3].

Many approaches can be taken to reduce or eliminate harmful environmental exposures including the following: personal and individual choice, voluntary market restrictions by the entity that is a source of environmental contaminants, market incentives or pressures on industries to remove harmful contaminants, or public policies that systematically address exposures through regulation. Development of public policies that can prevent or reduce harmful environmental exposures on a population level, or a public-health approach, is often the most efficient, equitable, and ethical means to address exposures to environmental contaminants. Many environmental contaminant exposures are externalities of production over which the individual has no control (e.g. power

*Environmental Impacts on Reproductive Health and Fertility*, ed. T. J. Woodruff, S. J. Janssen, L. J. Guillette, and L. C. Giudice. Published by Cambridge University Press. © Cambridge University Press 2010.

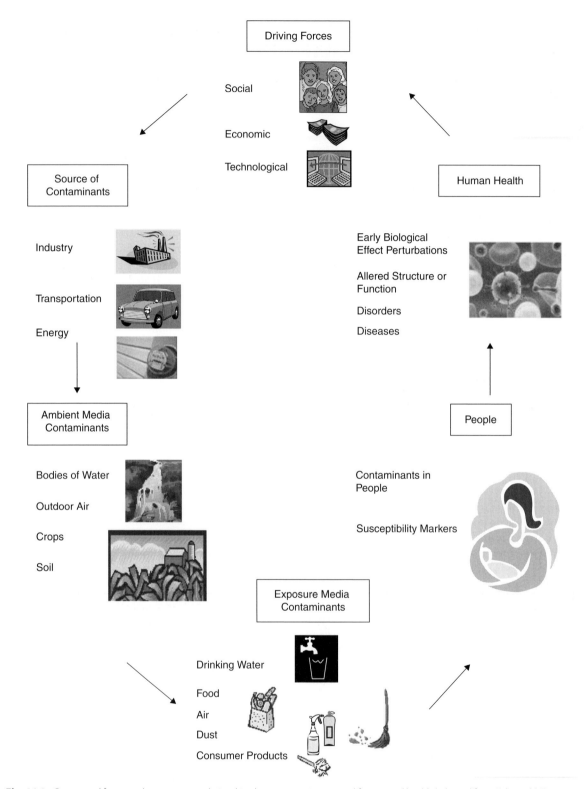

**Fig. 16.1.** Conceptual framework to represent relationships between environmental factors and health (adapted from Kyle *et al.* [2]).

plants, diesel trucks). Personal choice and market forces rely on personal and equal knowledge of facts and resources, which are asymmetrically distributed in the population. Public policy solutions, which can include mandates and market incentives, can be difficult to achieve because a number of external forces come to bear on the initiation, development, and implementation, such as special interests, politics, economics, feasibility, availability of alternatives, and conflicting science. All approaches to remove or reduce exposure to harmful chemicals, whether through personal, market-driven or government-based restrictions, are informed by some level of scientific knowledge that links exposures to the potential for human harm. The most effective approach has proven to be public policy solutions that are informed by scientific research (see example in Box 16.1).

### Box 16.1. Public policy and lead contamination.

The history of lead tragically illustrates how scientific understanding of toxicity can often take decades to result in policy change. While very high lead exposures were recognized to cause encephalopathy, coma, and death in children as early as 1900, it was not until the 1940s that childhood lead poisoning was also noted to cause persistent impairments in intellect, behavior, and sensory-motor function [4]. A specific toxic threshold for lead was established for the first time in the 1960s at 60 µg/dL, only modestly below the level at which encephalopathy occurs (80 µg/dL)[5]. It was only in the late 1970s, however, that lead was removed from indoor paint and gasoline. Interestingly, the decision to remove lead from gasoline was not driven by concern for public health but rather by requirements for reducing smog-producing emissions from cars. The conventional wisdom at the time was that removing lead from gasoline would not significantly impact blood lead levels. However, blood lead levels dramatically declined in step with the phase-out of lead from gasoline. Over the next 30 years, ongoing research has shown long-term neurological effects at progressively lower levels of exposure [6]. The "action level" for clinical interventions was most recently set at 10 µg/dL, the "official" 1990 standard that still holds today in many countries. However, despite studies demonstrating there is no threshold for harm and with observations of significant adverse effects occurring below a blood level of 10 µg/dL [7, 8], there have been no changes in the lead standard anywhere in the world.

This chapter will focus on how science is evaluated and used in decision-making for public policy measures and other actions that focus on reducing exposure to harmful environmental contaminants. We will briefly review the current statutory approaches to regulations and policy decisions, and will explore what is lacking and needed for more effective and protective policy decisions. Much of the science that has been described in earlier chapters can be used to inform public policies resulting in reduced exposure to environmental contaminants that may pose a risk to reproductive health. We will briefly discuss the current regulatory landscape in the USA and Europe that addresses the collection of and data requirements for environmental contaminants. Although significant and evolving theories on the impacts that environmental contaminants have on reproductive health exist, there are limitations in the current approach resulting in public policy lagging behind the state of the science. We will describe alternative policy options that can address these limitations. While other factors such as technological feasibility, costs, politics, and public opinion influence the development, passage, implementation, and enforcement of laws and regulations that address harmful exposures to environmental contaminants, a discussion of these are beyond the scope of this chapter.

## Defining the scope of the problem

The dramatic increase in industrialization over the past three centuries has changed the quality and quantity of human exposures to both natural and synthetic chemicals. In particular, there has been a dramatic rise in chemicals production in the USA since World War II, with an increase of more than 20-fold. The number of chemicals registered for commercial use has grown by over 30% since 1979 (Fig. 16.2) [3]. Manufactured and mined chemicals are now everywhere in our environment.

In the USA, as of 2006, the US EPA estimated there are approximately 75 000 chemical substances listed in the EPA's Toxic Substances and Control Act inventory [9]. While many of these chemicals are used in small quantities or within closed manufacturing systems, about 2800 are used or imported in high volumes (over 1 million pounds annually) [10]. In addition, there are also pesticides (with about 900 active ingredients and 2500 inert ingredients identified in the late 1990s), nuclear material, and chemicals in food (about 3000), and chemicals in drugs and cosmetics (about 5000) [11]. This brings the total number of chemicals to about 87 000, though it is difficult to ascertain the complete number of chemicals, because no single entity records the universe of chemicals used in the USA. Likewise, there is no international registry of chemicals in production or

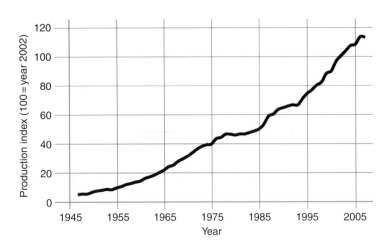

**Fig. 16.2.** Chemicals production in the USA from 1947 to 2007.

use. The European Chemicals Agency maintains a list of chemicals commercially available in the EU. There are currently over 100 000 chemicals on this list [12].

Common environmental pollutants include: pesticides and herbicides such as atrazine and chlorpyrifos; volatile organic compounds such as benzene, toluene, and chloroform; heavy metals such as lead, mercury, and arsenic; air contaminants such as carbon monoxide, ozone, particulate matter, and environmental tobacco smoke; and persistent organic pollutants, such as the dioxins, polychlorinated biphenols (PCBs), the pesticide dichlorodiphenyltrichloroethane (DDT) and its breakdown product dichlorodiphenyldichloroethylene (DDE) (see Chapters 1 and 2). Although some chemicals have been in commerce for several decades, the technology for measuring them in environmental or biological media has only recently been developed. In the past decade, additional environmental contaminants have emerged to include persistent chemicals used in common consumer products such as perfluorinated chemicals, flame retardants, and antimicrobial compounds. These chemicals all have in common that they are halogenated organic chemicals. In addition, this list of chemicals does not cover the emergence of novel manufactured materials such as nanomaterials, which are based on manipulation of matter at the scale of individual atoms or molecules [13]. Given the small scale, these materials are typically defined as having at least one dimension smaller than 100 nanometers and often have unique chemical and biological properties at this scale that differ from their normal-sized counterparts [13]. The number of materials and products that use nanomaterials is rapidly growing, yet there is currently no regulatory or policy structure to address potential health risks from these materials [13].

There are multiple sources of environmental contaminants (see Chapter 2), including industrial processes, transportation, building, and consumer products. These sources can emit or discharge environmental contaminants into air, water, food, and dust, to which humans are exposed through breathing, eating, drinking, and direct contact (e.g. personal-care products) [14–17]. For example, exposure to air pollution is ubiquitous and has been demonstrated through both monitoring and modeling studies to exist at concentrations that pose a risk to human health [18, 19]. Similarly, data from government agencies show there are multiple contaminants in drinking water [20, 21], and that there are contaminants in the food supply which come from both intended application (such as pesticides or food additives) [22] and from unintended applications (such as discharge or contaminants from water use) [23].

Data on sources of exposure are complemented by information on measured levels of environmental contaminants in people's bodies, referred to as biomonitoring data. Some European countries, such as Sweden, have been monitoring the presence of halogenated organic contaminants since the 1960s and have stored samples for future testing as new contaminants emerge [24]. There has been some biomonitoring in the USA since the 1970s for contaminants such as lead in children [25]; however, it was not until the early 2000s that more comprehensive data were published on levels of contaminants in the US population. The number of chemicals that have been measured in a representative sample of the US population has grown from 116 (years 1999–2000), to 148 (years 2001–2002), and then 275 for 2003–2004, and the number is expected to rise with further assessments [26]. The national data have been accompanied by more biomonitoring data produced by studies of individual populations, from both researchers [27–30] and non-governmental organizations [31–33]. Likewise, biomonitoring has expanded in the EU [34] and there are ongoing biomonitoring programs in Germany [35], Canada [36], and at the World Health Organization [37].

International studies show that many chemicals are detected in some portion of the population and a number of chemicals including perchlorate, bisphenol-A, phthalates, flame retardants (PBDEs), environmental tobacco smoke, and mercury are detected in almost every person sampled [38–40]. Thus, every person has multiple measurable contaminants in their body. For a number of these chemicals, the measured levels in people's bodies can be above levels of concern identified by the government or that have been identified as associated with adverse health outcomes in epidemiologic or animal studies, e.g. mercury [10], phthalates [41–43], and perchlorate [44–46].

While monitoring environmental contaminants in exposure media such as air and water has predicted changes in exposure to the population, data on biomonitoring has provided compelling and tangible evidence of human contact with environmental contaminants. Detecting environmental contaminants in people does not provide a prevention-oriented approach to reducing or eliminating harmful exposures. However, biomonitoring has prompted policy and regulatory actions. For example, the presence of the flame retardants, PBDEs, in breast milk was first revealed in 2000 after archived samples in Sweden were tested [24]. The testing revealed an exponential rise in levels from the 1970s. This revelation prompted a restriction on the use of PBDEs in Europe and an evening-off of levels in the population. Subsequent testing of PBDEs in the US population revealed that the levels of flame retardants were up to 40 times higher than European levels. United States flammability standards are more stringent than European standards resulting in the use of more chemicals in the USA in items such as upholstered furniture and subsequently higher levels of exposure in the US population [31]. This was a policy decision that – while intended to protect public health – has resulted in unintended and widespread exposure in the population with potentially adverse health impacts.

Although it is difficult to extrapolate these large study findings to an individual's health outcome, population level effects can be predicted. The extensive presence of measured environmental contaminants in the human population necessitates approaches that identify and mitigate exposure to harmful chemicals prior to discovering high levels of contaminants in people.

## Approaches to address toxicity from environmental chemical exposures and the role of policy

A critical component for informing and supporting public policies to address environmental contaminants is identifying whether and how a particular chemical or group of chemicals could adversely affect human health. One part of this process entails evaluating and using the available scientific information and data to assess a chemical's potential for human harm, which has generally been labeled as "risk assessment" [47]. The risk assessment is defined by using some or all of four separate steps: hazard identification (identifying potential health problems from chemical exposure); exposure assessment (determining the extent of human exposure, i.e. amount, duration, etc.); dose–response assessment (estimate of the magnitude of exposure and the probability of occurrence of adverse health effects); and risk characterization (assessing the magnitude and nature of the risk of harm to the human population) (Fig. 16.3) [47]. Although risk assessment is often associated with the quantitative assessment of the risks of an environmental chemical, this is actually only one part, and often the final part, of the assessment process.

While each step draws upon the data at hand, each step also requires making judgments and decisions starting with problem formulation [47] to deciding which data to use in the assessment, to how to account for unknowns and variability in the data, and ending with how to identify – both qualitatively and quantitatively – the potential for harm. For example, most of the data used to evaluate the potential for human harm comes from animal studies. To extrapolate the animal findings to potential effects in humans requires scientific-based judgments of how humans will respond compared with responses in animals.

The risk-assessment scenario assumes that there is a reasonable set of data for each step in the process; however there are many chemicals which lack data for key steps or have no data at all. This lack of data presents a dilemma for assessing chemicals with limited data, because in the risk-assessment process, the absence of data means no risk assessment will be done. If the public policy is based on "knowing" the hazard or quantifying the risk through risk assessment, then

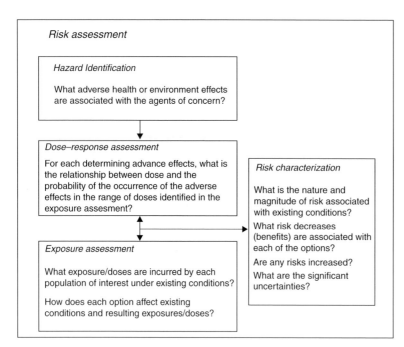

**Fig. 16.3.** Primary steps in risk assessment and risk characterization (adapted from National Research Council [47]; Office of Environmental Health Hazard Assessment [48]).

for unknown risks the default for likelihood of harm becomes essentially zero. For many chemicals we know that there is a small likelihood of a zero risk of harm. For example, if a chemical increased the risk of reproductive cancers in animals, even without supporting data, there is concern that this chemical would also contribute to other types of non-cancer reproductive effects (an example is diethystilbestrol; see Box 16.2). Furthermore, the numerical risk number is usually intended to cover risks to the full range of the population, including sensitive subpopulations such as children, those with pre-existing diseases, and genetic variability. There are often not enough data on all the extrinsic or intrinsic factors that can influence risk of chemical exposure. However, based on biological understanding and previous findings from other environmental contaminants, we known certain subpopulations, such as younger developmental ages, are more sensitive to chemical exposures. For example, the US EPA uses a factor to account for increased sensitivity of children to mutagenic (DNA-damaging) carcinogens based on findings from animal data for similar chemicals in this group. Given the body of knowledge, even if the experiment for a particular chemical has not been conducted to assess a particular aspect of the risk assessment, an assumptive value, or default, is used in place of data until data are obtained, because there is reasonable certainty that the value is not zero.

There are a variety of uses of risk assessment in the policy and regulatory process, such as identifying hazards for labeling, ranking hazards and risks from different chemicals for priority setting, setting standards for cleaning up contaminated waste sites, and setting national, state, or local standards for exposures to contaminants in sources such as air or drinking water. The scope, emphasis, and use of hazard identification and risk characterization will vary often based on the intended use of the information. Some policy approaches only use hazard identification, some require full risk assessments, and others may base decisions primarily on opportunities for exposure. Each approach evaluates the potential for environmental contaminants to adversely impact human health.

In this section, we present some of the typical types of scientific information that are used to identify potential human health hazards from environmental chemicals and what are some of the judgments/issues that arise when evaluating the information for use in the decision-making policy process.

## Identifying hazards

### Sources and interpretation of data on potential adverse health effects

Scientific data on the potential for chemicals to adversely influence health come from multiple sources, and generally fall within four broad categories: chemical structure activity relationships (using information on the chemicals' properties to assess potential for harm or to compare with known chemicals with similar properties), in vitro testing, in vivo animal testing or animal bioassays, and human studies. Within each of these areas multiple types of testing methodologies, strategies, and approaches are used. In vivo animal bioassays play a critical role in human health risk assessment as they are a preferable method to assess the potential for human harm and to develop strategies for prevention of harmful exposures. Unlike pharmaceuticals, environmental contaminants were not intended for human use, and so it is unethical to purposefully expose people to chemicals to assess for harmful effects. Given that there is general conservation of biological function across animal species, including humans, animal studies provide important insights into potential human harm.

However, there are limitations in how traditional toxicologic studies have been designed that decrease their utility for studying reproductive or developmental outcomes. Traditional toxicologic studies have tended to look for endpoints such as fetal death, severe birth defects, or the development of cancer under conditions of treatment using high doses of one chemical at a time. This methodology does not mimic human exposures to chemical contaminants which are often at lower levels and occur as mixtures over long periods of time and spanning critical windows of development. Animal studies using mixtures of chemical contaminants that affect the same physiologic system have found impacts at lower levels of exposure than testing done with single chemicals [49, 50]. Also, more subtle endpoints than previously considered in toxicological testing are associated with environmental contaminants (such as decreased testosterone levels and changes in gene expression). The advancement of scientific ability to evaluate early perturbations in the disease process increases the opportunity to identify potentially harmful chemicals using early biological markers of disease [3].

Animal bioassays have evolved to provide critical information on many different types of exposure scenarios (acute, chronic, early-life exposure versus later in life exposure) and endpoints (e.g. cancer, developmental, reproductive, and immunologic). However, interpreting the data for use in human health risk assessment is complicated by uncertainties in the data and the needs of the policy and decision-making process.

Policy and decision-making about exposures to environmental chemicals must be responsive to a number of extrinsic factors that influence the approach to evaluating the available science. These factors can include the involuntary nature of most exposures, the public's concern about potential harm, and the public health consequences of new or continued exposure to potentially harmful chemicals, all of which compel timely decision-making.

This creates a tension between efficient and timely prevention of harmful exposures and the pace and exactitude of scientific inquiry. The scientific process is a purposefully deliberate one that requires sorting through often-conflicting and incomplete studies to ascertain "true" relationships [51, 52]. Thus, there is a high emphasis on avoiding "false positives," and meeting this goal is a time- and resource-intensive process. The public policy process, alternatively, must balance the needs of the public and the consequences of continued or inadvertent exposure to potentially harmful chemicals. Thus, there is a higher emphasis on efficiently avoiding "false negatives," as delays in identifying harmful exposures have public health consequences. Consequently, the "level of proof" or extent of data necessary for a decision on whether a hypothesis is true or false in the laboratory setting is different than for deciding actions that can reduce or prevent harmful exposures among the public.

There are a number of characteristics of the human population that can influence the likelihood of "false negatives" or can underestimate risks based on data from animal bioassays or limited human epidemiologic studies (Table 16.1) [3]. These overlap with some of the features of the methods used in the scientific study of the relationship between environmental contaminants and health, which can influence the interpretation of the findings. For example, animal bioassays typically use animals that are of a single strain, relatively genetically homogeneous, and are usually exposed to one chemical at a time – at high doses and often – during adulthood. These features can influence the rate of "false negatives" in a broad sense, where different health endpoints, susceptible life stages, or populations may not be identified or the risks underestimated. There are some aspects that can contribute to "false positives." For example, exposures used in animal bioassays tend to be in the high-dose range to maximize the likelihood of observing a "true" response with a reasonable number of animals, and this may overestimate effects at the lower dose range. On balance, it appears that a higher proportion of these features increase the chances of finding

**Table 16.1.** Features of the human population that can influence risks from exposure to environmental contaminants.

| Feature | Definition | Example | Implications |
|---|---|---|---|
| Chemical background | Concurrent or pre-existing body burdens of environmental chemicals | Over 90% of the US population has measurable levels of plasticizers, pesticides, flame retardants, and perfluorinated chemicals | Exposure to an individual chemical in addition to other exposures can increase risk of subsequent disease |
| Biological background | Health status, as influenced by age, pre-existing disease, genetics, and other intrinsic biological factors | About 10% of adults are deficient in thyroid hormone; low thyroid hormone during pregnancy can cause neurodevelopmental harm in children | Chemical exposure has greater effect on people with pre-existing disease, genetic predisposition, etc. |
| Population variability and defining normal | An individual may have a smaller range of normal physiological function than would be observed over the whole population | Individual variability in normal thyroid hormone levels is smaller than the range of normal in the population | Chemical exposures which perturb physiologic systems within the "normal" population range may still have effects at the individual level |
| Small individual effects versus population effects | Chemical exposure may produce a small increase in risk or effect at the level of the individual but result in large shifts in effect at the population level | Observed prenatal phthalate levels slightly decreases the ano-genital distance in male babies | US population exposure to phthalates is ubiquitous, so small changes can shift the population distribution of the measurement, resulting in increased effects for a segment of the population |
| Periods of susceptibility | Exposure during vulnerable periods of development can pose a risk of irreversible effects, both in the short and long term, and diminished capacity for recovery | Exposure to solvents during pregnancy can result in miscarriage or preterm delivery or can cause permanent neurological damage to the fetus (e.g. fetal alcohol syndrome) | Exposures during susceptible periods can increase risk of permanent adverse effects that may manifest early or not until later in life |

a false negative [51]. While minimizing false positives can contribute to more comprehensive science, it can also have untoward consequences for public health as potentially harmful chemicals and exposures can go unidentified. In a public health context, an emphasis on reducing false negatives may be more important if the goal is to reduce harm.

---

**Box 16.2. Diethylstilbestrol**

Diethylstilbestrol (DES), a synthetic estrogen, provides a salient example of the need to evaluate science based on reducing false negatives over reducing false positives. Diethylstilbestrol was prescribed for women from the late 1940s through the 1970s [53]. When it was prescribed starting in 1947, it had undergone limited toxicologic investigation, and it was assumed to be safe, and was even promoted as being beneficial during pregnancy [53]. However, it was later discovered in 1971 that DES lead to vaginal clear-cell adenocarcinoma in the prenatally exposed daughters [54], a clear case of a false negative. Since the discovery of the prenatal effects of DES, there have been over 20 000 publications, yet there are still uncertainties about DES exposure and subsequent health effects [51]. At low levels of exposure, DES has been associated with the development of infertility, uterine fibroids, and even obesity [55–57]. Diethylstilbestrol serves as a model for the potential adverse effects of other estrogenic chemicals such as BPA and a cautionary tale for assuming the safety of chemicals with little supporting data.

---

Consequently, in the USA, there have been general policy principles used in the evaluation of scientific information – such as using animal data and applying public health defaults in the face of unknown information. While more science can increase the knowledge, it does not necessarily lead to better or more timely decisions, and vigorous debate over the science has often resulted in a delay in decision-making, even for the evaluation of chemicals with extensive information (e.g. dioxin, formaldehyde, trichloroethylene, etc.) [47].

Approaches in evaluating the science that acknowledge uncertainty while allowing for efficient and timely decision-making are critical to successful environmental health policy and decision-making. Some of these approaches can be qualitative, such as ascribing different levels of confidence for health hazard (e.g. cancer [52]), or quantitatively. There has been a movement since the early 1990s to apply a more "precautionary" approach to evaluating the weight of evidence of environmental chemicals and taking actions even when there are scientific uncertainties. The precautionary approach, first adopted into international policy as part of the Rio Declaration from the 1992 Rio Conference on the Environment and Development, essentially states that action should be taken if the science indicates serious or irreversible harm even if there is scientific uncertainty [58]. This approach, called the "Precautionary Principle," shifts the level of evidence required for chemical regulation away from definitive proof of harm to allow for policy actions that prevent possible harm even when there is uncertainty.

## Overview of chemical policy regulation

Throughout the world, there are varying degrees of oversight for chemical production, use and disposal. Developing countries have lagged behind other developed countries in banning some of the most toxic chemicals, and although international treaties have been negotiated to phase out some of the worst offenders (e.g. Stockholm Convention on persistent organic pollutants (POPs) or the Basel Convention on the transport of chemical waste), adoption and implementation of these treaties have been slow to non-existent. Chemical policy regulation continues to evolve throughout the world, and in this section we will highlight evolving North American and European chemicals policy.

## North American chemicals policy

In the USA, several different federal agencies have the authority to regulate chemical exposure depending on the source and location of exposure. Chemical exposure in the workplace is regulated by the Occupational Safety and Health Administration (OSHA), chemicals found in pharmaceuticals and personal-care products are regulated by the Food and Drug Administration (FDA), and chemicals that are found as outdoor environmental contaminants in media such as air or drinking water sources are regulated by the Environmental Protection Agency (EPA). The EPA also regulates chemicals used as pesticides in food and consumer products, which creates some redundancy in the regulation of single chemicals. For example, phthalates are found in the workplace; as yet, no workplace standards exist (OSHA). Additionally, some phthalates are approved as both food additives (regulated by the FDA) and as pesticide inert ingredients (regulated by the EPA). The scientific data required by each agency to regulate chemicals differ according to their federal statutes. The Toxic Substances Control Act (TSCA) authorizes the EPA to regulate chemicals under certain conditions while the Federal Food Drug and Cosmetic Act (FFDCA) authorizes the FDA to regulate chemicals only under their jurisdiction.

While the FDA statute requires that the safety of a chemical is demonstrated before approval, under the EPA's federal statute (TSCA), the EPA does not typically require chemical companies to submit sufficient toxicity information on new chemicals and they cannot require data on pre-1979 marketed chemicals unless a number of stringent criteria have been identified. As a result, there are large data gaps in the toxicity knowledge of the more than 87 000 chemicals in commerce in the USA, and since TSCA went into effect in 1979, the EPA has required toxicity testing data for fewer than 200 of these chemicals [59]. Moreover, of the tens of thousands of chemicals that existed in commerce prior to 1979, the EPA has evaluated only 2% for toxicity [59]. As a consequence of their limited ability to regulate chemicals under this statute, the EPA has restricted or banned only five chemicals or chemical classes, and the last regulation took place in 1990 [59]. A 2005 governmental review of this process concluded that programs that rely on voluntary submission of toxicity data have not provided sufficient information on the toxicity of chemicals and made several recommendations for providing the Agency with additional authority to assess the hazards of chemicals and control those of greatest concern [59]. Even though laws have been introduced, there have not yet been any substantive changes regarding how chemicals are regulated by the US government. However, individual states, such as California and Maine, are beginning to take action.

Although the FDA has a statute that requires safety information on chemicals prior to their approval, this has not prevented widespread exposure to potentially harmful chemicals. For some chemicals, such as bisphenol-A (BPA), approval as a food additive was first granted in the 1950s, before the toxicity of this chemical was fully understood. As a result, there has been widespread exposure in the population for several decades, As laboratory methods have become more sophisticated at detecting low levels of exposure, the current levels of exposure have been associated with developmental harm. Although required to establish the safety of a food additive before approving its use, the US FDA has not yet banned the use of BPA as a food additive and continues to assure the public that current levels of exposure are safe, despite scientific guidance to the contrary [60, 61].

Canada has a different chemicals policy from the USA that requires chemical companies to conduct testing of "new" (post-1994) chemicals based on production or import volume. Canada created a Domestic Substances List (DSL) Categorization, which examined information available on the roughly 23 000 previously unassessed chemicals that have been in commerce in Canada over the last two decades. Thus far, Canada has identified 200 substances that are of "high priority" [62] including persistent, bioaccumulative toxins and chemicals with a high likelihood of exposure. In contrast to the shortcoming of chemical policies in the USA, when evaluating the same scientific evidence, Canada has declared that bisphenol-A is a "dangerous substance" and has banned its use from baby bottles and placed restrictions on use in infant formula [63]. This difference in policy occurred because Canada uses a different weight of evidence when determining the safety of BPA. In April 2008, Canada's Health Agency concluded

> … bisphenol-A exposure to newborns and infants is below levels that may pose a risk, however, the gap between exposure and effect is not large enough.

Thus Canada has taken a more precautionary approach to regulating BPA by concluding the margin of exposure between effect and potential harm was not large enough to warrant continued exposure.

## European Union chemicals policy

The most comprehensive chemicals policy in existence is in the European Union where, since 2004, a set of directives targeting the management of chemicals and products produced or imported into the region have been enacted. As aforementioned, many of the European Union chemicals policies have been guided by the "precautionary principle," which has steered a number of directives in the EU including the following:

(1) The Cosmetics Directive, prohibiting the use of 1000 known or suspected carcinogens, mutagens, or reproductive toxicants in cosmetics (2004) [64].

(2) The Waste in Electrical and Electronic Equipment (WEEE) directive, requiring producers to take back products at the end of their useful life (2005) [65].

(3) The Restriction of Hazardous Substances in Electrical and Electronic Equipment (RoHS) regulation, prohibiting the use of lead, cadmium, mercury, and certain flame retardants in electronics sold in the EU [66].

(4) The Registration, Evaluation, Authorisation and Restriction of Chemicals (REACH) regulation of 2006 which requires producers and users of chemicals in commerce in Europe to register and provide public information on their chemical production, use, hazard and exposure potential. For chemicals identified as substances of very high concern, REACH will allow their use only if explicitly authorized [67].

While it will be many years before the full implementation of REACH, coupled with the directives that require product stewardship (WEEE) and restrict some hazardous substances (RoHS and the Cosmetics Directive), these chemical policies will make publicly available new information on chemical toxicity and will affect global markets. As a result, REACH has the potential to reduce chemical exposures worldwide, especially to some of the most toxic chemicals that are produced at high volumes. This new chemical policy will also require new substitutes to be tested for toxicity, and it has the potential to limit the current problem of replacing one toxic chemical with another. For example, as the PBDEs have been phased out of use, they have been replaced by other halogenated flame retardants that have similar persistent and bioaccumulative toxicities [68].

These new chemicals policies could result in a glut of toxic chemicals on the world market. In response, measures should be enacted to limit "dumping" of toxic chemicals from one country to another.

## Conclusion

Manufactured and mined chemicals are ubiquitous in the environment, in wildlife, and in humans. There is increasing growth of chemical manufacturing both in developed and developing countries, posing increased exposures to the human population. This increasing load, coupled with concerns about unexplained increases in many chronic diseases warrant close attention to environmental chemicals as a preventable risk factor of chronic disease. Making personal, market-based, and government-based decisions about exposures to environmental chemicals requires some type of knowledge about potential consequences of exposure. The current legal and regulatory structures in many countries do not typically require toxicity information for most chemicals – either those on the market or those proposed for manufacture. While scientific information is only one factor that plays a role in personal or public decision-making, it plays a critical role in making informed decisions.

Most forms of public policies and decision-making require some toxicological knowledge for informing actions, though scientific information is only one part of the process, as decisions and policies are also influenced by politics, economics, and other external forces.

While in the past it was often efficient to regulate within a country or region to protect local citizens, globalization of markets has shown that products and chemicals are increasingly moving among countries of the world, whether legal or not (e.g. lead in toys) and that while efforts within countries are important, ultimately internationally binding agreements are needed to ensure prevention of harmful exposures.

## References

1. Carson R. *Silent Spring*. Boston, MA: Houghton Mifflin CO, 1962.

2. Kyle AD, Woodruff TJ, Axelrad DA. Integrated assessment of environment and health: America's children and the environment. *Environ Health Perspect*, 2006; **114**: 447–52.

3. Woodruff TJ, Zeise L, Axelrad DA. *et al*. Meeting report: moving upstream-evaluating adverse upstream end points for improved risk assessment and decision-making. *Environ Health Perspect* 2008; **116**: 1568–75.

4. Needleman, HL. The future challenge of lead toxicity. *Environ Health Perspect* 1990; **89**: 85–9.

5. Needleman HL. The persistent threat of lead: medical and sociological issues. *Curr Probl Pediatr* 1988; **18**: 697–744.

6. Schwartz J. Low-level lead exposure and children's IQ: a metaanalysis and search for a threshold. *Environ Res* 1994; **65**: 42–55.

7. Jusko TA, Henderson CR, Lanphear BP. *et al*. Blood lead concentrations < 10 microg/dL and child intelligence at 6 years of age. *Environ Health Perspect* 2008: **116**, 243–8.

8. Lanphear BP, Hornung R, Khoury J. *et al*. Low-level environmental lead exposure and children's intellectual function: an international pooled analysis. *Environ Health Perspect* 2005; **113**: 894–9.

9. U.S. Environmental Protection Agency. *What is the TSCA Chemical Substance Inventory?* Washington, DC, 2006.

10. US Environmental Protection Agency. *America's Children and the Environment*. Washington DC, 2008.

11. US Environmental Protection Agency. *Endocrine Disruptor Screening and Testing Advisory Committee (EDSTAC) Final Report*. Washington DC, 1998.

12. European Chemicals Agency. *List of Pre-Registered Substances*. 2008.

13. Davies J. *Nanotechnology Oversight: An Agenda for the New Administration. Project on Emerging Nanotechnologies*. Washington, DC: Woodrow Wilson International Center for Scholars, 2008.

14. Environmental Working Group. *National Tap Water Quality Database*. Vol. 2008. Washington, DC: EWG, 2005.

15. Environmental Working Group. *Skin Deep Cosmetic Safety Database*. Vol. 2008. Washington, DC: EWG, 2007.

16. US Environmental Protection Agency. *Where You Live*. Washington DC, 2007.

17. US Food and Drug Administration. *Pesticides, Metals, Chemical Contaminants & Natural Toxins*. Washington DC, 2007.

18. US Environmental Protection Agency. *Air Quality Criteria for Particulate Matter*. Washington DC, 2004.

19. US Environmental Protection Agency. *Air Quality Criteria for Ozone and Related Photochemical Oxidants*. Washington DC, 2006.

20. Urbansky ET. Perchlorate as an environmental contaminant. *Environ Sci Pollut Res Int* 2002; **9**: 187–92.

21. Howd RA. Can we protect everybody from drinking water contaminants? *Int J Toxicol* 2002; **21**: 389–95.

22. Wormuth M, Scheringer M, Vollenweider M, Hungerbuhler K. What are the sources of exposure to eight frequently used phthalic acid esters in Europeans? *Risk Analysis* 2006; **26**: 803–24.

23. Sanchez CA, Crump KS, Krieger RI, Khandaker NR, Gibbs JP. Perchlorate and nitrate in leafy vegetables of North America. *Environ Sci Technol* 2005; **39**: 9391–7.

24. Noren K, Meironyte D. Certain organochlorine and organobromine contaminants in Swedish human milk in perspective of past 20–30 years. *Chemosphere* 2000; **40**: 1111–23.

25. Pirkle JL, Brody DJ, Gunter EW. *et al*. The decline in blood lead levels in the United States. The National Health and Nutrition Examination Surveys (NHANES). *J Am Med Assoc* 1994; **272**: 284–91.

26. National Center for Environmental Health. *Third National Report on Human Exposure to Environmental Chemicals*. Atlanta, GA: Centers for Disease Control and Prevention, 2005.

27. Toms LM, Harden F, Paepke O, *et al*. Higher accumulation of polybrominated diphenyl ethers in infants than in adults. *Environ Sci Technol* 2008; **42**(19): 7510–15.

28. Sathyanarayana S, Calafat AM, Liu F, Swan SH. Maternal and infant urinary phthalate metabolite concentrations: Are they related? *Environ Res* 2008; **108**(3): 413–18.

29. Adibi JJ, Whyatt RM, Williams PL. *et al.* Characterization of phthalate exposure among pregnant women assessed by repeat air and urine samples. *Environ Health Perspect* 2008; **116**, 467–73.

30. Petreas M, She J, Brown FR. *et al.* High body burdens of 2,2',4,4'-tetrabromodiphenyl ether (BDE-47) in California women. *Environ Health Perspect* 2003; **111**: 1175–9.

31. Zota AR, Rudel RA, Morello-Frosch RA, Brody JG. Elevated house dust and serum concentrations of PBDEs in California: unintended consequences of furniture flammability standards? *Environ Sci Technol* 2008; **42**: 8158–64.

32. Lunder S, Sharp R. *Mother's Milk: Record Levels of Toxic Fire Retardants Found in American Mother's Breast Milk.* Washington DC: Environmental Working Group, 2003.

33. Commonweal. *Taking It All In: Documenting Chemical Pollution in Californians Through Biomonitoring.* Bolinas, CA: Commonweal Biomonitoring Center, 2005.

34. European Human Biomonitoring. Homepage, 2008.

35. Human Biomonitoring Commission. *Health, and Environmental Hygiene,* German Environmental Agency, 2008.

36. Government of Canada. *Biomonitoring of Environmental Chemicals in the Canadian Health Measures Survey.* 2008.

37. World Health Organization. *Biomonitoring of Human Milk for Persistent Organic Pollutants (POPs).* WHO, 2008.

38. Calafat AM, Ye X, Wong LY, Reidy JA, Needham, LL. Exposure of the U.S. population to bisphenol A and 4-tertiary-octylphenol: 2003–2004. *Environ Health Perspect.* 2008; **116**: 39–44.

39. Centers for Disease Control and Prevention. *Third National Report on Human Exposure to Environmental Chemicals.* Atlanta, GA: CDC, 2005.

40. Ye X, Pierik FH, Hauser R. *et al.* Urinary metabolite concentrations of organophosphorous pesticides, bisphenol A, and phthalates among pregnant women in Rotterdam, the Netherlands: the Generation R study. *Environ Res* 2008; **108**: 260–7.

41. Main KM, Mortensen GK, Kaleva MM. *et al.* Human breast milk contamination with phthalates and alterations of endogenous reproductive hormones in infants three months of age. *Environ Health Perspect* 2006; **114**: 270–6.

42. Swan SH, Main KM, Liu F. *et al.* Decrease in anogenital distance among male infants with prenatal phthalate exposure. *Environ Health Perspect* 2005; **113**: 1056–61.

43. Hauser R, Meeker JD, Singh NP. *et al.* DNA damage in human sperm is related to urinary levels of phthalate monoester and oxidative metabolites. *Hum Reprod* 2007; **22**: 688–95.

44. Baier-Anderson C, Blount BC, Lakind JS. *et al.* Estimates of exposures to perchlorate from consumption of

45. Steinmaus C, Miller MD, Howd R. Impact of smoking and thiocyanate on perchlorate and thyroid hormone associations in the 2001–2002 national health and nutrition examination survey. *Environ Health Perspect* 2007; **115**: 1333–8.

46. Blount BC, Valentin-Blasini L, Osterloh JD, Mauldin JP, Pirkle JL. Perchlorate exposure of the US Population, 2001–2002. *J Expo Sci Environ Epidemiol.* 2007; **17**: 400–7.

47. National Research Council. *Science and Decisions: Advancing Risk Assessment.* Washington, DC: The National Academy Press, 2008.

48. Office of Environmental Health Hazard Assessment. *A Guide to Health Risk Assessment.* California Environmental Protection Agency, 2001.

49. Rider CV, Furr J, Wilson VS, Gray LE. A mixture of seven antiandrogens induces reproductive malformations in rats. *Int J Androl* 2008; **31**: 249–62.

50. Zoeller RT. Environmental chemicals as thyroid hormone analogues: New studies indicate that thyroid hormone receptors are targets of industrial chemicals? *Mol Cell Endocrinol* 2005; **242**: 10–15.

51. Gee D. Late lessons from early warnings: toward realism and precaution with endocrine-disrupting substances. *Environ Health Perspect* 2006; **114**: 152–60.

52. Woodruff T. Policy implications of endocrine-disrupting compounds. In Gore AC, ed., *Endocrine-Disrupting Chemicals: From Basic Research to Clinical Practice.* Totowa, NJ: Humana Press, 2007.

53. Ibarreta D, Swan SH. The DES story: long-term consequences of prenatal exposure. In Harremoes, DGP, MacGarvin M, Stirling A. *et al.* eds. *Late Lessons from Early Warnings: The Precautionary Principle 1896–2000.* European Environment Agency, 2001.

54. Herbst AL, Ulfelder H, Poskanzer DC. Adenocarcinoma of the vagina. Association of maternal stilbestrol therapy with tumor appearance in young women. *New Engl J Med* 1971; **284**: 878–81.

55. Goldberg JM, Falcone T. Effect of diethylstilbestrol on reproductive function. *Fertil Steril.* 1999; **72**: 1–7.

56. Newbold RR, Padilla-Banks E, Snyder RJ, Jefferson WN, 2007. Perinatal exposure to environmental estrogens and the development of obesity. *Mol Nutr Food Res* 2007; **51**: 912–7.

57. Baird DD, Newbold R. Prenatal diethylstilbestrol (DES) exposure is associated with uterine leiomyoma development. *Reprod Toxicol* 2005; **20**: 81–4.

58. Commission of the European Communities. *Communication from the Commission on the Precautionary Principle,* 2000.

59. US GAO. *Chemical Regulation: Options exist to improve EPA's ability to assess health risks and manage its chemical review Program.* G. A. Office, 2005.

human milk, dairy milk, and water, and comparison to current reference dose. *J Toxicol Environ Health A* 2006; **69**: 319–30.

60. CERHR. *NTP-CERHR Monograph on the Potential Human Reproductive and Developmental Effects of Bisphenol A,* 2008.

61. Food and Drug Adminstration, Scientific peer-review of the draft assessment of bisphenol A for use in food contact applications. FDA, 2008, pp. 17.

62. Government of Canada. *"Challenge" for Chemical Substances that are a High Priority for Action.* 2006.

63. Government of Canada. *Release of Final Screening Assessment Report and Proposed Risk Management Approach Document for Bisphenol A.* 2008.

64. European Union. *Cosmetics Directive.* Vol. 76/768/EEC, 2007.

65. European Union. *Waste Electrical and Electronic Equipment Directive.* Vol. 2002/96/EC, 2002.

66. European Union. *Restriction of Hazardous Substances Directive.* Vol. 2002/95/EC, 2002.

67. European Union. *Registration, Evaluation, Authorisation and Restriction of Chemicals.* Vol. EC 1907, 2006.

68. Betts K. New flame retardants detected in indoor and outdoor environment. *Environ Sci Technol* 2008; **42**: 6778.

# Conclusions – what does all this mean, and where are we going?

Shanna H. Swan, Patricia Hunt, and Linda C. Giudice

## Some important concepts

In this book, leaders in environmental health and science have summarized the most current information about environmental contaminants and exposures, and their relevance to reproductive health and reproductive disorders. Several themes emerge. One key theme is that exposure to environmental agents at all life stages – during embryonic and prenatal development, neonatally in childhood, adolescence, and adulthood – have the potential to adversely influence reproduction. Reproductive effects of these exposures include pubertal development, fertility, pregnancy outcome, and reproductive cancer risk. As discussed throughout this volume, timing, route of exposure, and dose are all important considerations in assessing risk of these exposures, as are synergistic effects of multiple chemicals, interactions with cofactors (e.g. nutrition or stress), and latency of effects.

Many chemicals that affect reproductive health are endocrine disruptors – mimetics or antagonists of naturally occurring steroid hormones, or chemicals that have the capacity to alter the metabolism, half-life, secretion, and excretion of endogenous hormones. These naturally occurring hormones are critical to a range of reproductive processes and are important in minimizing reproductive cancer risk. There is a wide range of mechanisms by which these endocrine disruptors may act, including binding to endogenous hormone receptors, promoting altered gene expression, direct mutation/alteration of DNA sequences, and epigenetic changes in histones or DNA that can result in transgenerational transmission of effects. While the human genome sequence was completed in 2000[1,2] the epigenome comprises the next generation of scientific advancement – the "second genome" [3] and is of critical importance in understanding effects of environmental contaminants on reproductive processes and reproductive health for exposed individuals, their offspring, and subsequent generations.

## Challenges

Attempts to link individual chemicals to specific reproductive outcomes – the way much of the research to date has been approached – may not be appropriate in this complex situation. Rather it is necessary to recognize that we are all exposed simultaneously to low doses of a large number of chemicals, many with the capacity to alter a range of reproductive outcomes, and recent work has shown these effects to be dose additive. On the other hand, most animal testing is conducted on chemicals singly and at higher doses, so that these testing scenarios are not appropriate to evaluate risks from realistic exposure scenarios in which the effective cumulative dose is actually not low. Exceptions include an isolated and well-defined high exposure (e.g. the pharmaceutical given to pregnant women, diethylstilbestrol (DES), which was a potent transplacental carcinogen) or a chemical disaster (e.g. massive dioxin exposure from a local factory in Seveso, Italy), or occupational exposures to specific chemicals. Such peak, isolated exposures provide unique insights into actions of endocrine disruptors, and DES is discussed extensively in this volume. However, multiple chemical exposures are ubiquitous, including from food and water, personal-care products (cosmetics, shampoo, deodorant, lotions), household dust, new linens, carpets, curtains, plastic shower curtains, tin and aluminum can linings, home furnishings, and pesticides. The issue of low- vs. high-level exposures is complex, and questions have arisen whether animal models, with which most toxicology studies are conducted, are really translatable to human exposures and human health outcomes.

*Environmental Impacts on Reproductive Health and Fertility*, ed. T. J. Woodruff, S. J. Janssen, L. J. Guillette, and L. C. Giudice. Published by Cambridge University Press. © Cambridge University Press 2010.

## Toxicity testing

Advances in health technologies to monitor biological actions of chemicals, along with advances in systems biology, including bioinformatics, computational technologies to quantify and characterize effects of thousands of chemicals on cellular functions, biochemical pathways and cellular components offer an opportunity to revolutionize toxicology testing. The US EPA established the National Center for Computational Toxicology to develop software and methods for predicting toxicity (http://www.epa.gov/ncct/). Also, the NIEHS has partnered with the NIH Chemical Genomics Center to conduct high throughput screening of multiple chemicals in a timely and cost-effective manner [4]. The optimal cell type for chemical screening of environmental contaminants remains to be determined, but the California Institute for Regenerative Medicine convened a workshop in Summer 2008 wherein human stem cells were considered an appropriate cell type for chemical screening [5]. The future of toxicology testing in the twenty-first century is summarized in a special report from the National Academy of Sciences (NAS) [6] that highlights the vision for toxicity testing in the future and is a "must read."

## Risk assessment

Regarding assessment of risk, the NAS has recently published a summary of special analysis of science and decisions: advancing risk assessment [7] that is particularly relevant to environmental risk assessment. In addition, a report by the National Academy of Sciences' panel on *Phthalates and Cumulative Risk Assessment: The Task Ahead* [8] recommends cumulative risk assessment. In addition, the uncertainty inherent to correlations, extrapolated studies from animals (wildlife and laboratory/experimental), and epidemiologic studies must be addressed. Importantly, assessment of risk must be linked to action(s) to be taken regarding the output of risk assessment [7].

## Public policy

In addition to understanding mechanisms underlying the actions of environmental contaminants on reproductive health, prevention of harm is of paramount importance, as is education of the public for preservation and maximizing reproductive (and other) health outcomes. Having rigorous scientific and epidemiology studies is essential in the translation to human health and risk assessment. To this end, the National Health and Nutrition Examination Survey (NHANES) provides periodic and regular monitoring of biomarkers of environmental contaminant measurements. The National Children's Study, launched this year, will provide unparalleled data collected by assessing prenatal exposures in 100 000 pregnant women nationally, and following their offspring with frequent assessments for up to 21 years. Also, responsible chemical policies, including inventories of chemicals in communities, states, and nationally, responsible disposal and re-use of chemicals, and educating a new workforce in research and education in green chemistry are all part of the future. Recently, the state of California has issued a set of Green Chemistry initiatives consistent with these goals [9].

## Summary

The task before us is large and the stakes are high. The health of our citizens, the health of future generations and, indeed, the continuation of our species depend upon the combined actions of scientists, legislators, community leaders, and individuals. To this end, we are responding to the challenge of assessing reproductive risk from widespread exposure to over 80 000 chemicals by embarking upon a new era of data collection, epidemiologic studies, mechanistic analyses, toxicity testing, green chemistry, and engaging the public and key stakeholders in understanding, controlling, and treating the threats to reproductive health.

## References

1. The Human Genome. *Nature*, 2001; **409** (6822): 813–958.
2. The Human Genome. *Science*, 2001; **291** (5507): 1304–51.
3. Jaenisch R, Bird A. Epigenetic regulation of gene expression: how the genome integrates intrinsic and environmental signals. *Nat Genet* 2003; (Suppl 33): 245–54.
4. Collins FS, Gray GM, Bucher JR. Toxicology. Transforming environmental health protection. *Science* 2008; **319** (5865): 906–7.
5. California Institute for Regenerative Medicine. *Stem Cells in Predictive Toxicology*. 2008.
6. National Research Council. *Toxicity Testing in the 21st Century: A Vision and a Strategy*. Washington, DC: The National Academies Press, 2007.

7.  National Research Council. *Science and Decisions: Advancing Risk Assessment.* Washington, DC: The National Academies Press, 2008.

8.  National Research Council. Committee on the Health Risks of Phthalates, ed. *Phthalates and Cumulative Risk Assessment: The Task Ahead.* Washington, DC: The National Academies Press, 2008.

9.  California Department of Toxic Substances Control. *California Green Chemistry Initiative: Summary of Recommended Policy Actions.* 2008.

# Index

243